HEARING CONSERVATION MANUAL

Fourth Edition

Alice H. Suter, PhD

Edited by: Elliott H. Berger, MS

Council for Accreditation in Occupational Hearing Conservation

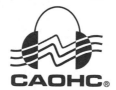

CAOHC®

Printed in the United States of America
CAOHC Executive Office
611 E. Wells Street
Milwaukee, WI 53202

Copyright 2002 CAOHC
ISBN 0-9723143-0-X

CAOHC Component Professional Organizations

American Academy of Otolaryngology – Head and Neck Surgery

American Association of Occupational Health Nurses

American College of Occupational and Environmental Medicine

American Industrial Hygiene Association

American Society of Safety Engineers

American Speech-Language-Hearing Association

Institute of Noise Control Engineering

Military Audiology Association

Foreword

The Council for Accreditation in Occupational Hearing Conservation (CAOHC) has been a leader in providing standards for occupational hearing conservation programs since its inception in 1973. The hearing conservation manual has been one of CAOHC's most important contributions to the field. This is the fourth edition and has significant updates and revisions from the third edition including new and improved questions and answers; updated photos and graphs; and website and print references.

There is updated and expanded regulatory information to include the Mine Safety and Health Administration (MSHA) as well as the Occupational Safety and Health Administration (OSHA). An especially helpful quick reference table comparing OSHA/MSHA/NIOSH regulations and recommendations is included in Chapter VI. In the incredible appendices you'll find OSHA and MSHA checklists, National Hearing Conservation Association (NHCA) guidelines for baseline revision, the most current worker compensation survey of North America, and three American National Standards Institute (ANSI) documents. The ANSI documents alone are worth more than twice the price of the manual!

The manual is designed to be used by CAOHC Course Directors (CDs) in teaching their courses and by Occupational Hearing Conservationists (OHCs) as a reference tool. But I believe everyone involved in hearing conservation at any level and to any degree will find this manual useful. It is an excellent resource for professional supervisors of OHCs (physicians and audiologists alike).

The field of occupational hearing conservation is a dynamic one requiring that practitioners regularly monitor changes in regulations, equipment, and procedures. Alice Suter has again shared her extensive knowledge and experience in the field of hearing conservation. Dr. Suter's career as a leader in hearing conservation is impressive. From 1973 to 1978, she served as a Senior Bioacoustical Scientist in the U.S. Environmental Protection Agency's Office of Noise Abatement and Control. Then, as Manager of the Noise Standard at the U.S. Department of Labor's Occupational Safety and Health Administration, she was the chief author of OSHA's Hearing Conservation amendment to the noise standard (29 CRF 1910.95). Dr. Suter joined the National Institute for Occupational Safety and Health (NIOSH) in 1988 as a Visiting Scientist and Research Audiologist. She is presently a private consultant in industrial audiology and community noise from her home in Ashland, Oregon. Dr. Suter holds fellowships in the American Acoustical Society (ASA) and the American Speech-Language-Hearing Association (ASHA), and has received honors from the National Hearing Conservation Association (NHCA), ASA, and the American Industrial Hygiene Association (AIHA).

The development of this manual has been a team effort. As its author, Dr. Suter has rewritten virtually the entire manual. In this process, she has consulted with numerous experts in the field. Additionally, Council members reviewed and supplied comments and additional materials, which have been integrated into the final document. I would like to acknowledge the efforts of Robert Bruce, David Chandler, Beth Cooper, Robert Goldenberg, Barbara Lechner, Susan Megerson, Gayle Rink, Myrna Stephens, Richard Stepkin, and Peter Weber. The project editor, Elliott Berger, deserves special recognition for his excellent guidance of this effort.

On behalf of CAOHC and hearing conservationists everywhere, I offer sincere thanks to Alice Suter for her outstanding contribution to the field of hearing conservation with the completion of this manual.

Theresa Y. Schulz, PhD
Chair/CAOHC Council

Introduction to the Fourth Edition

Alice Suter, PhD

Nine years have passed since the publication of the third edition of the CAOHC manual. For a while it didn't seem necessary to revise it because, after all, OSHA's regulation had not changed since 1983. But then it occurred to several of us that there had indeed been some important governmental events, as well as some interesting and beneficial changes in hearing conservation practices in the years between the third and present editions. Foremost among the governmental events are the revision of the NIOSH criteria for noise exposure published in 1998 and the MSHA noise regulation in 1999. Add to that a succession of OSHA interpretation and compliance letters, policies and standards from consensus organizations, as well as changes and improvements in instrumentation, and it was time to revise the manual again.

It appears to be a CAOHC tradition that the hearing conservation manual is revised in gradually increasing time increments. The first manual was published in 1978. The second edition of the CAOHC manual appeared in 1985, the third edition in 1993, and now the current edition in 2002. Each time important changes have been made.

Anyone familiar with the third edition will see that there have been many improvements in the present volume. Sections of the manual have been rewritten with an emphasis on providing current information in a "user-friendly" yet comprehensive manner. The text in Chapter VI has been expanded to include information about the NIOSH recommendations, the Americans with Disabilities Act (ADA), changes to OSHA's recordkeeping/recording requirements, and several pages devoted to the recent MSHA regulation. In addition, information has been updated and expanded on audiometric equipment and procedures for audiometric testing, noise measuring instrumentation, and hearing protectors. The Quiz questions have been modified and updated, and the answers may be found in an appendix at the end.

Many of the photographs are new to the manual, such as the series of otoscopic images in Chapter VII. The choice of audiometric, sound measuring, and hearing protection equipment reflects an attempt to represent a diversity of manufacturers, as well as the availability of suitable photos in the various categories. Of course, CAOHC does not recommend particular makes or models of equipment.

Readers will see that there have been significant changes to the appendices. The samples of forms have been eliminated and replaced with resource material that should be more generally useful. Examples are the list of websites in Appendix A, the list of OSHA interpretation and compliance letters in Appendix E, a checklist for the MSHA regulation in addition to the one for OSHA, and articles reprinted from the CAOHC *UPDATE* on hard-to-test workers and engineering noise control.

This book was designed to be used as a reference manual as well as a textbook. Hopefully, Occupational Hearing Conservationists (OHCs) will reread it periodically and refer to it whenever questions come up. But unfortunately (or perhaps fortunately), our field is constantly changing and progressing, and information that is on the cutting edge in 2002 may be obsolete by 2004. Government regulations and policies are good examples of this fact and Course Directors (CDs) and OHCs alike have the responsibility of keeping up with the field.

CDs will need to go beyond this manual and make sure that their information is current in all areas of hearing conservation when they teach their courses. Likewise, OHCs will need to be diligent about keeping up their knowledge base as well as their skills. They will need to follow their professional and trade journals, attend meetings when possible, and talk to government representatives, equipment vendors, and to each other to make sure they are current. Most importantly, OHCs will need to talk to their professional supervisors on a regular basis.

Occupational hearing conservation is a challenge for everyone involved: Management officials, workers, supervisors, union representatives, nurses, acoustical engineers, industrial hygienists, technicians, audiologists, physicians, everyone. As the focal point of the team, the OHC has a marvelous opportunity to meet the hearing conservation challenge head-on at the level where the action takes place. The OHC is the one who actually can conserve the worker's hearing. I hope this book will help in the process.

Alice H. Suter
Ashland, Oregon, 2002

Acknowledgment

Many people have contributed to the development of this manual in a variety of ways, and I would like to express my appreciation. I would especially like to acknowledge Elliott Berger, the editor, for reviewing the draft multiple times, for his astute comments, and for supplying numerous photos and drawings. Special thanks should go to Susan Megerson for her help with the MSHA regulation and her painstaking review of all the chapters. Thanks also to Theresa Schulz, CAOHC's current Chair, and to all the Council members who spent time and effort reviewing the first draft. CAOHC's Executive Director Barbara Lechner has provided helpful and good-natured administrative assistance, particularly in the arduous task of assembling the reviewers' comments onto one draft.

Although there have been substantial changes between the first two editions and the more recent two authored by me, I would like to acknowledge Maurice Miller, Jack Willeford, Richard Sweetman, and the others who drafted the original versions of several chapters, providing the structure on which the more recent editions are based.

Deanna Meinke deserves special recognition for sharing so generously of her materials, wisdom, and experience as an accomplished and dedicated hearing conservationist.

Finally, no acknowledgment would be complete without the name of my husband, Jack Hardesty, whose enduring support has been so important to me in nearly all of the major endeavors of my career.

Alice H. Suter

Editor: Elliott H. Berger

Elliott H. Berger, MS, is the Senior Scientist for Auditory Research at E•A•R / Aearo Company, where for over 25 years he has studied noise and hearing conservation, with an emphasis on hearing protection. He chairs the ANSI working group on hearing protectors, has been lead editor for two highly-regarded texts in noise and hearing conservation, and has also presented his research in over 60 articles and other text book chapters.

Project Coordinator: Barbara Lechner, Executive Director
Special Reviewers: Theresa Schulz and Susan C. Megerson
Copy Editors: Fran Kuecker and Cyd Kladden
CAOHC Publication Committee: Elliott H. Berger (Chair), Paul Brownson, Robert Bruce, Beth Cooper, Robert Goldenberg, Helen Young, Barbara Lechner

Dedication

This manual is dedicated to those who work in noisy conditions

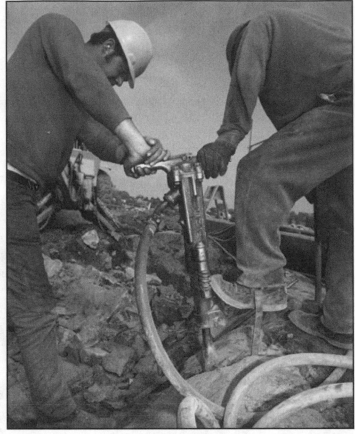

(Courtesy of Quest Technologies & Metrosonics, Inc.)

and to those who help conserve their hearing.

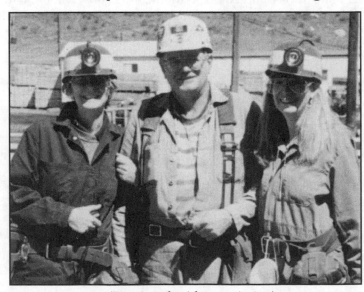

(Reprinted with permission)

Table of Contents

Appendices and Index

Chapter I

Occupational Hearing Conservationists: Their Mission, Training, and Role

Hearing is Priceless

Hearing is priceless. It is perhaps the most important function of the human sensory system. Without it, the vital interactions between people become degraded or lost. Helen Keller, the famous author who was both blind and deaf, used to say that blindness separates you from things, but deafness separates you from people. Noise in industry rarely produces the degree of deafness suffered by Helen Keller. But it does produce handicapping hearing loss, and these losses are permanent. Hearing aids may be of some help, but they can never "correct" the losses the way eyeglasses can usually correct faulty vision.

According to the Labor Department's Occupational Safety and Health Administration (OSHA), 5.2 million American workers in the manufacturing industries are exposed to average noise levels of 85 decibels (dB) and above. These noise levels may be considered potentially hazardous. According to the U.S. Environmental Protection Agency (EPA), more than 9 million American workers are exposed above these levels when all noisy jobs are considered, including those in the military, mining, construction, and transportation industries. OSHA estimates at least 1 million workers in the manufacturing industries alone have sustained job-related hearing loss, and about one-half million of these have moderate-to-severe hearing impairments. The problem is immense, but it is also preventable, and that is where you, the Occupational Hearing Conservationists (OHC), come in.

The Manual's Intent

This manual is intended to provide a text for training programs in occupational hearing conservation, and therefore, you, the OHC, will be its primary user. The best results will be achieved if you read it not only during the course, but afterward, once the basic areas have been explained. Later, you can use it as a reference and a tool for periodic brushing up.

Other members of the occupational health and safety team may also benefit from reading the manual. Occupational health nurses, who frequently take the role of OHC, are likely to be the principal users, but physicians, audiologists, industrial hygienists, safety specialists, noise control engineers, and safety and health technicians may also find it helpful. Representatives of management and worker organizations should also find it interesting and useful.

The manual's approach is to explain both the abstract and the practical in straightforward, down-to-earth language. The idea is not to make instant experts of its readers, but to provide a thorough, yet understandable explanation of the most important concepts and practices involved in occupational hearing conservation. The use of acronyms and abbreviations is kept to a minimum, but often-used terms, such as the Council for Accreditation in Occupational Hearing Conservation (CAOHC), will be abbreviated, and a list of abbreviations used in each chapter appears at the chapter's end. Technical terms that may be unfamiliar are printed in **bold** when they are first mentioned. For the sake of review and "digestion" of the material, a quiz is provided at the end of each chapter, and the answers can be found in Appendix Q. In addition, websites that have been mentioned in each chapter are reprinted at the chapter's end as well as in Appendix A. Appendix A also contains several additional websites that may be of interest.

Suggested readings are provided at the end of each chapter for those who would like further information on a particular topic, and some reprinted material of special interest is included. Frequent mention is made of the requirements of government regulations, and the manual is supplemented with some of the most important regulatory materials, such as the noise regulations issued by OSHA and the Mine Safety and Health Administration (MSHA), and a list of OSHA and MSHA interpretations. Readers should be cautioned, however, that this book does not hold all the answers. When in doubt, the best course is to ask a consultant, such as a noise control engineer, audiologist, industrial hygienist, physician who specializes in this area, or a government employee.

It is important to remember that occupational hearing conservation is a dynamic field, in that policies, procedures, and even regulations are subject to change. The reader should keep in mind that some of the documents reprinted or referenced here, such as the OSHA hearing conservation amendment and certain consensus standards, are not necessarily "etched in stone," and that they can be revised, amended, or updated. Usually, these events will be accompanied by public announcements. It is a good idea to stay current with occupational health and safety journals and magazines, to visit regulatory and other pertinent websites, or to call a government agency to make sure that the information printed here is current.

About CAOHC

In the late 1950s, representatives of four professional societies: the American Association of Industrial Nurses, the American Industrial Hygiene Association, the American Speech and Hearing Association, and the Industrial Medical Association, formed a group called the "Intersociety Committee." The group developed a syllabus outline called the "Guide for Training Audiometric Technicians in Industry," which was adopted in 1965.

One of the first courses was conducted for occupational health nurses under a federal grant to the New Jersey State Association of Industrial Nurses at the Middlesex County College in Edison, NJ. Five courses were given over a period of years, and trainees returned after a designated period of time to take a refresher course and to give feedback to the

instructors. Because of the program's success, the American Association of Industrial Nurses continued the training courses throughout the country.

During its formative years, the Intersociety Committee added the American Academy of Ophthalmology and Otolaryngology, as well as other new organizations. In 1972 the Committee took on the challenge of developing a national certification program for audiometric technicians, including exams, training schedules, and a manual. In 1973 the Committee officially changed its name to the Council for Accreditation in Occupational Hearing Conservation, or CAOHC, as it is known today.

CAOHC currently consists of two representatives from each of the following organizations:

American Academy of Otolaryngology—Head and Neck Surgery

American Association of Occupational Health Nurses

American College of Occupational and Environmental Medicine

American Industrial Hygiene Association

American Society of Safety Engineers

American Speech-Language-Hearing Association

Institute of Noise Control Engineering

Military Audiology Association

Each organization appoints its representatives for specified terms, and the Council[1] elects a Chair, a Vice-Chair, and a Secretary/Treasurer. The Council also employs an Executive Director to handle the many administrative matters.

CAOHC's principal activities revolve around the training and certification of OHCs. CAOHC defines the OHC as a person who is able to conduct the practice of hearing conservation, including a pure-tone air conduction hearing evaluation and other associated duties, under appropriate supervision. This individual can also function with other members of the occupational hearing conservation team.

The Council develops and periodically revises the syllabus, or course outline, and makes decisions about the minimum course length, the number and background of faculty members, and the certification procedures. To be eligible for certification, OHCs must complete the 20-hour course, pass an examination, and pay a certification fee to CAOHC, after which they will become Certified Occupational Hearing Conservationists (COHCs). Then, within 5 years of the date of their certification course (not

---

[1] CAOHC literally is the representative members of the organizations listed above. Sometimes the representatives are collectively referred to as "the Council."

the approval date of their application), they must complete a refresher course of at least 8 hours in length. Without the refresher course, the certification will expire, although CAOHC gives a grace period of up to 6 months if requested by an OHC for valid reasons, such as illness or difficulty in locating a course in a specific geographic area.

Another of CAOHC's most important activities is to train and certify Course Directors (CDs), and to approve their courses in advance. Certified Course Directors must attend a refresher workshop within 5 years of their certification, or justify their certification by continuing education units or through experience by giving at least 5 CAOHC-approved courses during the previous 5 years. More detailed information on certification requirements for both OHCs and CDs may be obtained by contacting CAOHC headquarters or visiting the CAOHC website at **www.caohc.org**.

CAOHC publishes a regular newsletter for OHCs, the *UPDATE*, giving useful information about the industry and the dates and locations of approved OHC courses. A periodic news alert called the *CABLE* is available on the CAOHC website for Course Directors only. In addition, CAOHC provides OHCs and CDs with practical responses to questions, a video curriculum titled "The Anatomy, Physiology and Diseases of the Ear," and, of course, this manual. See Appendix B for a listing of all materials available from CAOHC. Order forms for more copies of this manual and for the Anatomy video curriculum are available at the back of this edition.

One final benefit that should be mentioned is the recognition that comes with CAOHC certification. While it is possible to be trained in another program, most government and private authorities view CAOHC as *the* recognized authority on the training and certification of occupational hearing conservationists in the U.S. Both OSHA and MSHA encourage CAOHC certification as the best evidence that a technician is qualified, specifically mentioning CAOHC in their noise regulations.

State Requirements for "Support Personnel"

Many states within the U.S. set forth requirements for licensure for people who perform audiometric tests. While most states exempt audiometric technicians from licensure as an audiologist or an "Audiology Aide," this exemption is sometimes contingent upon supervision by an audiologist or by a physician. For example, Alabama and Arkansas currently exempt technicians if they are supervised by a physician, but not if they are supervised by an audiologist. Several states, such as Illinois, Maryland, and Tennessee exempt technicians who are certified by CAOHC. In

Ohio, unless they are supervised by a physician, audiometric technicians must be registered and licensed as Audiology Aides, although RNs and LPNs are exempt. Few problems along these lines have been brought to CAOHC's attention thus far, although it would be a good idea for OHCs to check first with their supervising professional and possibly with the licensure board in their own states to see if they need to register or be licensed. The website of the American Speech-Language-Hearing Association (ASHA) has information on state licensure, including "support personnel," at **www.asha.org**.

Course Outline

The material in this manual is intended to review and supplement the information provided by the instructors or CDs. The manual's content generally follows CAOHC's "Course Outline for Course Leading to Accreditation as an Occupational Hearing Conservationist." The current Course Outline is available on the CAOHC website. Course Directors may expand on this outline, but the basic essentials listed below must be covered. Each course must be approved by CAOHC in advance.

The training program spelled out in the Course Outline must equip the OHC with background knowledge and understanding of the following:

1. Responsibilities and limitations of the OHC.
2. Responsibilities of the other members of the hearing conservation team.
3. Parameters of sound as they relate to hearing conservation.
4. Basic anatomy and physiology as they relate to hearing conservation.
5. Types and causes of hearing loss.
6. Compensable hearing loss and state compensation legislation.
7. Federal, state, and military regulations pertaining to noise and hearing conservation.
8. Types of audiometric instrumentation.
9. Performance check and calibration of audiometric instrumentation.
10. Care and troubleshooting of instrumentation.
11. Pure-tone threshold testing and otoscopic screening techniques.
12. Recordkeeping.
13. Personal hearing protection devices.
14. Employee training and education in hearing conservation.
15. Basic concepts and principles of noise measurement and control.
16. Implementing a referral system.

There are certain activities that the course does not prepare an OHC to do. The course does not prepare the OHC to be an instructor of other hearing conservationists, an audiologist, a program manager, or a noise control engineer. Nor does the course prepare an individual (unless otherwise qualified) to interpret audiograms, conduct noise analyses, diagnose hearing disorders, administer a hearing conservation program, or be responsible for noise control problems.

The Course Outline gives specific requirements for the initial training course. The course must be conducted by a CAOHC-certified CD, and there must be at least three instructors (including the CD) representing three of the professional disciplines included on the Council. These disciplines include audiology, occupational health nursing, safety, industrial hygiene, occupational medicine, otolaryngology, and noise control engineering. In lieu of one required professional discipline instructor, a CAOHC-authorized video curriculum package may be substituted by the CD.

There must be at least one audiometric practicum instructor for every six students, and there must also be at least one audiometer for every three practicum students.

Each of the required topics must be covered by an instructor who is physically present during the presentation. The core topics have minimum time requirements, however the CD may spend more time and may add more topics at his or her discretion. The core topics at the time of publication are listed below. For the most current course requirements, see the CAOHC website.

1. Hearing Conservation in Noise.
2. Anatomy, Physiology, Diseases of the Ear, and Otoscopic Screening.
3. Hearing and the Physics of Sound.
4. Federal and State Regulations Relating to Noise and Hearing Loss.
5. The Audiometer and Test Environment.
6. Audiometric Techniques.
7. Supervised Audiometric Evaluations.
8. Review of Audiometric Evaluation.
9. Audiogram Review, Referral, and Employee Follow-up.
10. Principles of Noise Analysis and Noise Control.
11. Personal Hearing Protection.
12. Otoscopic Screening and Hearing Protection Fitting Practicum.
13. Employee Education and Motivation.
14. Recordkeeping.
15. Role of the Occupational Hearing Conservationist.
16. Additional Instruction/Practicum at Discretion of Course Director.
17. Review of Hearing Conservation Program.
18. Examinations.

There are also specific requirements pertaining to the refresher course, which must be completed within 5 years of the initial training course or previous refresher course. Otherwise, the OHC must complete another 20-hour training course to be eligible for recertification. The refresher course must also be approved in advance by CAOHC, it must be conducted by a CAOHC-certified CD, and the requirements for audiometric practicum instructors (one for every six students) and audiometers (one for every three students) are the same as for the full training courses. The topics that must be covered include:

1. Federal and State Regulations.
2. The Audiometer and Test Environment.
3. Audiometric Techniques.
4. Supervised Audiometric Testing.
5. Audiogram Review, Referral, and Employee Follow-up.
6. Personal Hearing Protection.
7. Employee Education and Motivation.
8. Recordkeeping.
9. Role of the OHC.
10. Additional Instruction/Practicum at Discretion of CD.

Role of the Occupational Hearing Conservationist

The OHC will usually be the focal point of the hearing conservation program. Even though the audiometric testing program must be supervised by a professional in the hearing field (an audiologist or physician), the OHC is usually the person who is most closely involved with noise-exposed workers and their activities.

The OHC will need to develop good communication skills since she or he will often be the one to identify the responsibilities of the different team members, define the roles of contractors, schedule meetings, and provide important links among hearing conservation professionals, management, and workers. The OHC must be prepared, on occasion, to spend extra time with workers to make sure that hearing conservation practices are adequately communicated and that workers' problems and constructive solutions are given the attention they deserve.

The OHC will, therefore, be a key member of the hearing conservation team. If the company is a large one, there may be a full-time medical director and a staff of physicians, nurses, industrial hygienists, safety engineers, and possibly an industrial audiologist. In this case the OHC's responsibilities may be limited to audiometric testing, coordinating the necessary follow-up, keeping the records, and fitting hearing protectors.

More likely, the team will be much smaller, or the OHC could even be a team of one, reporting directly to a company official, and using outside consultants for professional supervision and to fill the other roles. In either case, the OHC's role as liaison between workers and other members of the team, or between workers and management, is a vital one. If, for example, one worker has an infected earcanal and is unable to wear hearing protection, or another has an idea about controlling the noise of his or her machine, the OHC may well be the first person to hear about it. The OHC then needs to see that these situations are communicated to the proper authorities, and, to the extent possible, followed up appropriately.

Today, OHCs are working in a variety of settings. Many are employed by hearing conservation or occupational health service providers and find themselves traveling to a number of different companies in several counties or even across state lines. In addition to long hours on the road, these OHCs interact with a variety of company personnel and an assortment of different management styles. Other settings in which OHCs often work include occupational health clinics, government agencies, and military installations.

OHCs who complete the CAOHC training course *can* be responsible for the following activities:

1. Audiometric testing, including baseline, annual testing, and in some cases retesting.
2. Visually inspecting the ear to rule out any condition that might interfere with the test.
3. Taking a medical history.
4. Screening the audiograms and selecting problem audiograms for review by an audiologist or physician.
5. Referring to the appropriate sources for further testing or medical treatment.
6. Caring for and maintaining the audiometer, including a functional check before each use, and making sure that it gets calibrated at the appropriate times.
7. Recordkeeping.
8. Notifying employees of a standard threshold shift in a timely manner.
9. Educating, training, and counseling employees.
10. Selecting, fitting, and supervising the wearing of hearing protection devices.

Role of the Professional Supervisor

Following is an outline of the responsibilities of the audiometric testing program's professional supervisor, who must be an audiologist, otologist, or other physician. This person's role is to supervise the audiometric testing conducted by the OHC, recommend follow-up procedures, manage the audiometric database, and determine the work relatedness of an employee's hearing loss. OHCs are *not* (unless otherwise qualified) responsible for these activities:

1. Audiogram interpretation.
2. Diagnosis of hearing problems.
3. Any type of audiometric testing other than air conduction, such as bone conduction or speech audiometry.
4. Evaluation of hearing conservation program effectiveness.
5. Training of other OHCs.

A clear understanding of each person's role will enhance the effectiveness of the hearing conservation program.

CAOHC Certification

Upon completion of the training, the trainee may apply for certification as an OHC by submitting the official application form, along with proof of course completion and a fee that is set by the Council. Sometimes a CD will submit the trainees' applications as a group, along with the required fees. In either case, applicants must be listed on the CD's roster of successful students. They will then receive an official certificate, along with a certification number and a wallet I.D. card with their number and expiration date, and quarterly issues of the *UPDATE* newsletter.

OHCs who successfully complete the training course will have a credential that will be important in the recognition of their work by workers, employers, government personnel, and possibly by courts in the event that hearing loss litigation should arise. Once certified, the OHC is permitted and encouraged by CAOHC to evidence his/her certification by including the acronym "COHC" after his/her name.

CAOHC is an ongoing source of information and assistance. In addition to receiving regular publications, OHCs may contact CAOHC headquarters at (414) 276-5338 or access its website at **www.caohc.org**.

Quiz

1. Name four types of professionals who are likely to make up the hearing conservation team.
2. OSHA estimates _____ workers are exposed to average noise levels of 85 dB and above in the manufacturing industries.
3. What does CAOHC stand for?
4. Name at least five organizations that are members of CAOHC.
5. The OHC can be responsible for the care and maintenance of the audiometer. (True or False)
6. The OHC can be responsible for the diagnosis of hearing problems. (True or False)
7. Under what conditions may a video be substituted for one of the required professional disciplines in the certification course?
8. Name at least six activities that the OHC is being trained to carry out.
9. Name at least four activities that the OHC is not being trained to carry out.
10. To maintain their certification, OHCs must be recertified within five years of _____.
11. How is decibel abbreviated?

Abbreviations Used in Chapter I

ASHA	American Speech-Language-Hearing Association
dB	Decibel
CAOHC	Council for Accreditation in Occupational Hearing Conservation
CD	Course Director
COHC	Certified Occupational Hearing Conservationist
EPA	U.S. Environmental Protection Agency
MSHA	Mine Safety and Health Administration
OHC	Occupational Hearing Conservationist
OSHA	Occupational Safety and Health Administration
RN	Registered Nurse
LPN	Licensed Practical Nurse

Recommended Reading

Council for Accreditation in Occupational Hearing Conservation. "Q & A" (pamphlet).

Council for Accreditation in Occupational Hearing Conservation. (1998). *UPDATE* (newsletter), especially "The evolution of the Council for Accreditation in Occupational Hearing Conservation." *UPDATE*, 9(1).

Franks, J.R., Stephenson, M.R., and Merry, C.J. (1996). *Preventing Occupational Hearing Loss: A Practical Guide*. U.S. Dept. Health and Human Services, National Institute for Occupational Safety and Health. Cincinnati, OH.

Meinke, D. (1995). "State regulation of audiometric technicians in industry." *Audiology Today*, 7(2).

Websites

www.asha.org
American Speech-Language-Hearing Association

www.caohc.org
Council for Accreditation in Occupational Hearing Conservation

www.osha.gov
Occupational Safety and Health Administration

www.msha.gov
Mine Safety and Health Administration

Chapter II

The Effects of Noise and the Conservation of Hearing

The Need to Prevent Hearing Loss

Noise is one of the most pervasive of all the occupational hazards. Even though workers have put up with it for generations, noise is one of the occupational problems most frequently complained about. According to OSHA, about 5.2 million workers are exposed to daily average noise levels of **85 dBA**[2] and above in the manufacturing industries (OSHA, 1981). Of these, about 1.5 million are exposed to average levels of noise between 90 and 95 dBA, nearly 1 million experience levels between 95 and 100 dBA, and about 425,000 endure daily average noise levels above 100 dBA.[3]

The manufacturing industries are not the only occupations where hazardous noise exposures occur. The U.S. Environmental Protection Agency (EPA, 1981) surveyed noise exposure conditions in a variety of occupations and came up with the following estimates for workers exposed to daily average noise levels over 85 dBA:

Agriculture	323,000 workers
Mining	218,400 workers
Construction	513,000 workers
Military	976,000 workers
Transportation	1,934,000 workers
Manufacturing	5,124,000 workers
Total	9,088,400 workers

Since most of these estimates are more than 20 years old (with the exception of mining),[4] we can hope that there has been some improvement in the occupational noise environment. However, no surveys of noise exposure have effectively replaced these figures, and there is no reason to believe that they are not reflective of today's conditions.

OSHA estimates that slightly more than 1 million Americans have hearing losses sufficient to be considered a "material impairment of hearing"[5] from noise exposure in the manufacturing industries alone (OSHA, 1981). The total number of hearing-impaired workers is undoubtedly greater, when the noise-exposed workers in other occupations are also taken into account.

---

[2] An average noise level of 85 dBA is considered to be the approximate beginning of hearing hazard, although there is evidence that some of the more sensitive individuals will incur hearing loss from slightly lower noise levels. Likewise, some people can be exposed to average sound levels above 90 dBA without sustaining significant loss of hearing.

[3] A word about notation: The abbreviation **dB** stands for **decibel** and the term "**A**" means that the sound level has been filtered with the A-weighting network of the sound level meter. There will be more discussion of these terms in Chapter V.

---

[4] The recent estimate of the number of miners overexposed is calculated using Table 15 from the preamble to MSHA's final noise regulation (MSHA, 1999) and an MSHA technical report, IR 1224 (Seiler and Giardino, 1994).

[5] OSHA defines material impairment of hearing as an average hearing threshold level of 25 dB or greater at the frequencies 1000, 2000, and 3000 Hz. This should not be confused with OSHA's definition of standard threshold shift, which will be discussed in detail in later chapters.

Not too long ago noise-induced hearing loss was called "boiler-maker's disease" and many thought that it was an inevitable consequence of a noisy job. But, as many professionals have known for a long time, this condition is preventable. This is why the work of the hearing conservation team, and especially the OHC is so important. If hearing is protected from the beginning of employment, hearing impairment doesn't need to occur.

The Effects of Noise

At this point it would be useful to look at the various effects of noise. Although hearing loss is the most well-known adverse effect and probably the most serious, it is not the only one. Usually, preventing hearing loss will protect against most other effects, an additional reason for initiating and maintaining a good hearing conservation program.

Hearing Loss

Although noise-induced hearing loss is so common, it is often underrated because there are no visible effects, no bleeding, and in most cases, no pain. There is only a gradual, progressive loss of communication with family and friends, and a loss of sensitivity to the environment. Also, there is a cultural resistance, especially among men, to admitting that one has a hearing impairment, since people often associate it with getting old and infirm. Unfortunately, good hearing is usually taken for granted until it is lost.

Hearing Handicap:

Hearing loss may be so gradual that individuals do not realize what has happened until the impairment becomes handicapping. The first sign is usually that other people do not seem to speak as clearly as they used to. The hearing-impaired person will have to ask others to repeat, and he or she often becomes annoyed with their apparent lack of consideration. Family and friends will often be told, "Don't shout at me. I can hear you, but I just can't understand what you're saying."

As the hearing loss becomes worse, the individual will begin to withdraw from social situations. Church, parties, and movies begin to lose their attraction and the individual will choose to stay at home. The volume of the TV becomes a source of contention within the family, and other family members are sometimes driven out of the room because the hearing-impaired person wants it so loud.

One of the most serious and yet one of the least talked about consequences of hearing impairment is a reduction in the degree of intimacy between family members. It becomes more difficult for spouses and other family members to communicate with the hearing-impaired person. Communication between partners becomes less personal, there is less satisfaction with the relationship, and both members of the couple begin to feel lonely and isolated.

The hearing loss that naturally accompanies the aging process adds to the hearing handicap when the person with noise-induced hearing loss becomes older. Eventually, the loss may progress to such a severe stage that the individual can no longer communicate with family or friends without great difficulty, and then he or she is indeed isolated. A hearing aid may help in some cases, but, unlike vision and eyeglasses, the clarity will never be restored.

Hearing Loss From Occupational Noise:

Noise-induced hearing loss is usually considered an occupational disease or illness, rather than an injury, because its progression is gradual over time. On rare occasions, an employee may sustain immediate, permanent hearing loss from a very loud event such as an explosion or a very noisy process, such as riveting. In these circumstances the hearing loss is sometimes referred to as an injury and called **"acoustic trauma."** The usual case, however, is a slow decrease in hearing ability over a number of years. The amount of loss will depend on the level of the noise, the duration of the exposure, and the susceptibility of the individual worker. Since there is no medical treatment for occupational hearing loss, prevention is the only option.

Unlike many other occupational illnesses, the auditory effects of noise are well documented, and there is little controversy over the amount of **continuous** noise that causes varying degrees of hearing loss. **Intermittent** (on and off) noise also causes hearing loss. Periods of noise that are interrupted by periods of quiet can offer the ear an opportunity to recover and may therefore be somewhat less hazardous than continuous noise. This is true mainly of outdoor occupations, but not inside factories where quiet is rare. **Impulsive** noise, (often referred to as **impulse** or **impact** noise), such as the noise from gunfire and metal stamping,[6] also damages hearing. The amount of damage will depend mainly on the level and duration of the impulse, and it may be worse when there are other types of noise in the background.

Hearing loss from noise is often temporary at first. During the course of a noisy day, the ear becomes fatigued and the worker will experience a

---

[6] Impulsive noise in the factory is often called "impact" noise since it is usually generated by two objects hitting or impacting each other.

reduction in hearing known as **temporary threshold shift (TTS)**. Between the end of the workshift and the beginning of the next shift the ear usually recovers from much of the TTS. As evidence of this, workers will often say that the next morning when they start up the car, the radio will come on blaring, indicating that they were not hearing as well during the drive home from work the night before. After days, months, and years of exposure, the TTS becomes a **permanent threshold shift (PTS)** and new amounts of TTS begin to build on top of the now permanent losses. The OHC's job is to prevent hearing loss, even when it is in the TTS stage, and to catch these losses before they become permanent.

Ototoxins (Ear Poisons):

Experimental evidence indicates that several industrial agents are **ototoxic**, meaning toxic or poisonous to the ear. They can be damaging to the nervous system and produce hearing loss in laboratory animals, especially when they occur in combination with noise (see Franks and Morata, 1996 for a review of this work). These agents include (1) heavy metals, such as lead and trimethyltin, (2) organic solvents, such as toluene, xylene, and carbon disulfide, and (3) an asphyxiant, carbon monoxide. Recent research on industrial workers indicates that certain of these substances can increase the damaging potential of noise (Morata, 1998). The U.S. Army's hearing conservation program lists 13 potentially ototoxic substances, with carbon monoxide, styrene, trichloroethylene, toluene, and xylene as "high-priority ototoxins" (Dept. of the Army, 1998).

There is also evidence that certain drugs, which are already toxic to the ear, can increase the damaging effects of noise (Boettcher et al., 1987). Examples include certain antibiotics and cancer chemotherapy drugs. More information on these drugs will be presented in Chapter IV. The OHC should be aware that workers exposed to these chemicals or using these drugs may be somewhat more susceptible to hearing loss, especially when exposed to noise as well.

The information described above provides additional incentive for a carefully conducted hearing conservation program, even when noise levels are moderate, around 85 dBA.

Hearing Loss From Non-occupational Sources:

It is also important to understand that occupational noise is not the only cause of noise-induced hearing loss among workers. In addition to the non-noise-related hearing losses that will be discussed in Chapter IV, there are non-occupational sources of noise exposure. These sources of noise produce what some noise professionals call **sociocusis**, and their effects on hearing are virtually impossible to differentiate from occupational hearing loss. Their existence can only be surmised by asking detailed questions about the worker's recreational and other noisy activities. Examples of sociocusic sources could be woodworking tools, chain saws, unmuffled motorcycles, loud music, and, of course, guns. Frequent shooting with large caliber guns (without hearing protection) may be a significant contributor to noise-induced hearing loss, whereas occasional hunting with smaller caliber weapons is more likely to be harmless. Some would include military noise in the sociocusis category, but for soldiers and other members of the Armed Forces, this is occupational noise.

The importance of non-occupational noise exposure and the resulting sociocusis is that this hearing loss adds to the exposure that an individual might receive from occupational sources. It is also conceivable that a worker in an effective hearing conservation program, who engages in noisy recreational activities, could have a hearing loss that is entirely sociocusic, and yet the company might be blamed. But mainly for the sake of the worker's overall hearing health, OHCs should counsel workers to be sure to wear adequate hearing protection when they engage in noisy recreational activities.

Tinnitus and Hyperacusis

Tinnitus is a condition that frequently accompanies both temporary and permanent hearing loss from noise, as well as other types of sensorineural hearing loss. Often referred to as a ringing in the ears, tinnitus may range from mild in some cases to severe in others. People with tinnitus are likely to notice it the most in quiet conditions, such as when they are trying to go to sleep at night, or when they are sitting in a sound-booth taking a hearing test! It is a sign that the sensory cells in the inner ear have been irritated. It is often a precursor to noise-induced hearing loss and therefore an important warning signal. Some people are actually more distressed by tinnitus than they are by their hearing loss. Additional information is available from the American Tinnitus Association (ATA) at (800) 634-8978 or on its website, **www.ata.org**.

Hyperacusis, which is a greatly increased sensitivity to sound, is another consequence of noise exposure that is becoming more widely recognized today. It is most frequently related to a traumatic noise exposure, but it can also occur from the gradual exposure that is typical of a long-term noisy occupation. People with hyperacusis experience discomfort with certain sounds, to the extent that these noises can be painful, almost unbearable. This reaction may occur to sounds that most people would find quite moderate in intensity. Even though these people have sustained hearing losses, the margin between loud enough and too loud can become very narrow.

Communication Interference

The fact that noise can interfere with or "mask" speech communication and warning signals is only common sense. Many industrial processes can be carried out very well with a minimum of communication among workers. Other jobs, however, such as those performed by airline pilots, railroad engineers, armored tank commanders, and many others rely heavily on speech communication. Some of these workers use communication systems that suppress the noise and amplify the speech through electronics. Sophisticated communication systems are now available, some with devices that actually cancel some of the unwanted noise so that communication can take place more easily.

In many cases, workers just have to make do, straining to understand communications above the noise and shouting above it or signaling. Sometimes people may develop hoarseness or even **vocal nodules** or other abnormalities on the vocal cords from excessive strain. The OHC needs to be on the lookout for these kinds of problems and refer the individuals for medical care if necessary.

People have learned from experience that in noise levels above about 80 dBA they have to speak very loudly, and in levels above 85 dBA they have to shout. In levels much above 95 dBA they have to move very close together to communicate at all. Acoustical specialists have developed methods to predict the amount of communication that can take place in industrial situations — methods dependent upon various characteristics of the noise, as well as the distance between talker and listener.

It is also common sense that noise can interfere with safety, although there has been relatively little research on this problem. For example, high noise levels and the high incidence of accidents and fatalities in construction are most likely related. Studies have implicated noise and hearing loss in a large percentage of the injuries among shipyard workers (Moll van Charante and Mulder, 1990) and other types of jobs, such as equipment operators and laborers (Zwerling et al., 1997). There have also been numerous anecdotal reports of workers who have gotten clothing or hands caught in machines and have been seriously injured while their coworkers were oblivious to their cries for help. To prevent communication breakdowns in noisy environments, some employers have installed visual warning devices.

Another problem that is recognized more by noise-exposed workers than by hearing conservation professionals is that hearing protection devices may sometimes interfere with the perception of speech and warning signals. This appears to be true mainly when the wearers already have hearing losses and the noise levels fall below 90 dBA. In these cases, workers have a very legitimate concern about wearing hearing protection. It is important for the OHC to be attentive to the workers' concerns and to bring them to the attention of management. This kind of situation calls either for engineering noise control or for an improvement in the kind of protection offered, such as protectors built into an electronic communication system. Today there are hearing protectors available with a more "high fidelity" response that may improve workers' abilities to understand speech and warning signals. This topic will be explored further in Chapter X.

Effects on Job Performance

The effects of noise on job performance have been studied both in the laboratory and in actual working conditions. The results have shown that noise usually has little effect on the performance of repetitive, monotonous work, and in some cases can actually increase job performance when the noise is low or moderate in level. High levels of noise can degrade job performance, especially when the task is complicated or involves doing more than one thing at a time. Intermittent noise tends to be more disruptive than continuous noise, particularly when the periods of noise are unpredictable and uncontrollable. Interestingly, recent research indicates that people are less likely to help each other and more likely to exhibit antisocial behavior in noisy environments than in quiet ones. (For a detailed review of the effects of noise on job performance see Suter, 1992a.)

Annoyance

Although the term "annoyance" is more often connected with community noise problems, such as airports or race-car tracks, industrial workers may also feel annoyed or irritated by the noise of their workplace. This annoyance may be related to the behavior patterns described above. Sometimes the annoyance or aversion to noise is so strong that a young worker will look for employment elsewhere (if possible). After a period of adjustment, most will not appear to be bothered as much, but they may still complain about fatigue, irritability, and sleeplessness. The adjustment will be more successful if these young workers are properly fitted with hearing protectors and trained in how to use them from the start. Interestingly, this kind of information sometimes surfaces after a company starts a hearing conservation program and workers become aware of the contrast.

Extra-auditory Effects

As a biological stressor, noise can influence the entire physiological system. Noise acts the same way other stressors do, causing the body to respond in ways that may be harmful in the long run and lead to disorders known as the stress diseases. When facing danger in primitive times, the body would go through a series of biological changes, preparing either to fight or to run away (the classic "fight or flight" response). There is evidence that these changes still persist with exposure to loud noise, even though a person may feel "adjusted" to the noise.

Most of these effects appear to be transitory, but with continued exposure some effects have been shown to be chronic in laboratory animals. Several studies of industrial workers also point in this direction (Suter, 1992b). The evidence is probably strongest for cardiovascular effects, such as increased blood pressure and changes in blood chemistry. The scientific community, however, still has not come to agreement on the connection between noise and stress diseases.

The stress effects of noise are mediated by the auditory system, meaning that it is necessary to hear the noise for any adverse effects to occur. Therefore, properly fitted hearing protection will reduce the possibility of these effects just the way it does with hearing loss.

The Solution — Hearing Conservation Programs

Benefits of a Good Hearing Conservation Program

The benefits of effective hearing conservation programs are experienced both by employees and management. The primary benefit to workers, of course, is the prevention of noise-induced hearing loss. But hearing conservation programs can also detect hearing losses that may be due to causes other than workplace noise, and which might otherwise have gone untreated. Temporary hearing loss and tinnitus will also be reduced or eliminated, as will some noise-related safety hazards. As mentioned above, employees are less likely to feel fatigued and annoyed, and the possibility of stress-related illness will also be reduced.

Management will benefit from effective hearing conservation programs as well. Better labor-management relations should result from improved employee morale and the decreased likelihood of anti-social behavior resulting from annoyance and stress. Less noise and better hearing can lead to greater job satisfaction, productivity, and safety. Studies have shown that hearing conservation programs can actually result in reductions in accident rates, illnesses, and lost time (e.g., Cohen, 1976; Schmidt et al., 1982). Reducing the noise through engineering control can have a very positive effect, not only in the prevention of hearing loss but by reducing absenteeism and increasing productivity (Staples, 1981). Finally, the prevention of noise-induced hearing loss will reduce the risk of worker compensation payments and may help contain the costs associated with worker compensation insurance.

Establishing a Hearing Conservation Program

The first and probably most important step in establishing a hearing conservation program is to obtain the cooperation of the whole management team. Without its support, the program is not likely to succeed. Managers and supervisors need to understand the rationale for the program, the effects of noise on hearing, the requirements of applicable regulations, and the need for their participation in the program. All management personnel, even visitors, must be willing to display leadership by wearing hearing protectors in noisy environments at all times. Otherwise, workers will feel that protectors are a burden imposed only on hourly employees, and not considered important by management.

The next step is to enlist the support of the workers to be included in the hearing conservation program. If possible, they should be included in the planning of the program. These employees are usually the ones who know the most about factors that are important to the hearing conservation program, such as their work schedules, the sources of noise in their environments, whether improved maintenance could reduce the noise of their machines, and how the noise might be controlled.

If the employees are unionized, it is a good idea to enlist the cooperation of the local union president or safety representatives, and if possible, to include them in the planning of the hearing conservation program. If hearing protectors are to be worn, these officials should lead the way and help other workers through the adjustment period.

The early development of an engineering noise control plan is also an important step. Not only is noise control the most satisfactory ultimate solution, but all employees will be more inclined to accept the idea of hearing protectors if they are reasonably sure that they will not have to wear these devices forever. The OHC will not usually be the one who develops the noise control plan (unless otherwise trained), but he or she can stress the importance of such a plan with management.

Major Components of the Hearing Conservation Program

Further information on the development of hearing conservation programs, along with details about the program's components, will be discussed in upcoming chapters. At this time it would be useful to summarize the major components of the program. They are: noise measurement, engineering noise control, audiometric testing, hearing protection, employee training and education, recordkeeping, and program evaluation.

Noise Measurement:

Although relatively few OHCs will actually conduct noise measurements, this is an integral part of the overall program, and the OHC should be aware of the basic concepts. There are two principal types of industrial noise measurement: one is to assess employees' noise exposures and the other is to determine the amount of noise that is generated by specific machines. The first type of measurement can by performed by people with a variety of training, while the latter type of measurement is usually more complex and is generally performed by a **noise control engineer** or an **industrial hygienist**.

Employees' noise exposures are measured to determine whether they should be included in the hearing conservation program, and if so, to see what kind of hearing protection is needed. These measurements are performed with a **sound level meter** or a **noise dosimeter**. Another use for these measurements is, of course, to comply with OSHA and other governmental requirements.

It is always a good idea to inform employees about the initiation of a noise measurement program and enlist their cooperation. This will help safeguard the accuracy of the measurements, satisfy the provisions of certain regulations, and encourage good working relationships.

Engineering Noise Control:

Removing the source of noise by engineering means is the most effective long-term solution to the occupational noise problem. Sometimes this process is prohibitively expensive, but often it is quite reasonable, and occasionally it is surprisingly cheap. Here is where a noise control engineer or an industrial hygienist comes in but, as mentioned above, individual workers may have some very good ideas about the means of controlling the noise from their particular machines.

There are three principal approaches to noise control: controlling the **source**, the **path**, and the **receiver**. (See Appendix M for additional discussion.) One of the best approaches to controlling the

noise source is to redesign the process to be quieter. An example would be the mechanical ejection of parts instead of using compressed air. Design for quiet may also be written into a company's specifications for new equipment. Other examples of source noise control would be adding a muffler to a pneumatic tool or isolating a noisy machine to prevent the vibrations from radiating.

The transmission or path of a noise source can be controlled by the use of absorptive material on ceilings and walls, or by erecting barriers around an area, or noise-reducing curtains made of heavy materials such as loaded vinyl. These methods are particularly effective to control high-frequency noise. Finally the area immediately around the receiver can be quieted. This can be done by enclosing the receiver in a sound-treated control booth.

Audiometric Testing:

The **audiometric testing** program is probably the portion of the hearing conservation program where the OHC will be most involved, and there is a detailed discussion of this topic in Chapters VII and VIII. The OHC should become competent in giving a valid audiometric test, which includes the inspection of the worker's outer ear and earcanal, the administration of a **pure-tone, air conduction** audiometric test, taking care of and checking the calibration of the **audiometer**, performing an initial inspection of the **audiogram**, and instructing and counseling workers as necessary. OHCs must also understand the limitations of their capabilities and responsibilities and where the guidance and input of the supervising audiologist or physician is necessary.

There has been some controversy over the word "test," which commonly follows "audiometric" because it may lead people to think that this is a "pass/fail" situation. The word "evaluation" has been suggested as a substitute, but that implies a judgment on a continuum of good to bad, which is not appropriate either. The word "test" will continue to be used in this manual, but the OHC should be aware of this potential misinterpretation. She or he should never talk in terms of "passing" or "failing" the audiometric test, or "doing well" or "doing poorly." Instead, the test merely determines a person's hearing threshold levels.

It is also important to remember that audiometric testing does not actually *protect* workers, and therefore it should not become an end in itself. If it is done carefully, however, it is the most effective tool for determining whether the hearing conservation program is working. Conducting tests carefully means that the tests are done by conscientious, knowledgeable personnel, in sufficiently quiet audiometric test rooms, with well-calibrated equipment, and on well-instructed subjects. When all these conditions are met, audiometric tests can offer a lot of information about the status of an individual's hearing and also about the effectiveness of the hearing conservation program as a whole.

The purpose of audiometric testing in an occupational setting is to identify the progression of hearing loss so that measures can be taken to stop the loss. The best approach is to identify a temporary hearing loss before it becomes permanent. This is not done by testing an employee's hearing and filing away the record. It is done by obtaining a noise-free **baseline audiogram**, testing the employee periodically (usually annually), and comparing the results of the periodic test with the baseline. If a progression of noise-induced loss occurs, the OHC or professional supervisor needs to intervene with such steps as counseling, refitting of hearing protection, recommendations for noise control, and possibly providing quiet time during the day for recovery from TTS.

The baseline audiogram should always be performed after at least 14 hours away from noise exposure of any kind, and preferably pre-employment. The periodic or annual audiogram, however, should be performed *well into the work shift* so as to identify any temporary changes in hearing level before they become permanent. If there is no TTS this way, the OHC may be reasonably sure that the hearing protection is working adequately (or that the employee is not particularly sensitive to noise). If these testing and intervention methods are successful, they represent a truly effective prevention program, and this is what hearing conservation is all about.

Hearing Protection:

Hearing protection, along with engineering controls, is the other principal method of preventing noise-induced hearing loss. Here again, the OHC can play a very important role in making sure that the hearing protectors do the job they are expected to do.

Most managers should be aware that the company cannot simply hand out hearing protection devices and expect workers to benefit from them. There are a great many of these devices on the market, and they need to be tailored to an individual's working conditions and to the size and shape of the head or earcanal. But equally important, workers need to be trained in the fitting, care, and use of hearing protectors, and the OHC is usually the person to do this job. Hearing protectors that fit incorrectly may be quite uncomfortable, and sound is likely to leak around the edges of the protector and enter the earcanal unabated. This may lead to hearing protectors that provide insufficient **attenuation** (noise reduction), or protectors that are not worn at all.

The OHC should also be cautioned not to place too much reliance on the conventional **Noise Reduction Rating (NRR)** that appears on the package of the hearing protector. Studies of the use of hearing protectors over the past 20 years have shown that the noise reduction received in actual use is far less than the NRR would indicate. This may occur even when users have been taught how to fit the devices.

A recent improvement in the rating of hearing protectors is the use of the **NRR(SF)**,[7] which has been developed to give the users of hearing protectors a more realistic estimate of the attenuation that a specific protector may provide. Although no government agency is currently requiring the NRR(SF), some manufacturers are beginning to make these data available.

It is important for OHCs to help workers select the hearing protector with the correct amount of attenuation for their job. Bigger is not necessarily better, especially when people work in moderate levels of noise and need to communicate with their co-workers.

Supervision of the use of hearing protectors is critical to the success of the program. First, the OHC will want to make sure that the protectors are being used. But the OHC can also examine some of the protectors up close to see if they have been properly inserted (in the case of earplugs) or positioned (in the case of earmuffs). Also, the OHC may want to perform a quick check of the attenuation of earplugs using an audiometer. Chapter X will provide more details on all of these topics.

Employee Education and Training:

Not only are the education and training of employees required by OSHA's noise standard, but it makes good hearing conservation sense. Employees who understand the effects of noise on hearing are likely to be more conscientious about the hearing conservation program. They are more likely to leave noise control devices, such as mufflers and enclosures, intact, even though these devices may be cumbersome at times. They should also be more motivated to wear hearing protection, both on and off the job.

The OHC will often play a key role in worker education and training, and may be called upon to provide training for supervisors and foremen as well. The training programs may range from individual counseling to group question-and-answer sessions. Audiovisual materials, such as films, videos, and pamphlets may be used to supplement the training sessions, but none of these can replace personal, face-to-face contact.

---

[7] "SF" stands for Subject Fit, a process of testing the protector in the laboratory where the individuals being tested don the protectors themselves rather than having the experimenter place them.

The most important topics will be the effects of noise on hearing, and the selection, fitting, care, and use of hearing protection devices. Other topics, such as an explanation of the audiogram, the need to avoid noise exposure of any kind before the baseline audiogram, and the benefits of wearing hearing protectors during noisy recreational activities should also be covered.

Education and training programs will be discussed in more detail in Chapter XI.

Recordkeeping:

No matter how carefully the audiometric test is performed, if adequate records are not kept, it is an empty exercise. The only way to tell whether hearing levels are deteriorating is to compare records. Also, the only way to assess the need for hearing protectors or to relate an employee's noise exposure to his or her audiometric thresholds is to look at the records. These are only a few of the important reasons why valid, complete, and legible records need to be kept. Other reasons include government regulations, the need to be responsive to inspectors from OSHA and other government agencies, and the use of audiometric records for evaluating hearing conservation program effectiveness and in potential litigation.

In recent years, computers have made recordkeeping much less tedious and space-consuming than it used to be. OHCs who use microprocessor audiometers can keep their records with a minimum of clerical work. Computers can also be programmed to keep the data in the most convenient format, create letters to workers advising them about the status of their hearing, and perform calculations to identify the presence of a "standard" threshold shift.

Program Evaluation:

Although this topic is not currently specified in government regulations, it has become the focus of increasing concern in the professional hearing conservation community and among certain employers. The fact is that an employer may conscientiously comply with a government regulation, such as the OSHA hearing conservation amendment, and yet the employees may still suffer noise-induced hearing losses. There are certain methods by which the supervising professional, and sometimes the OHC, can evaluate the audiograms as a group to see whether workers are losing their hearing in a manner that exceeds the amount that is expected from the normal aging process. For example, a technical report, "Evaluating the Effectiveness of Hearing Conservation Programs Through Audiometric Database Analysis" (ANSI S12.13 TR-2002), provides statistical methods for program evaluation.

Most of these methods involve fairly large noise-exposed populations, but there are certain comparisons that can be made less formally with smaller groups. These methods will be presented in Chapter XII and the ANSI technical report reproduced in Appendix P.

References

ANSI (2002). Technical Report: Evaluating the Effectiveness of Hearing Conservation Programs Through Audiometric Database Analysis. ANSI S12.13 TR-2002. Acoustical Society of America, Melville, NY.

Boettcher, F.A., Henderson, D., Gratton, M.A., Danielson, R.W., and Byrne, C.D. (1987). "Synergistic interactions of noise and other ototraumatic agents." *Ear and Hearing, 8,* 192–222.

Cohen, A. (1976). "The influence of a company hearing conservation program on extra-auditory problems in workers." *J. Saf. Res., 8* (4), 146–162.

Department of the Army (1998). Pamphlet 40-501, *Medical Services: Hearing Conservation Program.* Washington, DC.

EPA (1981). *Noise in America: The Extent of the Noise Problem.* EPA/550/9-81-101. U.S. EPA, Washington, DC.

Franks, J.R., and Morata, T.C. (1996). "Ototoxic effects of chemicals alone or in concert with noise: A review of human studies." In A. Axelsson, H.M. Borchgrevink, R.P., Hamernik, P.-A. Hellstrom, D. Henderson, and R.J. Salvi, (Eds.), *Scientific Basis of Noise-Induced Hearing Loss.* Thieme, New York, 437–446.

Moll van Charante, A.W., and Mulder, P.G.H. (1990). "Perceptual acuity and the risk of industrial accidents." *Am. J. Epidemiol. 131*(4), 652–663.

Morata, T.C. (1998). "Assessing occupational hearing loss: Beyond noise exposures." *Scand Audiol, 27,* Suppl. 48, 111–116.

MSHA (1999). "Health standards for occupational noise exposure; final rule." 64 *Fed. Reg.,* 49573.

OSHA (1981). "Occupational noise exposure: Hearing conservation amendment." 46 *Fed. Reg.,* 4078–4179.

Schmidt, J.W., Royster, L.H., and Pearson, R.G. (1982). "Impact of an industrial hearing conservation program on occupational injuries." *Sound and Vibration 16*(1), 16–20.

Seiler, J.P., and Giardino, D.A. (1994). *The Effect of Threshold on Noise Dosimeter Measurements and Interpretation of Their Results.* Informational Report IR1224. Mine Safety and Health Administration, Pittsburgh, PA.

Staples, N. (1981). "Hearing conservation: Is management short changing 'those at risk'?" *Noise and Vibration Control Worldwide 12*(6), 236–238.

Suter, A.H. (1992a). "The effects of noise on task performance." Chapter 4 in *Communication and Job Performance in Noise: A Review.* ASHA Monographs No. 28. American Speech-Language-Hearing Association, Rockville, MD.

Suter, A.H. (1992b). "Noise sources and effects: A new look." *Sound and Vibration, 26*(1), 18–38.

Zwerling, C., Whitten, P.S., Davis, C.S., and Sprince, N.L. (1997). "Occupational injuries among workers with disabilities." *JAMA, 278*(24), 2163–2166.

Quiz

1. OSHA estimates more than _____ American workers in the manufacturing industries alone have a "material impairment" of hearing.

2. People will often resist talking about their hearing impairment because it is associated with getting old and infirm. (True or False)

3. Noise-induced hearing loss can usually be reversed by medical treatment. (True or False)

4. Sudden loud noise from gunfire or metal stamping is called _____ noise.

5. TTS stands for _____ and the OHC needs to catch these hearing losses before they become _____.

6. Name at least three agents besides noise that are toxic to the ear, especially when combined with noise exposure:_____.

7. Name four sources of non-occupational noise that could contribute to hearing loss. Can you think of some more?

8. The technical term for ringing or other noises in the ears is _____. Why is it an important warning signal?

9. What kinds of problems are caused by noise in addition to hearing loss? (Name at least four.)

10. Why is it important for management to wear hearing protectors in noisy environments?

11. Give at least two reasons why employees' noise exposures are measured? What kinds of equipment are used to make the measurements?

12. When is the best time to perform a baseline audiogram?

13. When is the best time to perform a periodic (annual) audiogram?

14. What are some of the potential benefits to the company management of a good hearing conservation program? (Name at least three.)

Abbreviations Used in Chapter II

ANSI	American National Standards Institute, Inc.
dBA	Decibels measured on the A scale of the sound level meter
EPA	U.S. Environmental Protection Agency
NRR	Noise Reduction Rating
NRR(SF)	Noise Reduction Rating, Subject Fit
OHC	Occupational Hearing Conservationist
OSHA	Occupational Safety and Health Administration
PTS	Permanent Threshold Shift
TTS	Temporary Threshold Shift

Recommended Reading

Berger, E.H. (2000). "Noise control and hearing conservation: Why do it?" Chapter 1 in E.H. Berger, L.H. Royster, J.D. Royster, L.H. Driscoll, and M. Layne (Eds.), *The Noise Manual, Fifth Edition*, American Industrial Hygiene Assoc., Fairfax, VA.

Burke, A. (Nov. 1996). "Have you heard? Noise isn't the only hearing hazard...." *Industrial Safety and Hygiene News*, 29–30.

Franks, J.R., Stephenson, M.R., and Merry, C.J. (1996). *Preventing Occupational Hearing Loss—A Practical Guide.* DHSS (NIOSH) Pub. No. 96–110. U.S. Dept. Health and Human Services, National Institute for Occupational Safety and Health, Cincinnati, OH.

Malcore, D. (1999). "Hyperacusis." CAOHC *Update, 10*(2), 1.

NIOSH (1998). "Criteria for a Recommended Standard: Occupational Noise Exposure: Revised Criteria, 1998." DHHS (NIOSH) 98–126. Dept. Health and Human Services, Public Health Service, Cincinnati, OH.

OSHA (1981). "Occupational noise exposure; Hearing Conservation Amendment, Section II Health effects," 46 *Fed. Reg.,* (11), 4081–4129.

Suter, A.H. (1992). "Noise sources and effects: A new look." *Sound and Vibration, 26*(1), 18–38.

Suter, A.H. (1992). "The effects of noise on task performance." Chapter 4 in *Communication and Job Performance in Noise: A Review.* ASHA Monographs No. 28. American Speech-Language-Hearing Association, Rockville, MD.

Website

www.ata.org
American Tinnitus Association

Chapter III

Anatomy and Physiology of the Human Ear

Homage to the Ear

When most people think of the ear, they think of the fleshy thing that sticks out on the side of the head. But internal to the visible ear is one of the most amazing accomplishments of nature. It is an extremely delicate, highly sensitive organ that operates with great efficiency. In a quiet environment it is sensitive enough, as the old saying goes, to hear the scratch of a mosquito's leg on a postage stamp. In fact, the motion of the eardrum may be smaller than the diameter of a hydrogen molecule, and yet the listener can still perceive it as sound (Stevens and Warshofsky, 1980). At the other extreme the ear can withstand sounds that are almost painfully loud, although sounds of this intensity can't be repeated often without causing damage.

These vibrations, whether they are thunderclaps or whispers, are the vibrations that eventually move the tiny membranes in the inner ear. The movements of the sensory mechanism of the inner ear, which then transmit this stimulation to the brain, are 100 times smaller than the kind of activity that takes place at the eardrum. This is undoubtedly one of the reasons why the physiological processes of the ear are difficult to measure. The introduction of the electron microscope, however, as well as other sophisticated technology, has added greatly to the current knowledge base.

One of the most useful characteristics of the intact hearing mechanism allows the listener to pick out the desired signal and suppress the unwanted sounds. An example of this benefit is the ability to "tune in" to someone whom you want to listen to and "tune out" the general din of a social gathering. People with **unilateral** (one-sided) hearing losses, or people with **sensorineural** (nerve-type) hearing losses in both ears have difficulty picking out the speech they want to hear from the unwanted noise. This is one of the most troubling aspects of hearing impairment.

Other useful characteristics of a healthy hearing mechanism are too numerous to mention, but any quick summary would include the following abilities (just to name a few): to communicate in all walks of life, to perceive warnings (like the sound of an approaching car), to diagnose the sound of a machine that has begun to malfunction, and to hear the distress cries of a baby during the night. Good hearing also enables us to enjoy music, the songs of birds and the summer breeze, and the voice of a loved one.

But most importantly, our hearing enables us to share the lives of our closest family members and friends through spoken conversation. In short, good hearing is priceless.

Hearing Sensitivity

The ability to hear can be measured in a variety of ways, but the OHC will mainly be concerned with measuring hearing sensitivity for **pure tones**.[8] The

---

[8] Pure tones are sounds that consist of one frequency only, without any additional tones, overtones, or noise.

chart or document on which the responses are recorded is the **audiogram**, and measurements in decibels (dB) are routinely taken for pure tones from 500 **hertz (Hz)** to 6000 or 8000 Hz. Reading horizontally across an audiogram: 500, 1000, 2000, 3000, 4000, and 6000 Hz are the minimum **frequencies** that are measured. This is considered the "practical" range of human hearing, although sounds can be heard both above and below this range. The human ear is least sensitive for very low- or very high-frequency sounds. For example, the sensitivity of the ear for a 1000-Hz tone is about 10 times greater than that for a tone at 100 Hz.

Pure-tone audiometric testing establishes a subject's **hearing threshold level**, which is the softest level of sound that can be detected for a given frequency. There are also tests using speech materials, such as sentences or word lists delivered by compact disk, tape, or live voice, as well as a variety of other pure-tone tests that assist in evaluating more complex auditory functions. These tests are used mainly by audiologists and will not be part of the OHC's duties.

The ear's comparative insensitivity to very low sound frequencies is actually a blessing. Otherwise, people would hear the vibrations of their own bodily activities, such as muscle contractions and the movement of bones. This would be not only a distraction, but it could interfere with the ability to hear important sounds. The range of sensitivity to frequency is from about 20 Hz to 20,000 Hz. However, sometimes people can hear frequencies as low as 8 to 10 Hz, and some people may hear as high as 40,000 Hz. This extreme range can be found mainly in young, normal-hearing adults, and these abilities tend to diminish with advancing age.

Everyone, if he or she lives to be old enough, will lose some hearing due to the aging process. But there is considerable variability in the aging ear. Some people begin losing hearing relatively early in life, while others may live into their 80s with good hearing. Just as body tissue loses its elasticity, so does the hearing mechanism lose some of its efficiency as it ages. This condition is, of course, influenced by many other factors during one's life span, such as drug use, disease, stress, noise exposure, and genetic factors.

Anatomy of the Ear

Figure 3-1 is a diagram of the ear, showing the three major divisions of the ear, the **outer** or **external ear**, the **middle ear**, and the **inner ear**. Note the relative size of the outer ear in comparison to the other structures.

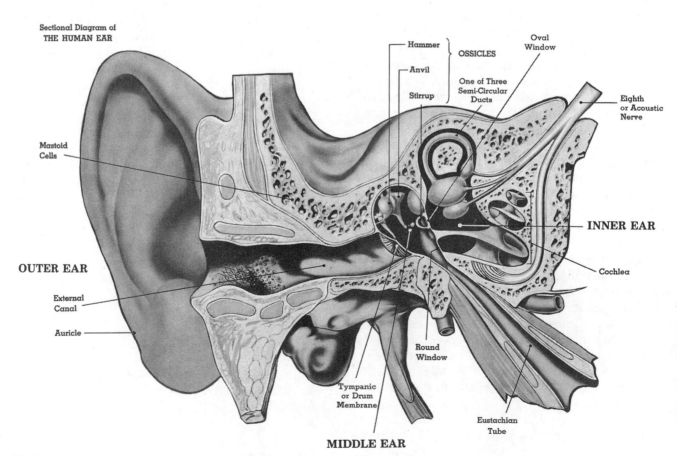

Sectional Diagram of
THE HUMAN EAR

Hammer

Anvil

Stirrup

OSSICLES

One of Three
Semi-Circular
Ducts

Oval
Window

Eighth
or Acoustic
Nerve

Mastoid
Cells

INNER EAR

Cochlea

OUTER EAR

External
Canal

Auricle

Tympanic
or Drum
Membrane

Round
Window

Eustachian
Tube

MIDDLE EAR

Fig. 3-1. Sectional diagram of the human ear. (Courtesy of the Sonotone Corp.)

The External Ear

The **pinna**, or **auricle** in medical terms, is the most visible and probably the least useful of all the parts in the auditory system. Its functions are to direct sound waves into the earcanal and to help in determining the location of a sound. The small cavity at the outer edge of the earcanal is called the **concha**. Sound waves enter the earcanal, the **external auditory meatus**, and proceed to strike the eardrum, the **tympanic membrane**. The tympanic membrane is the terminal point of the external ear and the beginning of the middle ear.

The external auditory meatus is about an inch long and one-fourth to one-third inch in diameter. It varies in size and shape among individuals, and some people even have differently sized earcanals in their right and left ears, which can be important when fitting certain hearing protectors. The exterior part of the canal is surrounded by cartilage, and the internal part is surrounded by the bony tissue of the **mastoid process**. The bony internal segment is quite sensitive because skin covers the bone directly, just as it does the shin-bone. Glands producing a brownish-colored earwax, or **cerumen**, are located in the external auditory meatus. The canal also contains hair and **sebaceous glands**, which lubricate the skin and help prevent foreign objects from getting into the ear. Earwax is produced continuously, and it is quite normal for the average person to have excess wax roll out of the ear once in a while. Wax is important to the earcanal because it traps debris and destroys bacteria. Occasionally, however, wax becomes lodged or "impacted" in the canal, where it can cause some temporary loss of hearing or interfere with the comfort and proper use of earplugs. In such cases it may be necessary to have the wax removed.

The Middle Ear

The middle ear, depicted in Figure 3-2, is frequently referred to as the **tympanic cavity**. In the middle ear, three tiny bones are held in place by muscles and ligaments, and these bones conduct the sound vibrations from the eardrum into the inner ear. They are popularly known as the **hammer**, the **anvil**, and the **stirrup**, and their technical names are the **malleus**, the **incus**, and the **stapes**. Taken together, these bones are known as the **ossicles**. Since they are attached to each other, they are referred to as the **ossicular chain**, and they form a bridge to the inner ear.

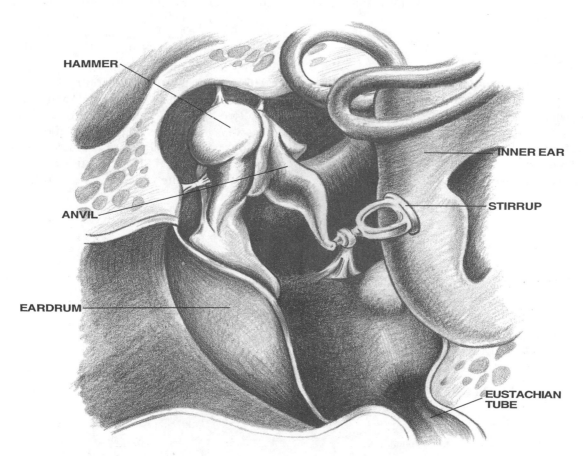

Fig. 3-2. Diagram of the tympanic cavity (middle ear).

In addition to conducting sound, another important feature of the middle ear is the **eustachian tube**, which connects the middle ear with the **nasopharynx**, the back of the nose and throat. The eustachian tube helps maintain an equal barometric air pressure on each side of the eardrum. For example, when ascending or descending in an airplane, rapid changes in barometric pressure are applied initially only to the outside of the eardrum. Eventually these pressure changes pass through the eustachian tube into the middle ear cavity to establish equal pressure on both sides of the drum. The eustachian tube may become temporarily closed due to swelling from colds or allergies, resulting in an uncomfortable pressure difference between the middle ear and the outside. Yawning can sometimes open the eustachian tube's entrance to the nasopharynx and give some relief.

The tympanic cavity is a small space, the entire cavity measuring only about one-half inch high and somewhere between one-twelfth and one-fourth inches wide. It may be viewed as a box with six sides: (1) The outer wall formed by the eardrum; (2) The inner wall formed by the bony division that separates the middle ear from the inner ear; (3) The front wall opening into the eustachian tube; (4) The back wall opening into the mastoid cells; (5) The roof separating the middle ear from the brain; and (6) The floor separating the middle ear from the jugular vein and the internal carotid artery.

The Inner Ear

The next stage in the auditory communication system is the inner ear, which is behind a bony wall forming the innermost side of the middle ear. There are two openings or "windows" in this wall. The stapes rests on the upper opening, the **oval window**, and the lower one, the **round window**, provides a sort of pressure release mechanism responding to the vibrations initiated by the stapes and spread through the inner ear. Because of its complex structure the inner ear is called the **labyrinth**. The labyrinth's chambers house the sensory mechanism for both balance and hearing. The **cochlea**, the sensory mechanism or "end organ" for hearing, is a snail-shaped membrane about 35 millimeters long when uncoiled. It is connected to the vestibular organ, which includes the three **semicircular canals** that assist in space-orientation and balance. These two organs are innervated and connected to the brain by the **eighth cranial nerve**. It is the cochlea, with its delicate "**hair cells**," that is most vulnerable to damage when the ear is exposed to excessive noise.

How the Ear Operates

When sound waves strike the tympanic membrane, the ossicular chain is mobilized and the stapes begins to move back and forth in the oval window. Because the oval window is much smaller than the tympanic membrane, the ossicles act as a mechanical transformer, increasing the sound energy reaching the inner ear by about twenty times.

The ossicular movement sets up vibrations in the fluids filling the inner ear, converting the sound from mechanical to hydraulic energy. The path of this movement is shown in Figure 3-3. Movement of the stapes causes the fluid in the **scala vestibuli** (vestibular duct) to vibrate, and these vibrations pass rapidly through the cochlear spiral and back along the **scala tympani**, (the tympanic duct). Within a fraction of a second, the sound wave reaches the round window membrane, where it is reflected back, if it has not died out already. Along the way, the waves impinge on the walls of the **cochlear duct**, which houses the actual sense organ, the organ of Corti. The pressure displacement is transferred to the organ of Corti's tiny hair cells,

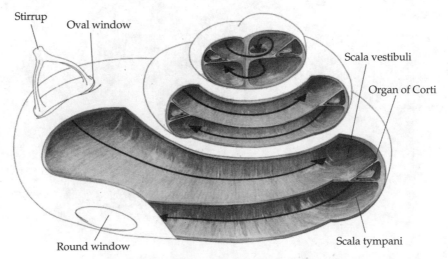

Fig. 3-3. Schematic of the cochlea showing the pathway of sound waves through the spiral. (Courtesy of Bilsom, a Bacou-Dalloz Company)

20

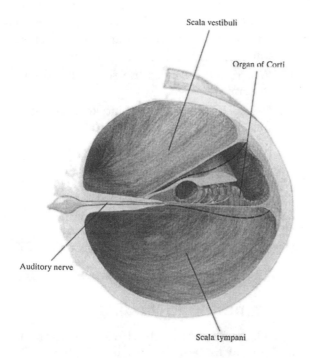

Fig. 3-4. Cross-section of a turn of the cochlea, showing the vestibular and tympanic ducts and the organ of Corti in between. (Courtesy of Bilsom, a Bacou-Dalloz Company)

Figure 3-4 shows a cross-section of one of the spirals or "turns" of the cochlea, showing the scala vestibuli, the scala tympani, and the organ of Corti in between. Sound vibrations in these two chambers cause the organ of Corti to vibrate, which, in turn, causes the tiny **cilia** or tufts at the top of the hair cells to bend very slightly. In response to this sensation, the hair cells send an electrical impulse to the brain via the eighth cranial or auditory nerve. Repeated overstimulation of the delicate hair cells by noise eventually causes their destruction, and the result is a gradual loss of hearing.

The next diagram, Figure 3-5, depicts an enlargement of the organ of Corti, showing the hair cells and their connection to the auditory nerve fibers. These drawings are, of course, greatly simplified.

The organ of Corti responds differently to tones of different frequency. In general, the area closest to the oval window sends high-frequency messages to the brain, whereas the areas further toward the tip or apex of the spiral respond to lower tones. One reason why noise-exposed people lose their hearing for the high tones first is that the sound conduction mechanism is most efficient and hence the ear is most sensitive at these frequencies, causing these nerve cells to wear out more quickly.

It is indeed a remarkable mechanism that the OHC will monitor!

which are seated on the basilar membrane. The hair cells then convert the hydraulic energy to neural (electric) energy.

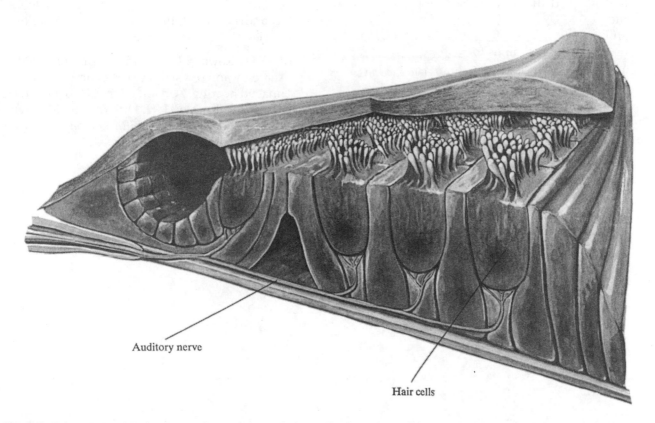

Fig. 3-5. Enlargement of the basilar membrane showing the hair cells, their cilia, and their connections to the auditory nerve. (Courtesy of Bilsom, a Bacou-Dalloz Company)

Reference

Stevens, S.S., and Warshofsky, F. (1980). "The machinery of hearing." Chapter 2 in *Sound and Hearing* (Revised ed.). Time-Life Books, Alexandria, VA.

Quiz

1. Three of the most useful abilities of human hearing are: _____ _____.

2. The chart on which hearing threshold levels are plotted is the _____.

3. The standard audiometric frequencies measured by OHCs are: _____ _____ Hz.

4. In addition to pure-tone testing the OHC may perform speech audiometry. (True or False)

5. The technical term for the eardrum is the _____. It is located at the beginning of the inner ear. (True or False)

6. The technical term for earwax is _____. It can sometimes interfere with the comfort and proper use of _____.

7. Inside the middle ear are situated three small bones called the ossicles, whose names are the _____, _____, and _____. The function of the ossicular chain is to _____.

8. The inner ear, or labyrinth, houses the mechanism for _____ as well as for hearing.

9. In the inner ear, the snail-shaped end organ for hearing is the _____.

10. The tiny _____ cells seated on the basilar membrane convert the hydraulic energy into _____ energy.

11. Which nerve carries the sound impulses to the brain?

12. Noise-exposed people tend to lose hearing first for the _____ tones.

Abbreviations Used in Chapter III

dB   Decibel

Hz   Hertz

OHC   Occupational Hearing Conservationist

Recommended Reading

Bess, F.H., and Humes, L.E. (1995). "Structure and function of the auditory system." Chapter 3 in *Audiology: The Fundamentals, 2nd Ed.* Williams and Wilkins: Baltimore, MD.

Newby, H.A., and Popelka, G.R. (1992). "What and how we hear," Chapter 2 in *Audiology, 6th Ed.* Prentice Hall, Englewood Cliffs, NJ.

Stevens, S.S., and Warshofsky, F. (1980). "The machinery of hearing." Chapter 2 in *Sound and Hearing* (Revised ed.). Time-Life Books, Alexandria, VA. (Out of print but available in libraries.)

Ward, W.D., Royster, L.H., and Royster, J.D. (2000). "Anatomy and physiology of the ear: Normal and damaged hearing." Chapter 4 in E.H. Berger, L.H. Royster, J.D. Royster, L.H. Driscoll, and M. Layne (Eds.), *The Noise Manual, Fifth Edition*. American Industrial Hygiene Assoc., Fairfax, VA.

Chapter IV

Hearing Disorders:
Their Causes and Management

Introduction

After introducing the human ear's structure and function, it is time to consider some of the things that may go wrong with this extremely complex structure. *The OHC will not be expected to diagnose hearing problems* (unless he or she has had professional training in otology or audiology). However, a basic understanding of the causes and treatments of different types of ear and hearing disorders will make the OHC's work more meaningful and provide a broader grasp of the OHC's role in the total process of preserving hearing. Some of the employees with whom the OHC comes into contact with will have complex auditory problems, and knowledgeable handling of these problems is very important.

Physicians specializing in diseases of the ears, nose, and throat are known as **otolaryngologists** and have had five to seven years of training and study after receiving the MD degree. The specialty is now called **otolaryngology—head and neck surgery** to reflect its involvement with major head and neck diseases such as cancer of the larynx, thyroid, and parotid glands, as well as plastic and reconstructive surgery of this area. Sometimes these doctors are referred to simply as ENTs (for ear, nose, and throat) physicians. Physicians who have specialized further and deal only with the ear are known as **otologists**. Their training has been similar, but with more focus on the ear in the postgraduate years. The OHC may wish to refer employees with various types of hearing loss or ear symptoms to otologists or otolaryngologists.

Another professional in this area is the **audiologist**, who specializes in the prevention, assessment, diagnosis, and rehabilitation of hearing impairments. Audiologists have either a master's or a doctoral degree in audiology, and may be certified by a professional organization, such as the American Speech-Language-Hearing Association or the American Board of Audiology. Practicing audiologists should also be licensed or registered by their state. The audiologist will often be the supervising professional of an audiometric testing program. The OHC should refer employees who are difficult to test or who have unusual audiometric configurations to an audiologist for more exhaustive clinical testing.

Hearing loss is divided into two main types. **Conductive** hearing loss is very common, in which there is a breakdown or obstruction in the transmission system in the external or middle ear. In most instances, these problems may be reversed and hearing is restored or stabilized by appropriate treatment. **Sensorineural**[9] hearing loss results from changes in the receptor hair cells in the inner ear or in the nerves carrying impulses to the brain. These losses are often permanent and are not usually correctable by medical or surgical means. Many people with this form of hearing loss will derive

---

[9] The term "sensorineural" is also written sensori-neural, sensory neural, or sometimes neuro-sensory. Occasionally the term "nerve loss" is used for this condition. This is usually a misnomer, since it is actually the cochlea and not the nerve that is the cause of the problem in most cases.

some benefit from hearing aids and hearing therapy or **aural rehabilitation**, such as auditory training and speech (lip) reading.

Conductive Hearing Loss

Conductive hearing losses impede the conduction of sound through the outer and middle ears. In the external ear conductive losses may be caused by something as simple as an obstruction of the external auditory canal by **cerumen** (earwax)[10] or a foreign object. Or they may result from perforations of the tympanic membrane (a ruptured eardrum). In the middle ear conductive losses result from numerous conditions caused by a build-up of fluid, or from defects or fixation of one or more of the ossicles. These problems may be the result of infection, either acute or chronic, or an injury. Also, some people are born with very small earcanals and a few have no canal at all. Occasionally, people have deformed outer ears, and there are many possible deformities of the middle ear. Aside from some of the cosmetic disadvantages, many of these conditions result in hearing impairment of the conductive type.

Conductive hearing losses are characterized by audiograms that are "flat" and depressed across the low- to mid-frequencies. They are sometimes accompanied by feelings of a "stuffy" head and a hollow-sounding voice, and occasionally by low-pitched tinnitus or head noises. These losses may be mild or they may be significant with people reporting difficulties in actually hearing as well as understanding others, but they are almost never profound. The good news is that conductive hearing losses usually respond well to medical treatment.

Problems of the External Ear

Otitis externa, external-ear infections, involve the skin of the earcanal. One type frequently seen is "swimmer's ear," in which there is widespread, painful swelling of the skin of the earcanal. This may be caused by moisture remaining in the ear for long periods of time and soaking the skin, resulting in a breakdown of its natural resistance.

If earcanals become dry and crusted, itching may result and people tend to pick at them with objects such as paper clips, hairpins, and pencils. This may bruise or break the skin and introduce infection. On rare occasions, workers may be allergic to the materials used in manufacturing earplugs and may develop an inflammation of the earcanal. Moisture

may collect around the earplug and create a predisposition to infection.

External-ear infections can be quite painful, but are easily treated by a general-practice physician or ear specialist. People with diabetes may have severe problems with otitis externa, and require special attention as soon as the problem is detected. Employees with external otitis should not wear earplugs, and should be careful about wearing earmuffs. Although there is little evidence that earplugs can actually cause infections, they can certainly produce further irritation, and the result may be quite painful. Sometimes earmuffs can be tolerated, but the OHC and the employee should make sure that the earcup does not rub against the affected area. Also, the lack of aeration and the potential for moisture build-up may cause problems underneath the muff. These employees should be referred for medical treatment as quickly as possible.

Disorders of the tympanic membrane may also lead to conductive losses. Perforations of the tympanic membrane are usually caused by infections in the middle ear, but they can also be caused by the insertion of a sharp object into the canal, or by a very intense sound, such as an explosion or blast. These intense exposures result in acoustic trauma that often causes sensorineural as well as conductive hearing loss. Surgical repair of a perforated or ruptured eardrum can be done by grafting tissue onto it, allowing it to heal normally.

The OHC may occasionally find a foreign object in the worker's earcanal during the otoscopic inspection. These patients should be referred to an otologist or otolaryngologist. Untrained personnel should not attempt to remove such an object since complications following inexpert attempts at removal may be worse than the problems caused by the object itself.

People with deformities of the external ear and earcanal can also pose special problems for the OHC, and need to be fitted for hearing protection with great care. Sometimes the use of earplugs will not be possible and earmuffs are the only solution. In the rare case where the earcanal is completely sealed or absent, protection may be unnecessary. Guidance from an otolaryngologist or audiologist would be useful here.

Another external-ear problem that OHCs should be aware of is collapsing earcanals. This is not a disease, but a problem that can seriously affect the accuracy of hearing tests for some employees. There is great variation in the sizes of earcanals, both in their length and diameter. Some people have large entrances from their pinnas to their canals, while most have average ones. However, a small percentage of people have unusually small earcanal openings, and with this group there is a good possibility that the pressure of earphones used in testing

---

[10] Cerumen is secreted by tiny sebaceous glands that line the earcanal. Its presence in the earcanal is natural and only rarely does it block the canal to the extent that it causes a hearing loss.

hearing can easily close off the entrance to the external meatus. When this happens, sound cannot pass directly from its source (the earphone) to the tympanic membrane because a portion of the passage has been squeezed shut. This kind of artificial hearing loss is caused by testing conditions that are not present during normal listening conditions, so a worker may be unaware of it as a problem. Collapsed earcanals are more likely to occur in older than in younger individuals, although they may occur in any age group. One lesson to be learned from this discussion is that the earphones should be positioned carefully and not "slapped on" for audiometric testing.

When an examination of a person's ears suggests the possibility of collapsing earcanals and a hearing loss is measured, this possibility should be recorded on the hearing test form. The person should be referred to an audiologist so that appropriate measures may be taken to prevent a false hearing loss from occurring during the hearing retest. The supervising professional can often suggest methods to ensure that the canal is open. These include the use of an insert earphone, a foam cushion behind the ear, or holding the earphone lightly against the pinna by hand.

Middle Ear Problems

In its healthy state, the middle ear may be considered an air-filled cavity in which air is being constantly absorbed and replaced. Air is replaced via the eustachian tube leading from the nasopharynx, the back of the nose and throat, to the front part of the middle ear. On swallowing or yawning, the tube is opened, and air passes into the middle ear. If the air is not periodically replaced in the middle ear, fluid forms, often as a result of negative pressure or a partial vacuum. This condition is probably the basis for most **otitis media** (middle-ear infections), and more serious chronic diseases of the middle ear and the mastoid area. In treating these infections, the physician must consider the possible role of allergy in causing the infection.

Treatment includes attempting to restore ventilation to the middle ear by way of the eustachian tube, with attention to any pathologies of the back of the nose, the adenoids, and sinuses. If this is not successful, ventilation may be reestablished by making an incision in the tympanic membrane and inserting a small tube, through which air will flow by way of the external earcanal. With such a tube, the fluid is usually absorbed quickly and the ear clears. These tubes are almost always temporary and may be expelled naturally in periods ranging from days to years, or they may be removed by the otolaryngologist after several months. In an adult, the presence of fluid or a conductive loss in one ear may signify a serious **lesion** (disease of a tissue or organ) in the nasopharynx. People with such conditions should be referred promptly to an otolaryngologist.

One complication of chronic otitis media is **cholesteatoma**. This is a skin-lined cyst that may originate in the middle ear or enter through a hole in the eardrum. By shedding surface cells that collect inside the cyst, it grows from the inside, expanding to destroy the bone and other structures around it. Generally, this results in a recurring, foul-smelling discharge. The disease is usually progressive, and, in most cases, cure requires surgical removal and repair. This may include the removal of bone and soft tissue and replacement of the diseased middle-ear structures by a prosthesis.

Another middle ear problem is **otosclerosis**, which is the new growth of a spongy bone material in the middle ear. It impedes the ability of the ossicles to conduct sound, and eventually causes the stapes to become fixed in the oval window. The resulting hearing loss is conductive at first, but in rare instances patients may develop a sensorineural component as the disease invades the inner ear. Otosclerosis is not uncommon in adults, and occurs twice as frequently in women as it does in men. Otologists treat this condition by removing the fixed stapes with great care and using a live tissue graft or other material to cover the defect in the oval window. They then insert a prosthesis to replace the missing stapes in the ossicular chain. Amplification with a hearing aid can be very useful in treating hearing loss from otosclerosis.

Other defects in the ossicular chain can be repaired by rearranging the bones to form a connection between the drum and the inner ear. Otologists may use tiny plastic or steel prostheses, or actual bones that have been banked or preserved.

Sensorineural Hearing Loss

Sensorineural hearing loss tends to be permanent in nature and is often accompanied by tinnitus. It poses difficulties in hearing and understanding speech, especially in a noisy background. People with sensorineural losses can have any degree of impairment, from very mild to completely deaf.

The most frequent form of sensorineural hearing loss that the OHC is likely to encounter is noise-induced hearing loss, which is usually characterized by a sloping configuration on the audiogram where high-frequency hearing is much more impaired than hearing in the low and middle frequencies. Such losses may be due to occupational or nonoccupational sources of noise exposure. They have been described in some detail in Chapter II. While noise-induced hearing loss is often temporary at first, it may become permanent fairly quickly, so the OHC must be diligent in identifying temporary losses and taking measures to prevent them from becoming permanent.

Another significant contributor to sensorineural loss is the aging process. This kind of hearing loss is called **presbycusis**, and its onset and magnitude vary greatly among individuals. Some people will have a noticeable amount of presbycusis at age 50, while others will have good hearing well into their 80s. Familial or genetic factors influence the extent of the loss. Other influences are the accumulation of all diseases and injuries of the ear, including the effects of exposure to noise. The aging of the hearing mechanism may be accelerated by the traumas of living in our "civilized" world. Hearing losses from noise and presbycusis appear to be additive, each contributing to the total hearing loss. This means that people with noise-induced hearing losses will become increasingly more hearing impaired as they become older.

Hearing loss may be hereditary or may develop from prenatal influences, such as rubella (German measles) in the pregnant mother, a host of viral and bacterial diseases, lack of oxygen to the fetus at the time of delivery, and various blood incompatibilities. Childhood illnesses, such as measles, mumps, scarlet fever, and a variety of viral infections can produce sensorineural hearing loss due to their toxic effect on the sensory cells in the cochlea. The hearing loss from mumps may be profound, but usually occurs in one ear only. Infections involving the spinal fluid, such as meningitis, can also cause severe sensorineural hearing loss. At any stage in life, sensorineural hearing loss can occur as a result of exposure to medications that are ototoxic (poisonous to the hearing mechanism). Examples of these drugs are certain antibiotics (the "Mycin" drugs), the "loop-inhibiting" diuretics, and some of the chemicals used in cancer chemotherapy.

Another source of sensorineural hearing loss is **Meniere's disease** or syndrome, which is caused by a build-up of fluid in the inner ear. Because Meniere's involves both the vestibular system as well as the cochlea, its symptoms include balance problems as well as hearing loss. The hearing loss usually fluctuates and is accompanied by a "dizzy" spell lasting from one to eight hours. It is also accompanied by tinnitus, which is usually described as "roaring" rather than the ringing sound commonly experienced by people with noise-induced hearing loss. Sometimes Meniere's affects only the cochlea with a fluctuating low-frequency hearing loss, but without dizziness. Medical and surgical treatments can give relief to some patients with Meniere's disease, but some degree of permanent hearing loss usually results.

Acoustic neuromas, tumors of the auditory nerve, occur in a small percentage of the population. They are potentially life-threatening and may be present for many years with hearing loss, usually on one side, as the only symptom. They are frequently associated with tinnitus and loss of balance. It is often the OHC who will identify a one-sided hearing loss and refer this potentially dangerous condition promptly to an otolaryngologist or otologist.

Mixed Hearing Losses

Sometimes a hearing loss will have both a conductive and a sensorineural component. This is referred to as a **mixed** loss. It can occur in the later stages of otosclerosis if the disease has invaded the inner ear. More often it is due to a combination of things, like a noise-induced hearing loss plus a middle-ear infection, or presbycusis plus impacted wax. If the conductive problem receives medical attention, then the hearing may improve, but the sensorineural component remains permanent.

Pseudohypacusis

Pseudohypacusis, sometimes called functional or non-organic hearing loss, has no demonstrated organic or physical cause. It may present itself audiometrically as either conductive or sensorineural hearing loss when there is actually no hearing loss or an existing loss is exaggerated. Pseudohypacusis may be the result of strong psychological causes over which the individual has no conscious control, or there may be a deliberate attempt to feign a hearing loss. Very specialized audiological assessment is required for diagnosis of this kind of condition. Pseudohypacusis may be suspected when a person shows great inconsistency in responding to audiometric tones during and between tests or whenever there is a large discrepancy between an individual's pure-tone test results and his or her ability to hear normal conversational speech. However, pseudohypacusis may exist in the absence of any such findings. It is very important to remember that inconsistent responses can result from factors other than pseudohypacusis, such as faulty equipment or even severe tinnitus. *The OHC should be careful not to label a hearing loss or an employee pseudohypacusic (or any related term),* but to describe the responses as inconsistent and refer the individual for further testing. These matters are discussed further in Chapter VIII.

Hearing Aids

Hearing aids have improved over recent years to the point where people with mild-to-moderate sensorineural losses may very well benefit from them. Current hearing aids are smaller, more versatile, and perform better than instruments of 20 or even 10 years ago. However, they average several hundred to several thousands of dollars, and they can never "correct" hearing the way eyeglasses can correct vision. Some people will swear by their hearing aids and not want to be without them. Others will experience considerable difficulty using them, especially in background noise, and still others will relegate them to the dresser drawer. A hearing aid can never compensate for the quality and precision of hearing that has been lost.

Quiz

1. Physicians specializing in diseases of the ear, nose, and throat are called _____.
   Those with further specialization in the ear are _____.
2. Under what conditions will the OHC need to diagnose hearing disorders?
3. An audiologist specializes in _____ _____.
4. Give three examples of outer or middle ear conditions that could cause a conductive hearing loss.
5. Under what conditions should a worker refrain from wearing earplugs?
6. What causes collapsed earcanals?
7. In what part of the auditory system does a sensorineural hearing loss occur?
8. Besides noise, one of the most frequent contributors to sensorineural hearing loss is _____, or the hearing loss from aging.
9. Name at least five possible causes of sensorineural hearing loss other than noise.
10. Why is it important for the OHC to identify a one-sided hearing loss and refer the individual to an ear specialist if he or she has not already received an examination for this condition?
11. A hearing aid can restore hearing to normal. (True or False)

Abbreviations Used in Chapter IV

ENT   Ear, nose, and throat
OHC   Occupational Hearing Conservationist

Recommended Reading

Bess, F.H., and Humes, L.E. (1995). "Pathologies of the auditory system," Chapter 5 in *Audiology: The Fundamentals*, *2nd Ed*. Williams and Wilkins, Baltimore, MD.

Newby, H.A., and Popelka, G.R. (1992). "Disorders of the auditory system." Chapter 3 in *Audiology*, *6th Ed*. Prentice-Hall, Inc., Englewood Cliffs, NJ.

Chapter V

Introduction to Sound

The Nature of Sound

Ordinarily, OHCs will not be responsible for taking noise measurements, unless they have been specifically trained. Despite this, it is helpful for the OHC to have a general knowledge about the nature of sound and noise, the basic concepts and definitions, and how sound works in the testing of hearing.

Everybody measures sound all the time without knowing it, by using their ears and categorizing their environments. That is how subjective judgments are made. For example, when the thunder gets sufficiently loud, a person needs to get home before the downpour starts. Or, one might think that a certain machine is very noisy, and it sounds different than it did last week. Another such judgment is that an audiometric tone is just barely loud enough to hear. So, sound may be considered subjectively, as just described, or it may be considered objectively, from a technical point of view. Both approaches are important. Those who measure sound generally use the objective approach. Those who measure hearing rely on the subjective approach when they ask workers to respond to the audiometric tones, but they know the value of the objective approach when discussing the audiometer's calibration or measurements of employee noise exposures.

Sound is caused by pressure variations in any "elastic" (movable) medium, like air, water, and solids.[11] These pressure changes may be in the form of vibration, such as the ringing of a bell or the vibration of the vocal cords, or turbulence, as in the release of compressed air or the explosion of a gun. A good example of a sound source is a tuning fork, which, when struck, sets air molecules into vibration (see Figure 5–1). In one cycle of this vibration the molecules push or bump against each other, then they move back toward the tuning fork to fill an empty space created by the movement of the tuning fork in the opposite direction, and finally back to their original places. Those molecules that have been bumped move on to bump other molecules, which move on to bump others, and so forth as the sound wave is propagated outward. In the meantime, the tuning fork continues to vibrate, perpetuating the pattern until it eventually dies down. The technical term for the pushing or bumping action is **compression**, and the term for the moving apart stage is **rarefaction**. It is important to remember that the actual air molecules do not travel very far at all, but it is the pressure wave that travels, sometimes for very long distances, as in thunder or an explosion.

---

[11] The speed of sound in air is 1128 feet per second on a standard day (normal barometric pressure and about 70 degrees F). In water sound travels about four times as fast, and in solids it travels quite a bit faster. For example, sound travels at 16,600 feet per second in steel.

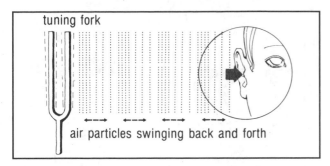

Fig. 5-1. Schematic drawing of the movement of sound through air. The sound source is a tuning fork on the left. Air particles are represented by dots, moving back and forth as the sound wave is propagated toward the listener. (From OSHA, 1980, *Noise Control: A Guide for Workers and Employers.* OSHA 3048. U.S. Dept. Labor, Washington, DC.)

Figure 5-2 shows what this movement would look like if it were graphed on a piece of paper. In the lower part of the figure the little dots represent the air molecules in their compression and rarefaction stages, and the upper part illustrates the resulting sound wave. After each compression phase and rarefaction phase, the wave passes through its original static position, which is represented by the horizontal line. The distance (A) between the crests of the curves is the wavelength of the sound.

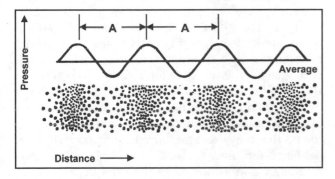

Fig. 5-2. Alternate compressions and rarefactions of a sound wave. The lower part of the figure shows the air molecules as little dots, and in the upper part as a graphic representation of the resulting sound wave. The distance (A) between crests of the curves is the wavelength of the sound. (From EPA, 1976, *About Sound.* EPA 550/9-76-100. U.S. Environmental Protection Agency, Washington, DC.)

The completion of one compression and rarefaction cycle is called one **cycle**. The faster these cycles occur, the higher the pitch of the sound will be, or technically, the sound's **frequency**. Sound frequency is quantified in terms of **cycles per second**, also called **hertz**, abbreviated **Hz**, after the German physicist Heinrich Hertz. The sound's **pitch** is the subjective perception of its frequency.

The more force used to move the air particles, the larger the pressure displacements will be. This is the sound wave's **amplitude**, which translates into **intensity** or **sound pressure level (SPL)**. Sound pressure level is the quantity measured with a sound level meter. The subjective perception of sound pressure level is **loudness**.

The properties of sound may be divided into three main categories: frequency, level, and temporal characteristics. Frequency and level have been mentioned above. The temporal properties of sound concern the way the sound is distributed in time; for example, whether it consists of short, rapid bursts of sound, or long periods of steady noise. All three of these categories will be discussed in the following sections.

Frequency

As stated above, the frequency of a sound wave is determined by the number of vibrations, or more exactly, the number of compression-plus-rarefaction cycles completed in one second. A sound with a frequency of 1000 Hz has completed 1000 compressions and rarefactions each second. You might think that this is a huge number of cycles to be produced in an awfully short time, and it must therefore be a very high-pitched sound. Actually, the human ear can hear sounds that are both much higher and much lower than 1000 Hz. The human ear is sensitive to frequencies as low as 20 Hz and as high as 20,000 Hz, as described in Chapter III. However, good hearing for frequencies in the range between 300 Hz and 4000 Hz is most important for understanding conversational speech.

Tuning forks and most conventional audiometers use a series of frequencies based on the musical scale in which middle C on the piano is equivalent to 256 Hz. The audiometric tones above this frequency, stated in octave intervals, are 512, 1024, 2048, 4096, 8192 Hz, etc. When one tone is an **octave** above another, its frequency is exactly twice that of the lower tone. The audiometers in use today have rounded off the frequency designations and produce tones at 500, 1000, 2000, 3000, 4000, 6000, and 8000 Hz. These frequencies are now the internationally recognized audiometric test tones. The 3000-Hz and 6000-Hz tones are sometimes called inter-octave points. They should always be tested in occupational hearing conservation programs because they, along with 4000 Hz, can reveal the early signs of noise-induced hearing loss.

When simple pressure changes are produced like the ones portrayed in Figures 5-1 and 5-2, the resulting sounds are referred to as **pure tones** because the variations in pressure occur at only one frequency. Pure tones are important to the OHC's work, since these are the stimuli that are produced by the audiometer. In the real world, however, there are few pure tones. Most sounds in our environment are **complex**, in that they contain sounds of many frequencies. Speech, music, and noise are all complex sounds.

Sound Level

Another important aspect of sound is the strength of the sound wave, stated as sound level, intensity, or sound pressure level. Each of these terms has its own technical definition. This manual will use the term "sound level" to describe environmental sound in general, and "sound pressure level" or "**A-weighted sound level**," as appropriate, when referring to levels measured by the sound level meter. Another designation, "**hearing level**," is used to describe the sound levels emitted by an audiometer.

There is an extremely large range of pressures that the ear can perceive as sound. The sound pressure that corresponds to a very loud sound may be more than 10 million times greater than the sound pressure of barely audible sounds. Instead of describing sounds as, for example, 10,000 times greater, or 1,000,000 times greater than a certain reference sound, an alternative method was developed that cut down on most of the zeros. This created a scale in **decibels**,[12] which expresses the tremendous range of sound pressures the human ear can experience in relatively few numbers. The decibel, abbreviated **dB**, is a unit, anchored to an arbitrary zero reference level, which expresses the magnitude of a measured sound relative to the reference sound. The decibel scale is logarithmic, not linear, like the scales used to measure distance and temperature.

In technical terms, sound pressure level in decibels is 20 times the logarithm to the base 10 of the ratio of the measured sound pressure to the reference sound pressure. This reference pressure has been standardized in acoustics as **20 micropascals**, abbreviated μ**Pa**.[13] It is roughly equal to the weakest sound pressure the human ear can hear at the frequency of greatest sensitivity, which is between 3000 and 4000 Hz. The measurements to establish this zero reference level were taken in young adults with excellent hearing and no history of ear disease or noise exposure.

A scale employing both decibels and micropascals is shown in Figure 5-3, along with some typical noise levels. Each time the sound pressure is increased ten times, the sound pressure *level* goes up by 20 dB. Because the decibel scale is logarithmic rather than linear, decibels cannot be added in the usual arithmetic way. For example, one machine producing 90 dB put next to another making the same amount of noise does not produce a sound level of 180 dB, but rather a total of 93 dB.

---

[12] Sound pressure levels were originally stated in terms of bels, named after Alexander Graham Bell. It proved to be more convenient to subdivide each bel into 10 divisions, and hence the decibel.

[13] Zero dB sound pressure level or 20 μPa can also be expressed as 20 micronewtons per square meter, 0.0002 dynes per square centimeter, or 0.0002 microbar.

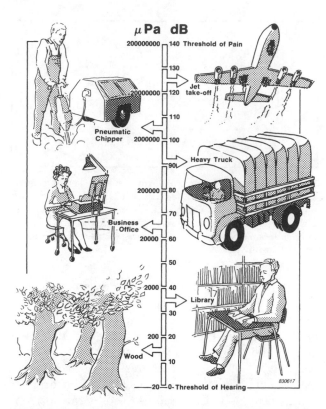

Fig. 5-3. Examples of some typical sound levels, expressed in micropascals, on the left side of the scale and decibels on the right. (From Brüel & Kjær, 1984, reproduced with permission.)

Figure 5-4 gives some examples of the sound levels emitted by various products, such as chain saws on the high end to refrigerators on the quieter end. These levels are stated in terms of ranges rather than single levels because some products within a category can be much noisier than others. They are also given as "A-weighted" sound levels. This means that they were measured using a certain filter in the sound level meter that excludes some low-frequency sound and very high-frequency sound, similar to the way the human ear perceives sound of medium intensity. A-weighted sound levels, often abbreviated **dBA**, are widely used in describing occupational and environmental noise.

Sometimes a different filter is used with the sound level meter, the **C-weighting network**, which does not exclude the high and particularly the low frequencies nearly as much. These measurements are stated in terms of **dBC** and are used to assess the amount of low-frequency noise in the worker's environment. Measurements in dBC are also used in determining the amount of attenuation needed for hearing protectors (to be discussed in more detail in chapters VI and X).

Although the level at which sounds become damaging to hearing is not shown on this scale, it is generally agreed that exposure to average sound levels between 80-85 dBA may cause some damage to hearing if they are experienced for many years. Some people who are particularly sensitive to noise may sustain hearing damage from long-term average levels of about 80 dBA, whereas others can withstand levels of 90 dBA for many years without any hearing damage. Individual susceptibility seems to play an important part.

Since the human hearing mechanism is most sensitive to sounds in the range between about 1000 and 4000 Hz, frequencies above and especially below this range require higher levels of sound pressure to become audible. Figure 5-5 shows the range of audible sounds as a function of frequency on the horizontal axis and sound pressure level on the vertical axis. Note that people can hear best in the middle-to-high frequencies, and not so well in the low frequencies. However, the human auditory system is well-suited for what it needs to hear. Speech sounds are clearly audible, as is music, and most necessary environmental sounds will also be audible for people with normal hearing.

Because people do not hear all frequencies equally well, a slightly different scale in dB is built into the audiometer. It is called the **hearing level scale**, abbreviated **HL**, or sometimes the **hearing threshold level (HTL) scale**. The HL scale was arrived at by testing a large group of young, normal-hearing people. It uses as its zero reference level the average sound pressure level at each audiometric frequency that was just audible to this group. These sound pressure levels have been standardized for purposes of audiometric testing, first in Europe and later in the U.S.

Those who use audiometers and talk about specific amounts of hearing loss need to remember that a certain level in decibels on the hearing level scale is not the same as sound pressure level. Zero dB hearing level has been "normalized" across frequencies, representing the average hearing threshold levels of young people for each frequency. This means that each frequency has a slightly different sound pressure level. For example, 0 dB HL at 500 Hz is actually 13.5 dB SPL, and 0 dB HL at 1000 Hz is actually 7.5 dB SPL. The OHC does not need to be concerned with the actual numbers, however, just the fact that the scale is slightly different, and that the audiometer uses HL and the sound level meter uses SPL.

Temporal Characteristics

Although frequency and level are the most commonly considered attributes of sound, no discussion would be complete without addressing the way the sound is distributed in time.

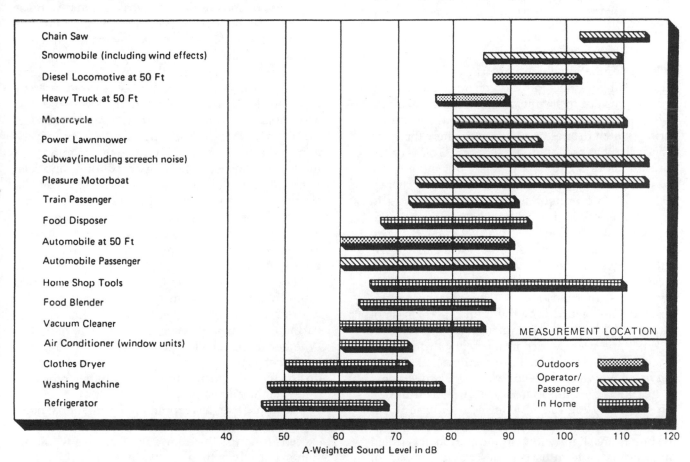

Fig. 5-4. Typical ranges of sound levels emitted by various products. (From EPA, 1978, *Protective Noise Levels*. EPA 550/9-79-100. U.S. Environmental Protection Agency, Washington, DC.)

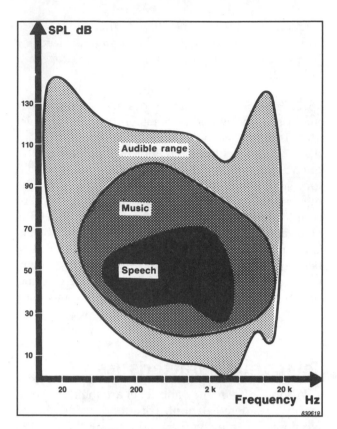

Fig. 5-5. The range of sounds heard by the normal human ear as a function of frequency (horizontal scale) and sound pressure level (vertical scale). (From Brüel & Kjær, 1984, reproduced with permission.)

Most occupational noise exposures, and virtually all exposures to noise in the general environment, are not constant over time. Some noises are remarkably steady, such as the noise from textile manufacturing, which drones on at approximately the same level as long as the looms are working. This is called **continuous** or **steady-state** noise. But more often, the noise will be less regular. Noise is often characterized as intermittent when large differences in sound level occur throughout the day, along with periodic interruptions of relative quiet between noise episodes. There is some evidence that intermittent noise is less hazardous than continuous noise because the ear has some time to recuperate during the quiet periods. However, in most factories, the noise level during the "quiet" periods is not sufficiently low to permit much, if any, recovery.

When the noise varies in level, but there are no significant quiet periods, it is sometimes called **varying** noise. Varying noise appears to be as damaging to hearing as continuous noise. A short-duration burst of fairly high level is termed **impulse** noise, and the best example is gunfire. Sometimes when the bursts are slightly longer in duration, it is called **impact** noise, a term used to describe the impact of solid objects, such as the sound of metal stamping. But because there are no official definitions for either

impulse or impact noise, the term "impulse" is often used to describe both types of noise. Impulse noise of moderate intensity appears to be no more damaging than continuous noise of equivalent intensity. But there is evidence that high-level impulses, especially when combined with continuous or varying noise, may be more hazardous to hearing than other types of noise.

Thus, a sound's **duration** is critical when judging its potential to damage hearing. This is true both in terms of the variation in sound level over a period of time, such as a day, and also the total duration over long periods of months or years. For example, an impulse noise, like the sound of a cap gun, can be startling and annoying, without necessarily being hazardous. But if this sound is repeated often (or if the listener's ear is very close to the gun), hearing loss may occur. Another example would be a worker's exposure to noisy machinery. If the worker is exposed for only one day to a machine that produces 95 dBA, he or she will probably not lose any hearing. If, however, this person is exposed for a working lifetime, then some amount of hearing loss is almost a certainty.

Duration may be measured in milliseconds or even microseconds, as in the duration of various kinds of gunfire. It is measured in hours and minutes when considering a worker's daily noise "dose," and in terms of years when assessing the potential for noise-induced hearing loss in groups of exposed people.

An important concept that involves noise duration is that of the **8-hour time-weighted average** exposure level, which is often abbreviated **TWA**. Most noise exposures fluctuate to some extent during the workday. For example, a worker may be involved in a very noisy activity for a few minutes, a moderately noisy one for five or six hours, and relatively quiet activities for the remainder of the day. To assess this person's noise exposure hazard, one can add up the amount of time spent at each noise level and compute the average exposure level for the day. Remember that decibels must be averaged logarithmically, not arithmetically. Because this process may be very laborious, it is almost always done automatically by a noise dose meter, or **dosimeter**. (More information will be presented on dosimeters and various measuring techniques in Chapter IX.) Whether these calculations are done with a sound level meter and a stop-watch or automatically by dosimeters, the resulting single number reflects a time-weighted average exposure level.

The term TWA, as it applies to occupational noise exposure, is "normalized" to 8 hours. If a workday exceeds 8 hours, the allowable exposure would be somewhat lower than the 90-dBA limit. Likewise, for a shorter day, the allowable exposure would be higher.

Sometimes a worker's daily noise exposure is expressed in terms of a **noise dose**, which is the percentage of an allowable noise exposure that the worker has experienced at a given point in time (usually the end of the work shift). The concept of noise dose takes into account two factors: the **permissible exposure limit (PEL)** for an 8-hour day, and the **exchange rate**. The PEL used in most U.S. government regulations is 90 dBA, so that a time-weighted average exposure level for eight hours at 90 dBA would yield a noise dose of 100 percent.

The exchange rate reflects the relationship between allowable exposure times and specific noise levels. OSHA and MSHA regulations specify a 5-dB exchange rate, meaning that an increase of 5 dBA is equivalent to a doubling of exposure duration. Thus, exposure to 90 dBA would be permissible for eight hours, 95 dBA for four hours, 100 dBA for two hours, and so forth. Most foreign countries, as well as the U.S. Department of Defense and the U.S. EPA, use a 3-dB exchange rate, which is somewhat more conservative. These concepts will be discussed in more detail in upcoming chapters.

References

Anon. (1984). *Measuring Sound*. Brüel & Kjær, Norcross, GA.

EPA (1976). *About Sound*. EPA/550/9-76-100. U.S. Environmental Protection Agency, Washington, DC.

EPA (1978). *Protective Noise Levels*. EPA 550/9-79-100. U.S. Environmental Protection Agency, Washington, DC.

Quiz

1. The OHC will usually be responsible for taking noise measurements. (True or False)

2. If the air molecules themselves do not move very far, what is it that does travel, sometimes long distances?

3. The aspect of sound that is perceived as loudness is called _____, and is quantified in terms of _____.

4. A sound's frequency is perceived by the ear as _____.

5. Why are the tones emitted by the audiometer called "pure tones"?

6. Why was 20 micropascals (20 μPa) chosen as the zero reference level for the sound level meter?

7. Name some of the noisiest products found outside the workplace.

8. What are the three most important properties of noise when hearing loss is considered?

9. Most occupational noise exposures fluctuate in level during the workshift. The logarithmic average sound exposure level normalized to an 8-hour workday is called the

_____

_____ exposure level, abbreviated _____.

10. The relationship between level and duration of an allowable noise exposure is called the

_____.

Abbreviations Used in Chapter V

dB	Decibels
dBA	Decibels measured on the A scale of the sound level meter.
dBC	Decibels measured on the C scale of the sound level meter.
HL	Hearing level
HTL	Hearing threshold level
Hz	Hertz
μPa	Micropascals
OHC	Occupational Hearing Conservationist
OSHA	Occupational Safety and Health Administration
MSHA	Mine Safety and Health Administration
PEL	Permissible exposure limit
SPL	Sound pressure level
TWA	Time-weighted average (sound level)

Recommended Reading

Anon. (1984). *Measuring Sound*. Available from Brüel & Kjær, 2815 Colonnades Ct., Norcross, GA.

Bess, F.H., and Humes, L.E. (1995). "The nature of sound." Chapter 2 in *Audiology: The Fundamentals, 2nd Ed*. Williams and Wilkins, Baltimore, MD.

Newby, H.A., and Popelka, G.R. (1992). "What and how we hear." Chapter 2 in *Audiology, 6th Ed*. Prentice-Hall, Inc., Englewood Cliffs, NJ.

Ostergaard, P.B. (2000). "Physics of sound and vibration." Chapter 2 in E.H. Berger, L.H. Royster, J.D. Royster, L.H. Driscoll, and M. Layne (Eds.), *The Noise Manual: Fifth Edition*. American Industrial Hygiene Assoc., Fairfax, VA.

Stevens, S.S. and Warshofsky, F. (1980). *Sound and Hearing (Rev. ed.)*. Time-Life Books, Alexandria, VA. (Out of print but available in libraries.)

Chapter VI

Standards and Regulations

Why Regulate?

Although the concept of regulation is not always popular, in the case of occupational safety and health, regulations are often necessary. There are few marketplace incentives to establish safety and health measures, and employers are often unaware of the benefits of such programs. You might think that workers could refuse to take noisy jobs, or quit and look elsewhere. But, in truth, most workers can't afford the luxury of shopping around for a quiet job.

While there are quite a few employers whose primary motivation for initiating hearing conservation programs is to protect the hearing of their workers, many others require economic or legal incentives to get them to act. Worker compensation for hearing loss should be an incentive for creating quieter workplaces, and the institution of hearing conservation programs can reduce future claims as well as insurance premiums. But, compared to the large number of workers who could be expected to have noise-induced hearing loss, relatively few file such claims and the dollar amounts are usually small. Thus, marketplace incentives do not appear to provide for safe and healthy workplaces, and consequently regulation by a government agency becomes necessary.

Development of Noise Regulations in the U.S.

Today there are numerous regulations for workers exposed to occupational noise. Various federal agencies, such as the Occupational Safety and Health Administration and the Mine Safety and Health Administration, as well as all three branches of the Department of Defense, have their individual noise regulations. In addition, many states have their own "state plans" with regulations that must be at least as stringent as the federal OSHA regulations.

Consensus Activities

Most of these governmental regulations did not exist a few decades ago. However, there was a great deal of activity among professional groups, and the result was a series of "consensus standards," which aided in the prediction of hearing damage that would occur from various levels and durations of noise exposure. The American Academy of Ophthalmology and Otolaryngology, the Industrial Medical Association, and the American Industrial Hygiene Association, among others, were involved in the development of these standards. By the end of World War II the clinical audiometer had been invented and noise-induced hearing loss was widely acknowledged. Most occupational health professionals knew that noise could damage hearing but there were differing opinions as to just how much noise caused how much hearing loss.

The Government Steps In

The first governmental noise standard was published by the Air Force in 1949, but it was not until 1955 that the Air Force issued a standard specifying maximum noise levels. The first civilian noise standard (or actually, regulation) was issued by the U.S. Department of Labor in 1969. It is known as the **"Walsh-Healey" noise regulation** because it was **promulgated** (legally set forward) under the authority of the Walsh-Healey Public Contracts Act, which had been enacted by Congress in 1935. In passing the Walsh-Healey Act, Congress had given the Labor Department the authority to regulate companies having contracts with the federal government, so the Walsh-Healey noise regulation applied only to these companies.

Also in 1969 Congress showed its concern over working conditions in the U.S. by passing the **Federal Coal Mine Safety and Health Act.** Shortly after that, in 1970, Congress enacted the **Occupational Safety and Health Act**, a monumental piece of legislation. Nowhere in the world had an elected body given its administrative arm such responsibilities and powers in the realm of occupational safety and health. The Act created the **National Institute for Occupational Safety and Health (NIOSH)** in the Department of Health, Education and Welfare (now the Department of Health and Human Services), and the **Occupational Safety and Health Administration (OSHA)** in the Labor Department.

NIOSH's job is to do the research, develop the criteria, and perform "Health Hazard Evaluations" in all areas of occupational safety and health OSHA then makes the regulations, enforces them, and conducts information and education programs. Both NIOSH and OSHA have special programs through which they provide consultation to employers at no charge. For miners, the **Bureau of Mines** does the research and development, and the **Mine Safety and Health Administration (MSHA)** in the Labor Department has functions similar to OSHA's.

At this point, a brief explanation of terminology would be helpful. First, the words **"standard"** and **"regulation"** are often used interchangeably. Strictly speaking, a standard is a specific requirement or set of requirements, often taking the form of guidelines that are developed by a consensus group, such as the **American National Standards Institute (ANSI)**. By contrast, a regulation is a rule or order prescribed by a government authority, which has the force of law. Regulations may incorporate standards to describe or clarify certain requirements. For example, OSHA's noise regulation incorporates some ANSI standards that deal with hearing testing equipment and calibration.

Next, it is important to understand the difference between **regulation** and **legislation**. Although these terms are also used interchangeably (by mistake), they have very different meanings. Congress or state legislatures enact legislation, and administrative agencies, such as OSHA, MSHA, and EPA do the regulating. Congress passes laws, like the Occupational Safety and Health Act, and appropriates money to fund the administration of these laws. The laws direct the administrative agencies to do all sorts of things, including the development and enforcement of regulations.

Rule Making for Noise

When a federal government agency decides to make a regulation or revise an existing one, the agency goes through a series of prescribed steps, known as the **rule-making** process. First the agency staff members develop extensive information on the subject and put it in a **docket**, a special file devoted to that regulation. Then they prepare a draft, called a **proposed standard** (really a proposed regulation). The proposal is published in the *Federal Register*, which is like the daily newspaper of the administrative arm of the federal government. Many companies, government agencies, and libraries subscribe to the *Federal Register*. The agency usually holds public hearings in conjunction with a proposal. Then, after much deliberation, the agency promulgates a **final standard** (regulation), which again is published in the *Federal Register*. Because employers may need some time to be able to come into compliance with the new regulation, the agency usually sets an **effective date** some months after the promulgation date. The effective date is the date on which the new regulation can be enforced.

OSHA's noise regulation is a good example of the rule-making process. In 1971 OSHA widened the application of the Walsh-Healey noise regulation beyond just federal contractors to virtually all companies in the U.S. In 1972, NIOSH published *Criteria for a Recommended Standard, Occupational Exposure to Noise*, commonly called the "noise criteria document." This document described the effects of noise in some detail, and made recommendations for a regulation that would help prevent noise-induced hearing loss. OSHA then began to revise its regulation using the NIOSH criteria document as a starting point. The process of committee work, proposal, public hearings, technical feasibility and economic impact reports, as well as meetings and docket analysis took nearly ten years. OSHA considered lowering the 90-dBA permissible exposure limit (PEL) to 85 dBA as NIOSH had recommended, but decided that the economic impact would be too great and the agency did not have the information it needed at the time to take this momentous step. Therefore, the Walsh-Healey regulation was kept intact and simply amended with comprehensive requirements for hearing conservation programs.

The promulgation of OSHA's hearing conservation amendment was announced in the *Federal Register* on January 16, 1981. The supporting documentation or **preamble** to the regulation contains a clear and concise description of the effects of noise on hearing (and other effects), as well as a detailed explanation of every provision of the regulation. This material is still applicable to most provisions of the regulation, and is listed in the Recommended Reading section at the end of this chapter.

It happened that the hearing conservation amendment came out shortly before a change in administration in Washington. The Reagan administration was not favorable to regulation in general, and delayed the amendment's effective date, meaning that it was legally in place but was not enforceable. OSHA did make most of the amendment's provisions effective later in 1981, but some provisions continued to be held back, more public hearings took place, and finally a revised version was promulgated in March of 1983. Because the regulation has not been revised since then, the 1983 version is the one that OSHA enforces and the one with which the OHC should be most concerned. The preamble to the 1983 version is also listed in the Recommended Reading section of this chapter so that the interested reader can see the rationale for the changes that took place between the 1981 and 1983 versions.

Even though many OHCs will be employed by the military or by companies covered by regulations other than OSHA's, the majority of American workplaces will be covered either by federal or state OSHA regulations. It is a good idea for all OHCs to be familiar with OSHA's noise regulation, since it tends to set the pace for all U.S. occupational noise regulations. OHCs should also become familiar with the more recent MSHA regulations, discussed later in this chapter.

The 1983 OSHA regulation is reprinted as Appendix C of this manual, and anyone who intends to participate actively in a hearing conservation program in the U.S. should be thoroughly familiar with its provisions. The regulation will be summarized here, and explanations of some of its provisions will be provided. However, readers are urged to study the actual regulation carefully so as to know exactly what is required by OSHA and what is not. *This is not to say that the OSHA regulation is the ultimate in hearing conservation; it is not.* There are many areas where it can be improved, and this manual will mention some of them. However, it is very important for the OHC to be able to give correct information to both managers and workers about what OSHA personnel will expect of them.

Appendix D of this manual contains a checklist that should help OHCs determine the extent to which their hearing conservation programs comply with the OSHA regulation. The checklist is reprinted from a NIOSH guide, *Preventing Occupational Hearing Loss: A Practical Guide,* issued in 1996 (Franks et al., 1996). Most of these recommendations stem from a lengthy effort to revise NIOSH's 1972 criteria document, which was published in 1998 as *Occupational Noise Exposure: Revised Criteria, 1998* (NIOSH, 1998).

The checklist in Appendix D contains the OSHA requirements, along with recommendations from NIOSH for many of the provisions. You will notice that NIOSH's recommended provisions are often more stringent than those of OSHA. There are at least two reasons for this. First, the role of NIOSH is to perform research and develop criteria that will be adequate to protect workers, regardless of economic feasibility. OSHA, however, takes feasibility into account when issuing regulations. Another reason is that the NIOSH recommendations are considerably more recent than OSHA's deliberations, so new research, information, and technologies have surfaced in the interim. While NIOSH's recommendations may or may not be accepted by OSHA in the future, they do constitute guidelines for "best practice," and certain companies and professionals in hearing conservation have begun to adopt them.

In the paragraphs below, the various provisions of OSHA's regulation will be discussed and clarified. The NIOSH recommendations pertaining to various provisions will occasionally be mentioned, so that readers may be aware of how OSHA's requirements may, in some cases, be improved upon. Later in this chapter a table from the recently revised *Noise Manual* published by the American Industrial Hygiene Association (AIHA) (and subsequent *Spectrum* article) has been reprinted as Table 6.1, which compares the hearing conservation regulations, interpretations, and recommendations of OSHA, MSHA, and NIOSH (Berger and Hager, 2000).

Enforcement

OSHA enforces the noise regulation by sending inspectors or **compliance officers** to high-hazard industries or companies where there have been complaints. If the company has violated or failed to implement any part of the regulation, the compliance officer may issue a **citation**, which may have penalties associated with it. Personnel in most OSHA offices will work with a company to help correct the violation.

The public may contact OSHA's Directorate of Compliance Programs with questions about any part of the regulation that may not be clear. OSHA responds with a letter clarifying the issue, and that letter becomes official OSHA policy. A list of these letters to date is given in Appendix E and the letters themselves are available on OSHA's website at **www.osha.gov/SLTC/noisehearingconservation/index.html.** It is a good idea to check this website periodically and make a note of current OSHA interpretations.

The "Walsh-Healey" Part of the OSHA Noise Regulation

As mentioned earlier, the provisions of the Walsh-Healey noise regulation remain virtually intact, even though it was amended in 1981. The regulation calls for a **maximum permissible exposure limit (PEL)** of 90 dBA, which is a **time-weighted average exposure level (TWA)**. There is a **5-dBA exchange rate**, meaning that the noise exposure level may be raised by 5 dBA each time the duration is cut in half. So, 95 dBA is permitted for 4 hours, 100 dBA for 2 hours, 105 dBA for 1 hour, 110 dBA for 30 minutes, and a maximum level of 115 dBA is permitted for 15 minutes.[14] Continuous noise of any duration is not permitted above 115 dBA. These levels must be achieved by means of **engineering controls** or **administrative controls**. Over-exposure can sometimes be controlled by rotating workers to quieter areas for a certain amount of time, a process known as administrative control.[15]

The OSHA noise regulation requires anyone exposed above the PEL to be provided with and to use hearing protection devices, which places the responsibility for compliance with this provision on workers as well as on their employers.

The regulation also recommends (but does not require) that workers not be exposed to impulse noise

exceeding a **sound pressure level (SPL)** of 140 dB. Unfortunately, the regulation does not define the term "impulse noise," and this has caused some controversy in the courts. But it does define continuous noise as levels whose maxima (highest levels) occur at intervals at least as often as one second, so that impulse noise is sometimes considered as noise with peak levels that occur less often than once per second, a definition by default.

Before it was amended, the regulation required that any employer who exposed employees to noise levels above the PEL must institute "a continuing, effective, hearing conservation program." Because no details about the hearing conservation program were given in the regulation itself, OSHA had difficulty enforcing this provision. OSHA did develop some policies during the 1970s, but enforcement was sporadic. It was not until 1981 that OSHA's requirements for hearing conservation programs were legally clarified in the form of the amendment, and then it was not until 1983 that the entire amendment became enforceable.

The Hearing Conservation Amendment to OSHA's Noise Regulation

The 90-dBA PEL, the requirements for engineering or administrative controls, the requirements for the provision and wearing of hearing protectors at TWAs above the PEL, and the recommendation for maximum impulse levels are found in sections (a) and (b) of the noise regulation. The rest of the regulation, sections (c) through (n), plus the appendices are usually referred to as the hearing conservation amendment. It is important for readers to understand that the hearing conservation amendment *did not replace* the Walsh-Healey noise regulation, but merely *amended* it. Thus, the requirements for engineering controls are technically still in place, although they have been modified by a compliance policy to be discussed later in this chapter.

Section (c) now states that employers must administer continuing, effective hearing conservation programs for any employees whose exposures exceed a TWA of 85 dBA. This level, which is one-half the dose of the 90-dBA level, does not change the PEL. It does not require employers to use engineering controls to reduce the exposure to 85 dBA (although some employers will choose to do that), but rather it is the trigger for a number of hearing conservation measures. OSHA calls this the **action level** and uses this practice in a number of regulations. In this regulation, 85 dBA is the same as 50 percent dose. The regulation's mandatory Appendix A explains how to compute employee noise exposure and to relate dose to TWA.

---

[14] The level and duration of noisy episodes usually vary during the work shift. To use a simple example, a worker's daily exposure may consist of three separate 15-minute periods at 105 dBA, two one-hour periods at 92 dBA, and the remainder of time at approximately 84 dBA. In this case the worker's dose would be 140% and the TWA would be approximately 92 dBA, which exceeds the 8-hour PEL of 90 dBA. For information on computing the noise dose and TWA, see Appendix A of the OSHA noise regulation reprinted in Appendix C of this manual.

[15] Administrative controls are not used very much because they often necessitate removing employees from the work for which they have been trained and substituting other, less trained workers. Union contracts sometimes prohibit them. Also, they have the disadvantage of spreading the exposure to workers who might not otherwise have been exposed to potentially hazardous noise. On the other hand, people sometimes refer to the practice of giving workers breaks in quiet rest areas or sound-treated lunch rooms as "administrative controls." These practices can be quite helpful in that they allow the ear some recuperation from TTS and can sometimes reduce the overall noise dose.

Noise Exposure Monitoring

The purpose of the noise exposure monitoring program is to identify employees who should be included in the hearing conservation program and to aid in determining the appropriate hearing protection for each employee. All employees exposed above a TWA of 85 dBA must be included in the noise monitoring program. The regulation does not specify how often they should be monitored, but they should be remonitored at least when there is a substantial change in the production process.

Area monitoring is allowable under some circumstances. This is the simplest kind of monitoring, where noise level readings are taken in different areas of the workplace, and the outcome is usually a "noise map" of the area. However, **personal monitoring** is required when workers are highly mobile, there are significant variations in the noise level, or when there is a significant impulsive component to the noise exposure. Personal monitoring involves measuring an individual worker's time-weighted average noise exposure or "dose" for an entire work shift. It may be carried out with a sound level meter and a stop-watch, but individuals who measure exposure will find it much more convenient to use a noise dosimeter, which makes the necessary calculations automatically.

The reason the regulation often requires personal monitoring is that area monitoring does not characterize the exposures of individual workers when they move around a lot, or when the noise levels vary substantially. The regulation states very clearly that "all continuous, intermittent, and impulsive sound levels from 80 dB to 130 dB"[16] must be included in the calculation of worker exposure or dose. This requirement means that impulsive noise must be integrated into the total dose, and not considered separately. The recommended ceiling of 140-dB peak SPL still stands, for which a separate measurement may be necessary. But for compliance with the amendment's monitoring provisions, *all* types of noise must be included in the calculation of dose.

There has been some confusion about the requirement to include all sound levels from 80 to 130 dBA in the dose, when the regulation prohibits exposure to continuous noise above 115 dBA. First the 115 dBA prohibition does not apply to impulsive noise, which often exceeds this level. But also, it is important to remember that there are times when noise levels will exceed OSHA's PEL ostensibly when the

control of these levels is infeasible or while controls are being installed. This does not excuse employers from recognizing and including these sounds when assessing employees' exposures to noise.

The noise monitoring section of the regulation also states that employees must be allowed to observe the monitoring and that they must be notified of the results. Just how the observation and notification procedures are carried out is left up to employers or those conducting the hearing conservation program.

Audiometric Testing Program

The audiometric testing program is the longest and one of the most important aspects of the amendment. It calls for audiometric tests to be made available to all employees whose TWAs equal or exceed 85 dBA. The regulation does not require all employees to take the test because employees may have personal reasons for not doing so. If large numbers of employees refuse audiometric testing, OSHA inspectors are likely to interpret this as a labor–management problem and urge both the company and the employees to work out their differences. The employer is always free to make audiometric testing a mandatory company policy.

Who May Test:

According to OSHA, those who may perform the tests are licensed or certified audiologists, otolaryngologists or other physicians, technicians (or OHCs) who are certified by CAOHC, or technicians who have "satisfactorily demonstrated competence in administering audiometric examinations, obtaining valid audiograms, and properly using, maintaining and checking calibration and proper functioning of the audiometers being used." This means that it is not mandatory for a technician to be certified by CAOHC, but in reality, there is no other nationally recognized certification program, and OSHA compliance officers will tend to look for CAOHC certification. Two states, Oregon and Washington, require CAOHC certification, and the new MSHA regulation requires certification by CAOHC or another organization offering equivalent certification.

The OSHA regulation goes on to say, "a technician who operates microprocessor audiometers does not need to be certified." This statement does not appear in the 1981 version. It is confusing because, technically, *no* technician *has* to be certified, but the statement makes it appear that technicians who use microprocessors do not need training and certification as much as those who use other types of audiometers, which is not true! OSHA's "clarification" of this requirement has failed to dispel the confusion. A 1983 interpretation maintains that the

---

[16] Section (c) of the regulation refers to 85 decibels measured on the A scale of the sound level meter using the "slow" meter response. After this section, wherever OSHA uses the term "decibels" or "dB" in the regulation, A-weighting can be assumed unless specified otherwise.

intent was that "audiometric technicians show competence in performing tests with the particular type of audiometer they would be using," whether or not they were certified (Vance, 1983). (And, of course, CAOHC certification is still the best way to demonstrate that competence.)

A technician who performs audiometric tests must be responsible to an audiologist, otolaryngologist, or other physician. The regulation does not define the term "must be responsible to," but leaves this relationship up to the technicians and the supervising professionals.

The Baseline Audiogram:

Under most circumstances a **baseline audiogram** must be performed within 6 months of an employee's first exposure to noise levels of 85 dBA or above. If a company relies on mobile audiometric test services, the company need only perform the baseline audiometric test within the first year of exposure, but employees must wear hearing protection at least during the second six months of exposure. Because of the importance of obtaining a baseline audiogram that is not contaminated by TTS from any source, employees must have at least 14 hours away from noise before having a baseline audiogram. The use of hearing protection may be substituted for this requirement, although NIOSH recommends against this substitution. Also, employers must counsel employees to avoid exposure to non-occupational noise before the baseline audiogram. Needless to say, the best time to perform a baseline (as opposed to an annual) audiogram is before any exposure to hazardous noise, and it is safer not to rely on hearing protection to achieve the necessary quiet.

The Annual Audiogram:

Every employee exposed to a TWA of 85 dBA or above must be provided with a new audiogram at least once a year. This **annual audiogram** may be administered at any time during the work shift, but the best time would be late in the shift so as to identify any TTS due to inadequate protective measures.

Audiogram Evaluation:

Audiograms are not to be taken and then merely filed away. Each audiogram must be compared to the current baseline audiogram. A technician can perform this comparison, but an audiologist or physician must review any **problem audiograms**. The regulation does not define the term "problem," but leaves it up to the professional reviewer. The person reviewing the audiograms must be provided with measurements of background noise levels in the audiometric test rooms and the records of audiometer calibrations, in addition to the baseline and annual audiograms.

The **National Hearing Conservation Association (NHCA)** has drafted two sets of guidelines on the issue of problem audiograms, one set for OHCs and the other for audiologist and physician reviewers. Although these guidelines may not be final at the time of this manual's publication, interested readers may check NHCA's website to see what hearing conservation professionals have in mind on this topic. It is important to remember that while NHCA's recommendations might be considered "best practice," they are not the same as an OSHA regulation or policy.

Standard Threshold Shift:

Although the term "significant threshold shift" is more descriptive, the term was changed to **"standard threshold shift" (STS)** between the 1981 and 1983 versions. The identification of STS is one of the primary purposes of the audiometric test program. It is a sign that a worker has begun to lose hearing and steps are needed to intervene. OSHA defines an STS as an average shift from baseline of 10 dB or more in the audiometric frequencies 2000, 3000, and 4000 Hz in either ear. Because it is an average, a threshold shift greater than 10 dB may occur at one frequency if a smaller shift occurs at another, and still be within the 10 dB limit. NIOSH recommends a different definition of STS (see Table 6.1), as does the **Department of Defense (DoD)**. *gradual decline in hearing from aging*

In making the STS determination, deductions for presbycusis may be included in the calculation. These amounts, which were originally supplied by NIOSH, are found in the tables of the 1983 OSHA regulation's Appendix F. If the OHC performs these calculations, it is important to follow the Appendix F procedures very carefully. Many professionals and certain state regulations (Oregon and Washington), as well as NIOSH and the DoD do not permit an adjustment for presbycusis in determining the existence of an STS.

Follow-up Procedures:

If the comparison of the annual audiogram with the baseline reveals an STS, the employee must be notified of this fact in writing within 21 days of the determination. However, the employee may be retested within 30 days of the annual test, and if the retest does not show an STS, the new test may be considered the regular annual test. Although OSHA does not require it, the retest should be conducted after a period of at least 14 hours away from noise to obtain threshold levels that are not influenced by TTS.

Comparison of U.S. Hearing Conservation Regulations and Recommendations

Elliott Berger and Lee Hager

Comparison of the various regulatory and "best practice" publications developed by agencies of the federal government is becoming important to hearing loss prevention professionals. The table which follows is intended to permit a quick comparison of the following requirements:

- US general industry (Hearing Conservation Amendment to the Occupational Safety and Health Administration [OSHA] Noise Rule, 29 CFR 1910.95, 1983)
- Mining (Mine Safety and Health Administration [MSHA] Health Standards for Occupational Noise Exposure, 30 CFR Parts 56 and 57 et al., 1999)
- The National Institute for Occupational Safety and Health (NIOSH) recommendations of the 1998 *Criteria for a Recommended Standard: Occupational Noise Exposure* (DHHS(NIOSH) Publication No. 98-126, 1998).

This table was developed originally for inclusion in the fifth edition of the American Industrial Hygiene Assocation's *Noise Manual*. Please note following caveats:

1. The MSHA regulation was published September 13, 1999 with a projected effective date of September 13, 2000. The reference is current as of June 2000, but litigation could result in changes before implementation. Check with MSHA (see web address below) for latest status.
2. The *Criteria Document* is a NIOSH recommendation intended to provide OSHA with evidence including new research as rationale for considering revision of an existing rule or development of a new rule. It is not a compliance document, but can be construed as a "best practices" guide.
3. Recordable or reportable hearing loss is addressed under OSHA in 29 CFR 1904 (not included in this analysis and was recently revised, see p. 46 this chapter), and directly in the MSHA rule.

✐ This analysis is not intended to be all-inclusive. Please check with the applicable agency for updates and current status. OSHA information is available at <http://www.osha.gov>; MSHA at <http://www.msha.gov>; and NIOSH at <http://www.cdc.gov/niosh>.

Issue	Description and Definition	OSHA 29 CFR 1910.95	MSHA 30 CFR Part 62	NIOSH Pub. No. 98-126
Action Level (AL)	The time-weighted average (TWA) exposure which requires program inclusion, hearing tests, training, and optional hearing protection	AL = 85 dBA TWA. AL is exceeded when TWA ≥ 85 dBA, integrating all sounds from 80 to 130 dBA.	Similar to OSHA, except integration is for all sounds from 80 *to at least* 130 dBA.	Does not have AL; rather has a single Recommended Exposure Limit (REL, see next row) for hearing loss prevention, noise controls, and HPDs.
Permissible Exposure Limit (PEL)	The TWA, which when exceeded, requires feasible engineering and (MSHA)/or (OSHA) administrative controls, and mandatory hearing protection.	PEL = 90 dBA TWA. PEL is exceeded when TWA > 90 dBA, integrating all sounds from 90 to 140 dBA, as inferred from Table G-16 of 1910.95(b).	Similar to OSHA, except integration range is explicit in the reg. (62.101, Definitions), and is for all sounds from 90 *to at least* 140 dBA.	REL = 85 dBA TWA. REL is exceeded when TWA > 85 dBA, integrating all sounds from 80 to 140 dBA
Exchange Rate	The rate at which exposure accumulates; the change in dB TWA for halving/doubling of allowable exposure time.	5 dB	Same as OSHA.	3 dB
Ceiling Level	The limiting sound level above which employees cannot be exposed.	No exposures >115dB SPL; generally interpreted as "*no unprotected* exposures" to give credit for HCP, HPDs and feasible engineering controls.	"P" code violation issued for any protected or unprotected exposures > 115 dBA SPL.	No protected or unprotected exposure to continuous, varying, intermittent, or impulsive noise >140 dBA.
Impulse Noise	Noise with sharp rise and rapid decay in level, ≤ 1 sec. in duration, and if repeated, occurring at intervals >1 sec.	To be integrated with measurements of all other noise, but *should* not exceed 140 dB peak SPL.	To be integrated with measurements of all other noise.	To be integrated with measurements of all other noise, but not to exceed 140dBA.

Continued

Issue	Description and Definition	OSHA 29 CFR 1910.95	MSHA 30 CFR Part 62	NIOSH Pub. No. 98-126
Monitoring	Assessment of noise exposure.	Once to determine risk and HCP inclusion; from there as conditions change resulting in potential for more exposure.	Mine operator must establish system to evaluate each miner's exposure sufficiently to determine continuing compliance with rule.	Every 2 years if any exposure ≥ 85 dBA TWA.
Noise Control	Investigation and implementation of feasible engineering and administrative control measures.	Feasible controls required where TWA > 90 dBA; subsequent compliance policy (which may be changed/revoked by OSHA at any time) permits proven effective HCP in lieu of engineering where TWA<100 dBA.	Feasible engineering and administrative controls required for TWA > 90 dBA; even if controls do not reduce exposure to the PEL, they are required if feasible (i.e. 3-dBA reduction). Administrative controls must be provided to the miner in writing and posted.	Feasible controls to 85dBA TWA. Administrative controls must not expose more workers to noise.
Hearing Protection	Exposure requirements and conditions for use of hearing protection devices (HPDs).	Optional for ≥ 85 dBA TWA; mandatory for > 90 dBA TWA, or for ≥ 85 dBA TWA for workers with STS. Protect to 90 or to 85 with STS. Choices must include a "variety" which is interpreted as at least 1 type of plug and 1 type of muff.	Use requirements same as OSHA, but amount of protection not specified, and choices must include 2 plugs and 2 muffs. Double hearing protection (muff plus plug) required at exposures >105dBA TWA.	Mandatory for ≥ 85 dBA TWA; must protect to 85. Double hearing protection (muff plus plug) recommended at exposures >100 dBA TWA.
Evaluation of Hearing Protector Effectiveness	Method of assessing adequacy of HPDs	Use manufacturers' labeled NRRs to assess adequacy, but subsequent compliance policy stipulates 50% derating of NRRs to compare relative effectiveness of HPDs and engineering controls.	No method included in standard. Preamble to regulation indicates that compliance guide will follow with suggested procedures.	Labeled NRRs must be derated by 25% for muffs, 50% for foam plugs, and 70% for other earplugs unless data available from ANSI S12.6-1997 Method B.
Supervisor of Audiometric Testing	The person who conducts or who is responsible for the conduct of audiometric testing and review.	Licensed or certified audiologist, otolaryngologist, or other physician	Licensed or certified audiologist, or physician.	Audiologist or physician.
Audiometric Technician	The person who conducts audiometric testing and review.	Must be responsible to supervisor (see above). CAOHC certified, or has demonstrated competence to supervisor. When microprocessor audiometers used, certification not required.	Must be under direction of supervisor (see above). Must be certified by CAOHC or equivalent certification organization.	Must be under direction of supervisor (see above). Must be certified by CAOHC or equivalent certification organization.
Audiometry	Initial and ongoing hearing tests used to assess the efficacy of hearing conservation measures.	Required annually for all workers exposed ≥ 85 dBA TWA. Baseline test within 6 months of exposure; 12 months if using mobile testing service, with HPD in the interim	Same as OSHA but audiograms at miner's discretion.	Required for all workers exposed ≥ 85 dBA TWA. Baseline test pre-placement or within 30 days of exposure. Best practice is to test workers exposed > 100 dBA TWA twice per year.
Quiet Period Prior to Baseline Audiogram.	Period of non exposure to workplace noise required prior to baseline audiogram.	14 hrs.; use of HPDs acceptable as alternative.	Same as OSHA.	No exposure to noise ≥ 85 dBA for 12 hrs.; HPDs can not be used as alternative.
Background Noise	Permissible noise in audiometric test chamber during testing.	Levels specified as 40 dB @ 500 and 1000 Hz, 47 dB @ 2000 Hz, 57 dB @ 4000 Hz, and 62 dB @ 8000 Hz.	According to scientifically validated procedures.	Per ANSI S3.1-1999 or latest revision; 19 dB more stringent than OSHA at 500 Hz, and 13 to 25 dB more stringent at other frequencies.

Continued

Issue	Description and Definition	OSHA 29 CFR 1910.95	MSHA 30 CFR Part 62	NIOSH Pub. No. 98-126
Audiogram Review and Employee Notification	Required actions following audiograms.	Not specified unless STS is detected; see STS follow up.	Audiograms must be reviewed within 30 days and feedback in writing for each miner within 10 days thereafter.	Not specified unless STS is detected; see STS follow up.
STS (OSHA/MSHA — *Standard* Threshold Shift; NIOSH — *Significant* Threshold Shift)	A change in hearing compared to an earlier (baseline) hearing test that requires follow-up action.	≥ 10-dB average shift from baseline hearing levels at 2000, 3000 and 4000 Hz in either ear.	Same as OSHA.	≥ 15-dB shift for the worse from baseline at any test frequency, in either ear, confirmed with follow-up test for same ear/frequency.
STS Retests	Follow-up audiogram that is permitted or required when initial STS is detected.	May obtain retest within 30 days and substitute for annual audiogram.	Same as OSHA.	Must provide confirmation audiogram within 30 days.
STS Follow-up	Required actions when an STS is detected.	Notify worker within 21 days; unless STS is not work-related, must fit or re-fit employee with HPDs and select higher attenuation if necessary, refer for audio/otological exam if more testing needed or problem due to HPDs, and inform employee of need for exam if problem unrelated to HPD usage is suspected.	Within 30 days of receiving evidence or confirmation of STS, unless STS is not work-related, must retrain the miner, provide miner an HPD or a different HPD, and review effectiveness of any engineering and administrative controls to correct deficiencies.	Notify worker within 30 days; must take action such as explain effects of noise, reinstruct and refit with HPDs, provide additional training in hearing loss prevention, or reassign to quieter area.
Baseline Revision	Procedures for revising the baseline audiogram to reflect changes in hearing.	Annual audio substituted for baseline when STS is *persistent* or thresholds show significant improvement.	Annual audio substituted for baseline when STS is *permanent* or thresholds show significant improvement.	Annual audio substituted for baseline when confirming audiogram validates an STS.
Presbycusis or Age Correction	Adjustments for hearing levels for anticipated effects of age.	Allowed.	Same as OSHA.	Not allowed.
Recordable or Reportable Hearing Loss	Amount of hearing loss triggering reporting requirements on workplace injury/illness logs.	*By OSHA CFR 1904.10: work related STS, ≥ 10 dB shift at 2000, 3000, and 4000 Hz in either ear, provided that the shift plus the baseline threshold totals ≥ 25 dB above audiometric zero. Age corrections allowed for determining existence of STS but not to determine if average hearing level ≥ 25 dB.	≥ 25-dB average shift from baseline, or revised baseline, at 2000, 3000, and 4000Hz in either ear.	Not indicated.
Training and Education	Description of the annual training and educational component of the hearing conservation program.	Annual for all employees exposed ≥ 85 dB TWA on effects of noise, HPDs, and purpose and explanation of audiometry.	Same as OSHA, except must begin within 30 days of enrollment in HCP, and include description of mine operator and miner's responsibilities for maintaining noise controls.	Same as OSHA, but must also include psychological effects of noise, and roles and responsibilities of both employers and workers in program.
Warning Signs and Postings	Requirements to post signs for noisy areas or to post regulations.	Hearing conservation amendment shall be posted in workplace.	No requirements for posting reg., but when administrative controls are utilized the procedures must be posted.	Signs must be posted at entrance to areas with TWAs routinely ≥ 85 dBA.
Record Retention	Specification on retention of data, and transfer requirements if employer goes out of business.	Noise surveys for at least 2 yrs., hearing tests for duration of employment, with requirement to transfer records to successor if employer goes out of business.	Employee noise exposure notices and training records for duration of enrollment in HCP + 6 months, and hearing tests for duration of employment + 6 months, with requirement to transfer records to successor mine operator.	Noise surveys for 30 yrs., hearing tests for duration of employment + 30 yrs., calibration records for 5 yrs, with record transfer per 29CFR1910.20(h).

Table 6.1. Comparison of U.S. Hearing Conservation Regulations and Recommendations. From Berger, E., and Hager, L., (2000). NHCA, *Spectrum*, 17(3).   *Revised July 2002.

If the retest shows the STS to be genuine (or if there is no retest), employers are obliged to take certain actions, unless a physician determines that the shift is not work-related. First, employees not using hearing protection must be fitted with these devices and trained to use them. (This generally applies to employees who are exposed to noise levels between 85 and 90 dBA). Employees already using protectors must be refitted and retrained, and, if necessary, provided with protectors offering greater attenuation.

In some cases additional testing will be necessary, and in these cases it is OSHA's policy that the employer must bear the expense. For example, employees whose test results are inconsistent or who appear not to be able to take the test should be referred for an audiological or otological evaluation. Also, employees must be referred for medical attention if the OHC suspects that a pathology of the ear is caused or aggravated by the wearing of hearing protectors.

In other cases, employees need to be informed of the need for medical attention if an ear pathology is suspected that is unrelated to the wearing of hearing protection. In these cases the employer is not required to bear the expense.

Revising the Baseline Audiogram:

OSHA allows the employer to substitute an annual audiogram for the baseline when the reviewing professional determines that an STS is **persistent** (permanent). This is to prevent the identification of the same STS and the subsequent notification of the employee year after year, in cases where an employee's hearing thresholds have stabilized. In addition, an annual audiogram may be considered the new baseline when thresholds have significantly improved. This might happen if the baseline had been contaminated by TTS or if the worker had a conductive hearing loss that had subsequently been treated. The regulation does not define a significant improvement, but once again leaves this up to professional judgment. The NHCA has developed guidelines for revising the baseline audiogram in the case of improved hearing thresholds (see Appendix K and discussion in Chapter VIII).

There may be instances where the hearing in both ears has deteriorated, yet only one ear shows an STS. In a 1996 interpretation, OSHA has allowed employers to revise both baselines when this occurs, but recommends that the thresholds for each ear be assessed and revised independently since this method is more protective and provides a clearer indication of how each ear is affected by noise (McCully, 1996).

Audiometric Test Requirements:

OSHA requires audiograms to include the frequencies 500, 1000, 2000, 3000, 4000, and 6000 Hz as a minimum, with tests taken separately for each ear. Audiometers must meet the specifications of a standard developed by the American National Standards Institute (ANSI), (S3.6, 1969).[17] OSHA gives detailed requirements for pulsed-tone and self-recording audiometers in the regulation's Appendix C, which include specifications for audiometers and methods for scoring audiograms taken with self-recording audiometers. Since self-recording audiometers are rarely used in occupational hearing conservation any more, these instructions are no longer pertinent except when the OHC is confronted with archived audiograms, in which case he or she may refer to OSHA's Appendix C to see if they were scored correctly.

Audiometer Calibration:

The **functional operation** of the audiometer must be checked before each day's use. The main purpose of the functional check is to make sure that the audiometer is working properly, that undistorted sound is coming out of the appropriate earphone, and that the sound pressure levels are accurate. In addition to a careful listening check, the OHC should use an electronic device to check the sound pressure levels, or, lacking that, can test someone with known, stable hearing threshold levels. This latter practice is sometimes referred to as a "biological check." Deviations of 10 dB or more in the audiometer's desired output trigger the next stage of calibration.

An **acoustic calibration** must be performed at least annually. This procedure is not so much a calibration, where the audiometer's settings are actually changed, but a calibration check. The test frequencies and specifications are listed in the regulation's Appendix E. The OHC will not usually be required to perform the acoustical calibration check unless otherwise trained.

The third step is the **exhaustive calibration**, which must be performed at least every two years or if triggered by an acoustic calibration. This calibration should be performed by a specially trained individual or in an appropriate laboratory.

Noise Levels in Audiometric Test Rooms:

Audiometric tests must be conducted in rooms that are at least as quiet as the sound levels specified in the regulation's Appendix D. However, the OHC

---

[17] ANSI S3.6 (1969) has since been revised twice and the latest version is dated 1996. OSHA requires that employers at least meet the specifications of the 1969 version, but it is always good practice to comply with the latest revision whenever possible.

uld be aware that these sound levels originated n ANSI standard that is now over 40 years old and has been revised three times since the 1960 standard to which OSHA refers. They are not adequate to permit testing to audiometric zero, and many workers will complain about interfering noise unless the room is quieter. This is one of the places where the OHC should try to improve upon the OSHA regulation and use more appropriate criteria. NIOSH recommends using the levels published in the 1991 ANSI standard, although it has since been revised again in 1999. (This subject will be discussed in more detail in Chapter VII.)

Hearing Protectors

Mandatory Use:

All employees who are exposed to noise levels at or above the PEL (a TWA of 90 dBA) must wear hearing protectors. Also, employees exposed to levels between 85 and 90 dBA must wear them if they have experienced an STS or if they have not yet had a baseline audiogram and they have worked in noise for more than 6 months.[18]

Mandatory Provision But Non-mandatory Use:

OSHA requires that employers supply hearing protectors to all employees exposed to TWAs of 85 dBA or above, but does not require their use by employees unless the TWA reaches 90 dBA, or one of the two other conditions mentioned above becomes true.

Employer's Duties:

It is not enough for employers merely to hand out hearing protectors to their employees. They must ensure that the protectors are properly fitted initially, they must provide training in the use and care of all hearing protectors, and they must supervise the correct use of these devices. That means that they must observe the protectors in actual use, and, as best they can, make sure that the devices are working as they should.

Workers must be given a variety of suitable protectors from which to choose. Since the regulation does not define "a variety," OSHA policy has been that the

employer should offer at least one type of plug and one type of muff (preferably more), but the emphasis is on "suitable" (Hillenbrand, 1983; Miles, 1983).

Attenuation:

Hearing protectors must attenuate employees' exposures to a TWA of at least 90 dBA, unless an employee has experienced an STS, in which case the hearing protector must attenuate to at least 85 dBA.

Acceptable methods for assessing the attenuation of hearing protectors are given in the OSHA regulation's Appendix B. Although the employer is given a choice of methods, the simplest and most commonly used method is the Noise Reduction Rating (NRR). An EPA regulation requires the manufacturers of hearing protectors to print the NRR on the package of the protector. To estimate the TWA beneath the protector, OSHA requires the employer to subtract the NRR from the employee's C-weighted workplace TWA. If the C-weighted TWA is not available, the employer may use the A-weighted TWA, but must subtract a 7-dB penalty from the NRR as a safety factor since the NRR is not intended for use with A-weighted measures.[19] More details on hearing protectors and the use of the NRR will be given in Chapter X.

The adequacy of hearing protector attenuation must be reassessed whenever there is a change in process or employee exposure that might necessitate greater attenuation. Although the OSHA regulations do not require it, attenuation should also be reassessed when the employee's noise exposure has decreased to the point where substantially less attenuation is needed. There will be more discussion about the disadvantages of over-protection in Chapter X.

Training Program

The OSHA regulation requires that all employees whose TWAs equal or exceed 85 dBA be part of a training program, and that the training be conducted at least annually. Workers must be trained in (1) the effects of noise on hearing, (2) the purposes and procedures of audiometric testing, and (3) the purpose of hearing protectors, the advantages, disadvantages, and attenuation of various types, and instructions on selection, fitting, use, and care of these devices.

---

[18] The OHC should remember that a company can make a policy that differs from the OSHA regulation as long as it is at least as protective. For example, the company can require that all employees exposed to TWAs above 85 dBA wear hearing protectors from the moment they start work until they receive their baseline audiograms. Or, for that matter, the company can require that wearing hearing protectors above a TWA of 85 dB is mandatory for everyone.

[19] The C-weighting network is relatively "flat" across the frequency spectrum and does not filter out low-frequency sound as does the A-weighting network. Most sound level meters can measure C-weighted sound levels, and many noise dosimeters also have this capacity. Since obtaining a TWA with a sound level meter and stop-watch is such a cumbersome exercise, most people will prefer to use the dosimeter for this purpose. If the dosimeter does not have the capability of measuring C-weighted noise levels, one can use the A-weighting network and subtract the necessary 7-dB penalty from the NRR.

The training program does not need to be carried out all at one time. For example, if the employer or the OHC prefers, training on the effects of noise could take place at a scheduled safety meeting and training on audiometric testing could take place at the time of testing. The training on hearing protectors should occur when the protectors are first issued and again when they are checked at various times during the year.

Recordkeeping

OSHA requires employers to keep records of noise exposure measurements and audiometric tests. The regulation gives details about the kinds of information to be kept with the audiogram, including information on the calibration of the audiometer, measurements of background sound levels in the test room, and the employee's most recent noise exposure assessment. Noise exposure measurements must be kept for at least two years, and audiometric test records must be kept for the duration of a worker's employment. Once again, the OHC should improve upon these requirements by keeping more detailed records and by keeping them significantly longer. There will be more discussion of good recordkeeping practices in Chapter XII.

The regulation gives employees, former employees, and their representatives access to their records, and requires that employers that cease doing business transfer these records to the new employer.

OSHA also requires that the employer post a copy of the noise regulation in the workplace, and make a copy available to affected employees and their representatives if they request it. OSHA has interpreted this requirement to mean that the regulation should be readily available for employees without having to ask for it and notice of its location should be posted centrally (Shepich, 1998).

Policies

Both OSHA and MSHA have issued policies after promulgating their noise regulations. Unlike the actual regulations, these policies often take the form of interpretations when the regulation's meaning is not clear and when the preamble has not clarified a particular section. Policies are created without going through the official rule-making process, and therefore are not always legally enforceable. They may be changed at any time and they sometimes reflect the politics of the moment. Although they are meant primarily for the agency's staff members, they are all available to the public, and they can be helpful in resolving ambiguities or issues on which the regulation is silent. Interpretation letters are available on OSHA's website (see list in Appendix E of this manual). MSHA's

primary source of interpretations is its "Program Policy Letter (P00-IV-4/P00-V-3): Noise Enforcement Policy," available on the MSHA website. Specific MSHA policies will be discussed, along with the MSHA regulation, in later sections of this chapter.

OSHA Policies

The purpose of most OSHA policies is to aid the compliance officers in enforcing OSHA regulations. Certain policies are issued as "instructions," others as "guidelines," and others are contained in books or manuals. The **Field Inspection Reference Manual**, designated CPL 2.103, sets official policy and guidelines for OSHA inspectors and is updated periodically. The **Technical Manual** contains guidelines only (without official policy), and is more technical in nature. Both documents are available on OSHA's website and can be helpful in ascertaining the expectations of OSHA personnel when they inspect a company's hearing conservation program.

In addition to the policies mentioned above, an important example of an OSHA policy is OSHA Instruction CPL 2-2.35 dated November 9, 1983. This policy tells compliance officers not to issue citations to companies for lack of feasible engineering controls unless (1) workers' exposures exceed a TWA of 100 dBA, or (2) the company does not have an "effective hearing conservation program." OSHA gives no formal definition of an effective hearing conservation program, but it is usually interpreted to mean that workers are not losing their hearing. (The inspection documentation is somewhat vague on this issue.) To assess the relative effectiveness of hearing protectors and engineering controls in such a program, the compliance officer "**derates**" the NRR by 50%. This means that only half of a protector's NRR is considered when assessing its adequacy relative to engineering controls, but not when assessing its general acceptability. (This policy is somewhat confusing, for both OSHA enforcement officers and industry representatives.) Sections of the policy are referenced in the *Field Inspection Reference Manual* and a series of questions and answers relating to the policy can be found among OSHA's interpretations and compliance letters (see Miles, 1994). The reader should understand that this policy is contrary to section (a) of the noise regulation, although it will remain official policy until OSHA withdraws it or until it is successfully challenged in court. At least one state, North Carolina, has not adopted the policy in its OSHA program.

OHCs should be aware that these policies may change at any time. The best course is to keep current on these kinds of matters by reading professional journals and newsletters, and by checking websites, especially OSHA's. CAOHC's newsletter *UPDATE* is a helpful source of information on these

...ds of issues. When in doubt, call OSHA's Office ...nformation in Washington, DC for a referral to a knowledgeable staff member.

Recording Work-Related Hearing Loss on the OSHA Form 300

The current version of OSHA's noise regulation makes no mention of an employer's duty to record a hearing loss on OSHA's **Form 300** (formerly Form 200), the **"Log of Work-Related Injuries and Illnesses."** Requirements for maintaining this log of injuries and illnesses are covered under a separate OSHA regulation (29 CFR 1904). Until recently, OSHA's policy had been to require employers to record on the Form 300 a work-related shift in hearing threshold level of 25 dB averaged over the frequencies 2000, 3000, and 4000 Hz in either ear, with adjustments for presbycusis allowed (Whitmore, 1994).

In 2001, OSHA issued a revision of its recordkeeping regulation, which covers a variety of recordkeeping requirements (OSHA, 2001), and in 2002 issued a final rule for recording hearing loss, section 1904.10, "Recording criteria for cases involving occupational hearing loss" (OSHA, 2002). The new rule requires employers to record a **work-related STS**, a 10-dB average shift from baseline (or the revised baseline) in either ear at 2000, 3000, and 4000 Hz if the shift plus the employee's baseline hearing thresholds at those same frequencies totals 25 dB or greater above audiometric zero. For example, an STS would have to be recorded if an employee's baseline thresholds, prior to the STS, averaged 15 dB or greater at the frequencies 2000, 3000, and 4000 Hz. If, in fact, the STS were as much as 15 dB, then baseline hearing thresholds need average only 10 dB and the loss would still have to be recorded since the average loss at these frequencies would equal 25 dB. Age corrections may be used but are not required, and may only be used when determining whether or not an STS has occurred and not when determining if the employee's current average hearing level is 25 dB or greater in relation to audiometric zero.

OSHA gives employers the opportunity to retest within 30 days before recording a work-related STS. If the retest confirms the STS, the hearing loss must be recorded within 7 calendar days of the retest. If the retest does not confirm the STS, then the case need not be recorded. Of course, the OHC should be aware that if a retest is not conducted, confirmation of the STS is assumed and the case should be recorded within 37 calendar days (i.e. 30 days for retest window plus 7 days for the recording requirement). In addition, if later testing reveals that the recorded STS is not permanent, the entry may be erased or lined-out.

OSHA defines work relatedness as follows: "If an event or exposure in the work environment either caused or contributed to the hearing loss, or significantly aggravated a pre-existing hearing loss, you must consider the case to be work related." If a physician or other licensed health care professional determines that the hearing loss is not work-related or has not been signifciantly aggravated by occupational noise, the employer is not required to record the loss on the OSHA Form 300.

The new recordkeeping rule is not a policy but an actual regulation and therefore carries more weight. The new rule is due to become effective on January 1, 2003. There is, however, one element of the new rule that is not yet final as of this printing, and that is the exact location where the employer must record the hearing loss. OSHA is considering adding a separate column for hearing loss on the Form 300. Until OSHA makes its final decision about whether or not to have a separate column, employers must record the hearing loss in Column M5, "All other illnesses."

Readers should note that OSHA's requirements for recording hearing loss on the Form 300 have done nothing to change the noise regulations's definition of STS.

OHCs would be wise to check OSHA's website for up-to-date information.

OSHA State Plans

Many states have their own OSHA programs, meaning that they promulgate their own regulations and have their own enforcement staffs. Under most circumstances, they are not bound by the federal regulations as long as their own regulations are at least as protective as the federal ones. An exception to this provision is the new recording rule detailed in the preceding paragraphs, where OSHA's federal regulation preempts any state's recording requirements.

At this time there are 23 states, along with Puerto Rico and the Virgin Islands, that have their own programs. They are: Alaska, Arizona, California, Connecticut,[20] Hawaii, Indiana, Iowa, Kentucky, Maryland, Michigan, Minnesota, Nevada, New Mexico, New York, North Carolina, Oregon, South Carolina, Tennessee, Utah, Vermont, Virginia, Washington, and Wyoming.

For a state to have its own program, its "State Plan" has to be approved by the federal OSHA. Some of the state programs have been in effect since 1973, while others are relatively new. Most state-plan states have noise regulations that are identical with the federal regulation. The California and Kentucky regulations have minor differences, and Oregon and Washington differ from the federal reg-

---

[20] The Connecticut and New York plans cover only state and local government employees. Enforcement in the private sector is conducted by federal OSHA.

ulation in several ways.[21] The enforcement policy in North Carolina differs from the federal policy in that North Carolina does not allow employers to rely on hearing protectors and other elements of the hearing conservation program rather than engineering or administrative controls.

Most of the states have what they call "On-Site Consultation Agreements," through which they provide free consultation to employers. For information about state programs call the local OSHA office or the OSHA office in the state capitol.

Construction

Although OSHA's noise regulation for general industry does not cover construction workers, there are separate regulations that do. One regulation, 29 CFR 1926.52, is very similar to the old "Walsh-Healey" noise regulation, and another, 29 CFR 1926.101, merely requires the use of hearing protectors above the PEL and that they be fitted or determined individually by "competent persons." The hearing conservation amendment does not apply to construction workers, but contractors bear some responsibility for protecting the hearing of their workers. Construction regulation 29 CFR 1926.52 requires "continuing, effective hearing conservation programs" for workers exposed above the 90 dBA PEL. An OSHA policy has defined this requirement as including (whenever feasible) (1) noise exposure monitoring, (2) installation of engineering, work practice, and administrative controls for excessive noise, (3) provision of individually fitted hearing protectors with adequate noise reduction rating, (4) employee training and education, (5) baseline and annual audiometry, (6) procedures for preventing further occupational hearing loss when such an event has been identified, and (7) recordkeeping (Clark, 1992).

---

[21]California's Table N-1 is somewhat more detailed than the federal Table G-16 and the state did not adopt OSHA's non-mandatory Appendix G. Kentucky requires testing at 8000 Hz. Oregon requires CAOHC certification for audiometric technicians, does not provide an exception for mobile test vans from the requirement for completing baselines within 6 months, does not allow audiograms to be adjusted for presbycusis, and requires all industries, including construction, to implement the hearing conservation provisions. The Washington noise regulation has six main differences: (1) Hearing protectors must attenuate to 85 dBA for all workers; (2) Hearing protectors must be worn by all workers with TWAs of 85 dBA, in areas where noise levels are greater than 115 dBA, or where impulse/impact noise levels exceed peak sound pressure levels of 140 dB; (3) A written description of the training program must be maintained; (4) Warning signs must be posted in areas where workers may be exposed at or above 115 dBA; (5) Employers must prepare and submit a written noise control compliance plan when requested by the state; and (6) There is no provision for adjustments for presbycusis. OHCs in these states should obtain copies of the state regulations and should be thoroughly familiar with them.

Two states, Oregon and Washington, do not exempt construction from the general industry noise regulation, and would, therefore, require compliance with their state hearing conservation regulations. Enforcement of these provisions in the construction industry by Oregon and Washington, as well as enforcement of the above policy on the federal level, has not been aggressive. Despite this, interest in hearing conservation for construction workers has been growing among professionals and in certain worker organizations (Suter, in press; see also the website of the Laborers' Health and Safety Fund of North America: **www.lhsfna.org/**).

Mine Safety and Health Administration (MSHA)

Like OSHA, the Mine Safety and Health Administration (MSHA) is another agency within the U.S. Department of Labor that is concerned with occupational noise, as well as other health and safety hazards, in this case as it affects miners. Until recently there were separate noise regulations for coal mines and metal/non-metal mines. In 1999, MSHA issued a single comprehensive noise regulation that applies to all kinds of mining (MSHA, 1999). Although there are substantially fewer noise-exposed workers in mining than in general industry (about 200,000 vs. more than 5 million), the promulgation of a new regulation for mining has generated considerable interest in the hearing conservation community. At this time, many mine operators are looking for ways to initiate noise control and audiometric testing programs.

The new MSHA noise regulation is reprinted as Appendix F in this manual. All OHCs who are involved with hearing conservation programs for miners should become thoroughly familiar with its provisions. Appendix G contains a checklist, reprinted courtesy of Associates in Acoustics, by which OHCs can verify compliance with the MSHA regulation. As with OSHA regulations, explanations and interpretations are available in the preamble to the MSHA noise regulation, published in the *Federal Register* (MSHA, 1999). In addition, MSHA has provided on its website a detailed set of interpretations in the form of questions and answers, Program Policy Letter (P00-IV-4/P00-V-3) "Noise Enforcement Policy" (Nichols and Teaster, 2000).

The new MSHA regulation is similar to OSHA's in its basic requirements, such as the 90-dBA PEL, the 5-dBA exchange rate, and the 85-dBA action level, as well as many of the audiometric testing, training, and hearing protector provisions. However, several exceptions to these similarities are discussed in the summary that follows. Most of the major differences are highlighted here, but the reader should always rely on the regulations themselves in the final analysis. Table 6.1 has been provided to aid in the comparison of the OSHA and MSHA regulations, as well as the NIOSH recommendations.

Permissible Exposure Level (Section 62.130)

Like section (b)(1) of the OSHA regulation, MSHA calls for feasible engineering or administrative controls for employees who exceed the 90-dBA TWA. Unlike OSHA, MSHA has no policy that exempts mine operators from the requirements for engineering or administrative controls, even if miners wear hearing protectors and participate in other aspects of the hearing conservation program. Also, MSHA states clearly that no miner may be exposed at any time to sound levels exceeding 115 dBA, regardless of the use of hearing protectors.

The term "feasible," as it applies both to engineering and administrative controls, is defined in MSHA's Program Policy Letter as incorporating three factors: (a) the nature and extent of the exposure; (b) the demonstrated effectiveness of available technology; and (c) whether the committed resources (costs) are wholly out of proportion to the expected results. MSHA's policy defines "demonstrated effectiveness" as a reduction in noise exposure levels of at least 3 dBA.

The mine operator must post any administrative controls that are being used on the mine's bulletin board and provide a copy to affected miners.

Noise Exposure Assessment (Section 62.110)

PEL:

In assessing compliance with the PEL, all sound levels between 90 and 140 dBA[22] must be included in the noise dose or TWA, and determinations must reflect the miner's full work shift. These provisions are more explicit than OSHA's requirement for the PEL.

Action Level:

Like OSHA, all sound levels between 80 and 130 dBA must be included for compliance with the 85-dBA action level.

---

[22] As with the OSHA regulation, MSHA permits employers to set the dosimeter's lower threshold only slightly below 90 dBA to assess compliance with the PEL. Although this is allowed, it is not considered "best practice" because it assumes all levels below 90 dBA contribute zero percent to the noise dose. Common sense tells us that noise levels below 90 dBA are not harmless. Also, for accuracy of measurement, professionals in acoustics recommend setting the dosimeter's lower threshold at least 5 dB below the criterion level, which in this case would be 85 dBA.

Dual Hearing Protection Level:

One entirely new aspect of MSHA's noise regulation is the requirement that mine operators must provide miners with dual hearing protection (meaning the concurrent use of an earmuff and earplug) at a TWA of 105 dBA or the equivalent dose of 800%.

Noise Monitoring:

The mine operator must establish a system of monitoring to evaluate each miner's noise exposure sufficiently to determine compliance. There is no discussion of personal versus area monitoring or requirements for repeated monitoring. Employees must have the opportunity to observe the monitoring and mine operators must give miners advance notice. The notification requirements are somewhat more specific than OSHA's, in that miners must be notified in writing when their exposures equal or exceed the action level, or exceed the PEL or dual protection level. Notification must take place within 15 days of the exposure determination and must include any corrective actions being taken.

The actual noise monitoring provisions are "performance oriented," leaving the details of noise measurement practice to mine operators or their contractors. In fact, it is MSHA's policy that if a mine operator enrolls all miners at a particular mine in the hearing conservation program, noise exposure monitoring is not necessary. However, the mine operator must still notify all miners in writing that they are overexposed.

In its interpretation document, MSHA stated that its inspectors will use a 2-dBA error factor, meaning that the agency will not issue citations until doses reach 66% for the action level, 132% for the PEL, and 1056% for the dual hearing protection level. The 2-dBA error factor also applies to the 115-dBA ceiling level, and MSHA has stated that a citation will not be issued until a level of 117 dBA is exceeded for 30 consecutive seconds.

Hearing Protectors (Section 62.160)

As in the OSHA regulation, MSHA requires miners to be provided with hearing protectors when their noise exposures equal or exceed the action level, but MSHA states that miners must be able to choose from at least two types of earmuffs and two types of earplugs. They must also be allowed to choose a different hearing protector if wearing the selected protector is not possible because of a medical pathology of the ear. Mine operators must ensure that the hearing protector is in good condition and fitted and maintained in accordance with the manufacturer's instructions.

MSHA's regulation is silent on the evaluation of hearing protector attenuation and there is no discussion of the NRR or other rating methods, although the Policy Letter states that either the NRR or another scientifically accepted indicator of noise reduction is required. The Policy also allows the use of noise-canceling earmuffs under certain conditions (but not as an engineering control), and disallows the use of hearing aids as hearing protectors.

In answer to a question about whether miners must use hearing protectors continually throughout the entire shift, the Policy allows the wearing of hearing protectors to be discontinued in quiet places or in circumstances where the equipment causing the excessive noise exposure is not running.

Audiometric Testing (Sections 62.170–62.175)

Similar to the OSHA regulation, MSHA requires mine operators to "offer the opportunity" for audiometric testing, but does not require miners to take the test. MSHA interprets this requirement by stating that mine operators must inform miners that audiograms are available but does not specify how miners are to be informed. Posting audiometric test dates and locations where all affected miners can see them will be acceptable. If a miner declines the audiometric test when it is first offered, but changes his or her mind at a later date, the mine operator is required to offer the test again.

A new baseline audiogram may be established for a miner who has been away from the mine for more than six consecutive months, but one cannot be established due only to changes in enrollment status in the hearing conservation program.

Audiograms conducted in accordance with OSHA's hearing conservation amendment are fully acceptable under MSHA's new regulation.

Audiometric Test Procedures (Section 62.171)

Rather than spell out detailed requirements for audiometers, test rooms, and calibration, as in OSHA's Appendices C, D, and E, MSHA requires testing to be "conducted in accordance with scientifically validated procedures." The mine operator must compile an audiometric test record, which must include a copy of all of the miner's audiograms and results of any follow-up examinations, in addition to the types of information required by OSHA. Audiometric test records must be kept for the duration of the miner's employment plus six months.

Evaluation of Audiograms (Section 62.172)

MSHA's requirements for audiogram evaluation are similar to OSHA's in many respects, but MSHA

explicitly states that a qualified technician may make the determination that an audiogram is or is not valid, whereas OSHA only implies it by requiring the supervising professional to review "problem audiograms." Also MSHA requires that neither the technician nor the supervising professional may reveal to the mine operator any audiometric finding or diagnosis unrelated to occupational noise without the written consent of the miner. The mine operator must obtain the results and interpretation of the audiograms within 30 days of conducting the audiogram, and this requirement is not contingent on an STS, as it is in the OSHA regulation.

Follow-up (Section 62.173 and 62.174)

MSHA requires that a retest must be provided within 30 days of a finding that an audiogram is invalid (Section 62.172). Follow-up evaluation is contingent upon the failure to obtain a valid audiogram rather than on the occurrence of an STS. If a valid audiogram cannot be obtained because of a medical pathology that is due to or aggravated by a miner's exposure to noise or wearing hearing protectors, he or she must be referred for an audiological or otological evaluation, at no cost to the miner. If the reason for the invalid audiogram is not occupationally related, the supervising professional must inform the miner of the need for a follow-up exam, but the mine operator does not bear the expense. Again, findings or diagnoses that are unrelated to occupational noise or hearing protection must not be revealed to the mine operator without the miner's written consent.

Follow-up procedures in the event of an STS are similar to OSHA's, with the additional requirement that the mine operator must review the effectiveness of any engineering and administrative controls to identify and correct deficiencies.

Notification and Reporting (Section 62.175)

This section contains a requirement for notifying the miner of the results of an audiometric test or follow-up evaluation, including an interpretation of the audiometric test, any finding of an STS or a reportable hearing loss, or the need and reasons for any further evaluation.

MSHA defines a reportable hearing loss as an average change of 25 dB or more at 2000, 3000, or 4000 Hz in either ear, relative to the miner's baseline audiogram. Such a loss must be reported to MSHA unless a physician or audiologist has determined that the loss is not work-related. A revised baseline may be used for this purpose only if the audiogram indicates a significant improvement over the original baseline (see Section 62.170[c][2]).

Training (Section 62.180)

MSHA's requirements for an annual training program are similar to OSHA's with the addition of a section that explains the mine operator's and the miner's respective tasks in maintaining noise controls. The mine operator must certify the date and type of training given each miner. The Policy Letter states that an audiometric testing service provider may conduct the training, but the agency will not accept certification by a service provider. The mine operator must provide the certification. A record of this certification must be kept for the duration of the miner's enrollment in the hearing conservation program plus 6 months.

Records (Section 62.190)

This section requires mine operators, upon written request, to provide records to miners or their representatives within 15 days of the request, including training certifications and noise exposure determinations as well as audiograms. The first copy must be supplied at no cost.

Mine operators must transfer the records to a successor mine operator, as with OSHA, but there is a specific requirement that the successor must use the baseline audiogram or revised baseline, as appropriate, to determine the existence of an STS or reportable hearing loss.

Appendix

The MSHA regulation has only one appendix, which consists of four tables. Table 62.1 lists reference durations for A-weighted sound levels, similar to OSHA's Table G-16a, although MSHA's table stops at 115 dBA, with the caveat that 115 dBA must not be exceeded. Table 62.2 gives noise dose in percent and the equivalent TWA. Again, this table is similar to OSHA's Table A-1, except that dose begins at 25% with an equivalent TWA of 80 dBA, while OSHA's begins at 10% and a TWA of about 73 dBA, and MSHA's table extends to 3200% for a TWA of 115 dBA, while OSHA's stops at 999% and a TWA of about 107 dBA.

Tables 62.3 and 62.4 contain the same age correction values as OSHA's Appendix F.

MSHA Resources

Personnel at MSHA have developed several useful documents since the promulgation of the noise regulation. Most of these documents are available on the "Resources Page" found on MSHA's website or accessed directly at **www.msha.gov/1999noise/noiseresources.htm**. These include a *Compliance Guide* written expressly for mine operators and miners, an *Audiometric Testing Reference Guide* intended for mine operators, contractors, audiologists, physicians, and others who conduct or evaluate audiometric tests, and a *Guide to Conducting Noise Sampling*, intended for personnel who monitor miners' noise exposures. There is also a list of hearing protectors with their NRRs. These data are simply compiled by MSHA from the manufacturers' literature and are not validated by MSHA.

Differences Among OSHA, MSHA, and NIOSH

Table 6.1 summarizes the differences among the OSHA, MSHA, and NIOSH provisions. This table was published in Chapter 16 of the 5th edition of the AIHA *Noise Manual* (see Suter, 2000) and in *Spectrum*, the newsletter of the National Hearing Conservation Association (Berger and Hager, 2000).

As mentioned above, NIOSH revised its criteria document for noise in 1998, based on new research and the availability of information (see NIOSH, 1998). Although the NIOSH provisions are recommendations and therefore not mandatory, many professionals and some of the larger companies have implemented them whenever possible. Some of the NIOSH recommendations have been mentioned above, but probably the most important differences between NIOSH and OSHA are the PEL[23] (OSHA 90 dBA, NIOSH 85 dBA), and the exchange rate (OSHA 5 dBA, NIOSH 3 dBA).[24]

NIOSH also publishes educational materials and information, as well as research reports and "Health Hazard Evaluations" performed at the request of companies with occupational safety or health problems.

Other Agencies With Occupational Hearing Loss Regulations

OSHA and MSHA are not the only agencies with noise regulations, although most of the other federal agencies, with the exception of the Department of Defense, have noise regulations that are fairly similar to OSHA's. For example, in the Department of Transportation, the Federal Railroad Administration regulates the noise exposure of railroad workers, and the Bureau of Motor Carrier Safety regulates the noise exposure of truck drivers. Many of the federal

---

[23] The NIOSH criteria document refers to it as an "REL" (recommended exposure limit).

[24] The 3-dBA exchange rate is more protective than the 5 dBA exchange rate in that it allows smaller increases in exposure level with every doubling of exposure duration. It is used by most European countries, several Canadian provinces, and two out of three branches of the U.S. armed services.

agencies, such as the National Aeronautics and Space Administration, the Department of the Interior, and the Department of Energy have noise programs to protect their own employees from hazardous noise exposure. Some of these programs are mandatory and others take the form of recommendations.

An interesting example of a federal noise program that differs from OSHA's is the U.S. Coast Guard guidelines, which apply to crews on board U.S. commercial vessels (Coast Guard, 1982). The guidelines recommend the evaluation of crew members' 24-hour exposures, a criterion level (similar to a PEL) of 82 dBA, the wearing of hearing protectors at 85 dBA, and an action level of 77 dBA, where hearing conservation programs should be initiated. All of these noise levels are measured and averaged over a 24-hour period.

The best way to obtain information on noise programs and regulations in any government agency is to call its public information office or check the agency's website.

OHCs should keep in mind that federal noise recommendations or regulations may be changed at any time, but, of course, regulations must follow public rule-making procedures and so there is usually plenty of advance notice.

The Department of Defense

The military has traditionally been a noisy occupation. Perhaps because military personnel need to perform well in crises, or perhaps because the various branches of the military have been known for their extensive research programs, hearing conservation in the military has often been on the leading edge over the years.

The Department of Defense (DoD, 1996) has a single general regulation that applies to all three of the U.S. Armed Services, and each branch has its own particular noise regulation. The DoD issues "Instructions" periodically on various matters, including safety and health, to be used by all three branches. A revised Instruction, DoD 6055.12, was issued on April 22, 1996 for hearing conservation programs. A copy of the instruction can be found on the website of the Defense Technical Information Center (see websites at end of chapter). It requires heads of all departments to establish and maintain hearing conservation programs when TWAs equal or exceed 85 dBA, and it requires an exchange rate at least as protective as 4 dBA and "strongly recommends" the use of a 3-dBA exchange rate.

Because the primary means of reducing exposure to hazardous noise is engineering controls, the 85-dBA TWA (using either the 3-dBA or 4-dBA exchange rate) is considered a PEL. The required aspects of the hearing conservation program are:

- Noise measurement and analysis
- Safety signs and labels
- Noise abatement when feasible
- Fitting, training in, and use of hearing protectors
- Education of noise-exposed personnel
- Audiometric testing
- Personnel assignments that may include hearing sensitivity criteria
- Access to information, training materials, and records
- Recordkeeping
- Program performance evaluation

Although each branch of the service may promulgate its own rules, they must be at least as stringent as the current DoD Instruction. The only major differences among the three regulations is that the Navy uses the 4-dBA exchange rate, while the Army and the Air Force use 3 dBA.

Worker Compensation for Hearing Loss

No discussion of federal and state regulations would be complete without mentioning the subject of worker compensation for hearing loss. Although not all OHCs will be involved in the administrative procedures surrounding this issue, it helps to have some knowledge of the subject. Also, the fact that some workers do receive compensation for noise-induced hearing loss in most jurisdictions provides added incentives for the OHC to keep careful and detailed records.

The principle behind the worker compensation system is that the employer automatically assumes liability for injuries and illnesses that are work-related, and the employee gives up the right to civil suit. Theoretically, neither the employer nor the employee needs an attorney once work-relatedness is established, but, in practice, attorneys are usually employed. The more specific the worker compensation statute or criteria, the less litigation is necessary.

Unfortunately, there are nearly as many statutes and procedures for filing and awarding compensation claims for hearing loss as there are states in the U.S. (including the U.S. territories) and provinces in Canada. In addition, certain workers are covered by different types of statutes. The U.S. Department of Labor administers the **Federal Employee's Compensation Act (FECA)** for civilian federal employees and the **Longshore and Harbor Workers Compensation Act** for people working on the docks. Military personnel are compensated for hearing loss by the **Veterans Administration**. Railroad workers and merchant seamen are not covered by worker compensation programs. Consequently, these workers may file lawsuits in civil courts, but they must prove employer negligence. Product liability suits for noise-induced hearing loss also take place in civil courts and the litigation is usually more complex and involves higher awards.

Because each jurisdiction has a slightly different twist to its statute or procedure, it is important that OHCs be familiar with the rules of their own state, territory, province, or other venue. Also, these statutes and procedures are continually changing, so OHCs must keep up with worker compensation issues through their professional and trade organization publications and websites, or worker compensation boards. Another good source of information is the U.S. Chamber of Commerce in Washington, DC, which publishes an "Analysis of Worker Compensation Laws" every year. The compensation office in the OHC's own jurisdiction will usually be the most accurate source of information.

Reprinted as Appendix I in the back of the manual is a survey of worker compensation practices conducted by Susan Megerson and her colleagues, from Chapter 18 of the 5th edition of the AIHA *Noise Manual* (Dobie and Megerson, 2000). In addition to listing the impairment formulas used by each U.S. jurisdiction, the survey includes Canadian provinces. It contains some useful information, such as whether the jurisdiction considers tinnitus, reductions for presbycusis, improvement with a hearing aid, and failure to utilize hearing protection in granting an award. It also lists the maximum amounts of compensation that each jurisdiction could give for hearing losses in one or both ears. At the time of publication, the maximum amount for hearing loss in both ears ranged from a high of $152,600 in Iowa to a low of $9,000 in Rhode Island.

The reader should be aware of certain caveats, however. First, not every jurisdiction provided complete and consistent response to the survey, so the information should not be considered definitive. Next, the fact that maximum awards may amount to over $100,000 bears little relationship to reality, since these amounts are for "total" hearing loss in both ears, which is usually considered to be an average hearing threshold level of 92 dB in the frequencies 500, 1000, 2000, and 3000 Hz. Noise-induced hearing loss that severe is almost non-existent. The average worker compensation award for hearing loss is considerably less, probably under $10,000, although the exact figure is not currently available. Also, as mentioned above, the reader should be aware that these statutes may be updated at any time, so some of the information in Appendix I may already be outdated.

It would be helpful for the OHC to have a general familiarity with the formulas used to calculate the degree of hearing handicap. Most states use the formula published by the American Medical Association in 1979, referred to as the **AAO-79 formula**, which uses the average hearing threshold level at 500, 1000, 2000, and 3000 Hz. A few states use the older, 1959 "**AAOO**" formula, which uses only 500, 1000, and 2000 Hz, and some use their own individual formulas. Quite a few states use "**medical evidence**," meaning that the physicians (and sometimes audiologists) involved will testify as to the amount of handicap the worker has incurred, without reference to a formula. Most of the formulas consider hearing handicap to begin at a "**low fence**" or average hearing level of 25 dB for the frequencies of 500, 1000, 2000, and 3000 Hz, below which the worker is considered to be 0 percent handicapped. Three states, Illinois, New Jersey, and Wisconsin, use a 30-dB low fence, and Oregon includes the 4000 Hz and 6000 Hz frequencies in its formula. The growth of handicap with increasing hearing loss is usually $1\frac{1}{2}$ percent per decibel of hearing loss, with a "**high fence**," or 100 percent handicap (often referred to as "total" hearing loss), at 92 dB.

There are a number of requirements and other considerations that vary among jurisdictions' rules that may be of interest. Several of these rules impose restrictions on the ability of workers to file claims for hearing impairment. For example, many jurisdictions require waiting periods away from noise exposure ranging from 3 days to 6 months before employees may file claims. In addition, several have a statute of limitations, after which the worker's claim will not be considered. Some jurisdictions penalize claimants or even deny their claims if there is proof that they failed to use hearing protection. Also, some require proof of exposure to a minimum noise level (usually 90 dBA) for a claim to be awarded. One rule that significantly penalizes the claimant is a deduction for presbycusis, and many jurisdictions now employ this practice, even though historically, use of the low fence has been considered by some to account for the effects of aging.

Other rules may have the effect of increasing the amount of the claim. The majority of jurisdictions compensate for work-related tinnitus, although the condition usually has to be accompanied by a hearing impairment. Most jurisdictions will provide a hearing aid, if needed, to the worker whose claim for hearing loss has been awarded, and a few will take into account the claimant's self-assessment of hearing handicap in determining the amount of the award.

The Americans with Disabilities Act (ADA)

One relatively new development that may be of interest to OHCs, as well as to supervising professionals, is the **American with Disabilities Act (ADA)** of 1990. Although much of the emphasis is on providing access to people confined to wheelchairs and having similar disabilities, the Act also applies to people with hearing impairments. The Act is administered and enforced by the U.S. Department of Justice and information about it is available on the internet at the ADA's home page: **www.usdoj.gov/crt/ada/adahom1.htm**.

Regulations issued under the authority of the ADA require employers not to discriminate in their hiring or promotion practices against a person with a disability if the person is otherwise qualified for the job. Employers may ask all applicants about their ability to perform a job and even have them demonstrate this ability before being hired. Employers may also require a medical examination. If the person is qualified, then the employer is obligated to make "reasonable accommodation" to the person's limitations, as long as these accommodations do not impose an "undue hardship" on the operation of the business. Undue hardship is defined as a significant difficulty and/or expense. Employers may determine that a person poses a significant risk of harm to the health or safety of that individual or others, and this risk cannot be eliminated or reduced by reasonable accommodation. This determination must be based on an individual assessment of that particular person's abilities and the specific functions expected of anyone in that job.

Reasonable accommodations for a hearing-impaired person may involve a variety of adjustments, some of which are already commonly used, like fax machines, personal computers, e-mail capabilities, and the addition of lighting. Others, such as assistive listening systems (amplification), telecommunication devices for the deaf (TDD), captioned videotapes, visual warning signals, and vibrating pagers can often be installed at relatively modest expense. In some cases interpreters using sign language may be necessary. The type and extent of these accommodations depend upon the abilities and preferences of the hearing-impaired employee and the technical skills and responsibilities of the job.

Title II of the Act covers state and local governments, and Title III applies to businesses and commercial facilities. Regulations developed under these sections of the Act are available at the Department of Justice ADA website. Examples of these regulations are Title III section 4.3400 concerning TDDs and sections 7.5160 and 7.5161 dealing with alarms and detectable warnings. Technical assistance manuals and other materials are available from the ADA's publications website: **www.usdoj.gov/crt/ada/publicat.htm** and also from the ADA Information Line at 1-800-514-0301.

References

Berger, E.H., and Hager, L. (2000). "Comparison of U.S. hearing conservation regulations and recommendations." *Spectrum, 17*(3), National Hearing Conservation Association, Denver, CO.

Clark, P.K. (1992). "Occupational noise, including hearing conservation, in construction work." OSHA Standards Interpretations and Compliance Letters, 8-4-92.

Coast Guard (1982). "Recommendations on control of excessive noise." Dept. of Transportation, U.S. Coast Guard, Navigation and Vessel Inspection Circular no. 12–82.

Dobie, R.A., and Megerson, S.C. (2000). "Workers' compensation." Chapter 18 in E.H. Berger, L.H. Royster, J.D. Royster, D.P. Driscoll, and M. Layne, (Eds.), *The Noise Manual, Fifth Edition*. American Industrial Hygiene Assoc., Fairfax, VA.

DoD (April 22, 1996). Department of Defense Instruction no. 6055.12.

Franks, J.R., Stephenson, M.R., and Merry, C.J. (1996). "Preventing occupational hearing loss—a practical guide," U.S. Dept. Health and Human Services, NIOSH, Cincinnati, OH.

Hillenbrand, B. (1983). "Ear muffs and ear plugs are not both required if one offers protection." OSHA Standards Interpretations and Compliance Letters, 9-30-83.

McCully, R. (1996). "Baseline audiograms." OSHA Standards Interpretations and Compliance Letters, 2-23-96.

Miles, J.B. (1983). "One type of muff and plug available for employee hearing protector selection." OSHA Standards Interpretations and Compliance Letters, 10-17-83.

Miles, J.B. (1994). "Questions and answers relative to the noise standard." OSHA Standards Interpretations and Compliance Letters, 5-8-94.

MSHA (1999). "Health standards for occupational noise exposure: Final rule." Mine Safety and Health Administration, 30 CFR Part 62, 64 *Fed. Reg.*, 49548–49634, 49636–49637.

Nichols, M.W., and Teaster, E.C. (October 5, 2000). "Noise enforcement policy." Program Policy Letter No. P00-IV-4/P00-V-3. Mine Safety and Health Administration.

NIOSH (1972). "Criteria for a recommended standard: Occupational noise exposure." U.S. Dept HEW (NIOSH) 73-11001. Dept. Health and Human Services, Public Health Service, National Institute for Occupational Safety and Health.

NIOSH (1998). "Criteria for a recommended standard: Occupational noise exposure: Revised criteria, 1998." DHHS (NIOSH) 98-126. Dept. Health and Human Services, Public Health Service.

OSHA (1981). "Occupational noise exposure: Hearing conservation amendment." Dept. Labor, Occupational Safety and Health Admin., 29 CFR 1910.95 46, *Fed. Reg.*, 4078–4179.

OSHA (1983a). "Occupational noise exposure: Hearing conservation amendment; final rule." Dept. Labor, Occupational Safety and Health Administration, 29 CFR 1910.95 48, *Fed. Reg.*, 9738–9784.

OSHA (1983b). OSHA Instruction CPL 2-2.35, Nov. 9, 1983. "Guidelines for noise enforcement." Dept. Labor, Occupational Safety and Health Administration.

OSHA (2001). "Occupational injury and illness recording and reporting requirements; Final rule." Dept. Labor, Occupational Safety and Health Administration, 66 *Fed. Reg.*, 5916–6135.

OSHA (2002). "Occupational injury and illness recording and reporting requirements; Final rule." Dept. Labor, Occupational Safety and Health Administration, 67 *Fed. Reg.*, 44037–44048.

Shepich, T.J. (1998). "Posting of the occupational noise exposure standard." OSHA Standards Interpretations and Compliance Letters, 2-9-88.

Suter, A.H. (2000). "Standards and regulations." Chapter 16 in E.H. Berger, L.H. Royster, J.D. Royster, D.P. Driscoll, and M. Layne, (Eds.) *The Noise Manual, Fifth Edition.* American Industrial Hygiene Assoc., Fairfax, VA.

Suter, A.H. (in press). "Construction noise: Exposure, effects, and the potential for remediation, a review and analysis." *Amer. Ind. Hyg. J.*

Vance, L. (1983). "Methods of training for microprocessor audiometer technicians." OSHA Standards Interpretations and Compliance Letters, 8-4-83.

Whitmore, B. (1994). "Recording of a hearing injury." OSHA Standards Interpretations and Compliance Letters, 6-27-94.

Quiz

1. Explain the difference between the missions of NIOSH and OSHA.

2. Which is OSHA's function: legislation or regulation?

3. OSHA's noise regulation calls for a PEL of _____, an exchange rate of _____, and an action level of _____.

4. If a worker is exposed to noise for only two hours in an eight-hour workshift, what is the maximum average level the worker may be exposed to during that period and be within OSHA's PEL?

5. According to the OSHA regulation, what must employers and employees do if the PEL is exceeded?

6. Under what circumstances does OSHA allow area noise monitoring for compliance with its regulation?

7. Both the OSHA and MSHA noise regulations require all employees exposed over the action level to take audiometric tests. (True or False)

8. Under both OSHA and MSHA, how soon after the beginning of an employee's noise exposure must the baseline audiogram be performed? When is the best time to perform the baseline?

9. According to OSHA, who must review "problem audiograms?"

10. What is OSHA's definition of standard threshold shift (STS)? What is MSHA's definition? Can you give the NIOSH definition? (See Table 6.1 if necessary.)

11. If the annual audiogram shows an STS with respect to the baseline, according to OSHA, the employee must be notified in writing within _____ days of the determination.

12. What are the employer's duties under MSHA when a miner has an STS?

13. In the daily calibration of the audiometer, what is the purpose of the "functional check?" Is this the same as the biological calibration check?

14. When employees are exposed to time-weighted average noise levels between 85 dBA and 90 dBA, the wearing of hearing protectors is not mandatory unless _____ _____.

15. The hearing protector rating that appears on the protector's package is the _____, abbreviated _____.

16. How often do noise-exposed employees need to be trained? Does all of the training need to be carried out at the same time?

17. The policies issued by OSHA and MSHA may interpret and clarify the noise regulation, but they do not have the weight of a regulation and may be changed without going through the rule-making process. (True or False)

18. MSHA requires dual protection at a TWA of _____ dBA or the equivalent dose of _____ %.

19. MSHA allows a qualified technician to determine whether or not an audiogram is valid. (True or False)

20. In addition to OSHA and MSHA, name at least three other government agencies that have occupational hearing loss regulations or programs.

21. The low fence used in most worker compensation formulas is a hearing threshold level of _____ dB, and the high fence is _____ dB.

22. Under the ADA, employers must make "reasonable accommodation" to a person's limitations, regardless of whether doing so imposes an undue hardship on the operation of the business. (True or False)

23. An example of a reasonable accommodation for a hearing-impaired person would be a visual warning signal. (True or False)

Abbreviations Used in Chapter VI

AAO	American Academy of Otolaryngology
AAO-HNS	American Academy of Otolaryngology—Head and Neck Surgery
AAOO	American Academy of Ophthalmology and Otolaryngology
ADA	Americans with Disabilities Act
AIHA	American Industrial Hygiene Association
ANSI	American National Standards Institute
CAOHC	Council for Accreditation in Occupational Hearing Conservation
dB	Decibels
dBA	Decibels measured on the A scale of the sound level meter (or dosimeter)
DoD	U.S. Department of Defense
EPA	Environmental Protection Agency
FECA	Federal Employee's Compensation Act
Hz	Hertz
MSHA	Mine Safety and Health Administration
NHCA	National Hearing Conservation Association

NIOSH	National Institute for Occupational Safety and Health
NRR	Noise Reduction Rating
OHC	Occupational Hearing Conservationist
OSHA	Occupational Safety and Health Administration
PEL	Permissible exposure limit (OSHA) Permissible exposure level (MSHA)
SPL	Sound pressure level
STS	Standard threshold shift
TDD	Telecommunication devices for the deaf
TTS	Temporary threshold shift
TWA	Time-weighted average exposure level

Recommended Reading

Dobie, R.A., and Megerson, S.C. (2000). "Workers' compensation." Chapter 18 in E.H. Berger, L.H. Royster, J.D. Royster, D.P. Driscoll, and M. Layne, (Eds.), *The Noise Manual, Fifth Edition.* American Industrial Hygiene Assoc., Fairfax, VA.

Nichols, M.W., and Teaster, E.C. (Oct. 5, 2000). "Noise enforcement policy." Program Policy Letter No. P00-IV-4/P00-V-3. Mine Safety and Health Administration.

NIOSH (1998). "Criteria for a recommended standard: Occupational noise exposure: Revised criteria, 1998." DHHS (NIOSH) 98–126. Dept. Health and Human Services, Public Health Service, Cincinnati, OH.

OSHA. (Jan. 16, 1981). "Summary and explanation of the standard." Occupational Noise Exposure: Hearing Conservation Amendment. 46 *Fed. Reg.*, 4131–4161.

OSHA. (March 8, 1983). "Summary and explanation of actions taken." Occupational Noise Exposure; Hearing Conservation Amendment; Final Rule. 48 *Fed. Reg.*, 9742–9772.

OSHA Interpretations, Noise Standard (see website below).

Suter, A.H. (2000). "Standards and regulations." Chapter 16 in E.H. Berger, L.H. Royster, J.D. Royster, D.P. Driscoll, and M. Layne, (Eds.), *The Noise Manual, Fifth Edition.* American Industrial Hygiene Assoc., Fairfax, VA.

Websites

www.usdoj.gov/crt/ada/adahom1.htm.
Americans with Disabilities Act (ADA)
home page at the Department of Justice

www.usdoj.gov/crt/ada/publicat.htm
Americans with Disabilities Act (ADA)
Publications website

www.aiha.org
American Industrial Hygiene Association (AIHA)

www.dtic.mil/whs/directives/corres/html/
605512.htm
Defense Technical Information Center
(for DoD Instruction 6055.12)

www.hearingconservation.org
National Hearing Conservation Association
(NHCA)

www.cdc.gov/niosh
National Institute for Occupational Safety
and Health (NIOSH)

www.lhsfna.org
Laborers' Health and Safety Fund of North
America

www.msha.gov
Mine Safety and Health Administration (MSHA)

www.msha.gov/regs/complian/ppls/2000/
PPL001V4.htm
MSHA Program Policy Letter

www.msha.gov/1999noise/noiseresources.htm
MSHA Resources

www.osha.gov
Occupational Safety and Health Administration
(OSHA)

www.osha.gov/SLTC/noisehearingconservation/
index.html
(scroll to Standard Interpretations and
Compliance Letters and click on SEARCH)
OSHA Interpretations

www.osha-slc.gov/dts/osta/otm/otm_iii/
otm_iii_5.html
OSHA Technical Manual, Section III Chapter
5—Noise Measurement

www.osha-slc.gov/Firm_osha_data/100007.html
OSHA Field Inspection Reference Manual, Section
7, Chapter III: Inspection (see section C.3.b)

Chapter VII

The Audiometric Testing Program

Purpose of Audiometric Testing

Despite what some may think, the audiometric testing program itself does not conserve hearing. It can be a very useful tool in the hearing conservation program, helping the OHC and other members of the team to know when to counsel and educate employees, when to refit and readjust hearing protectors, and when to recommend engineering or administrative controls. But the audiometric test itself is simply a tool that can signal the need for other measures. It is a vital and extensive part of the program, but it is always important to remember the purpose of the test.

The purpose of the audiometric testing program is to make sure that employees are not losing their hearing, to identify progressive noise-induced hearing losses before they become handicapping, and to identify temporary losses before they become permanent so that remedial steps can be taken. A side benefit of the audiometric testing program is that medical problems of the ear and hearing losses unrelated to occupational noise may also be identified and referred for treatment to a physician or audiologist, as appropriate. In addition, audiometric testing provides a continuing record of an individual's hearing status in case it is needed for medico-legal purposes, which benefits employees and employers alike.

The audiometric testing program accomplishes its purpose only if the testing is of sufficient quality. Audiometry in an industrial setting is not just "hearing screening," where certain individuals are identified and given a follow-up clinical test. Audiometry for purposes of hearing conservation uses audiogram comparisons as its method of operation. Therefore, reliable and valid audiometry is essential. If, for example, a baseline audiogram is not done properly, then future audiograms do not have an adequate reference point and an employee may lose hearing without the threshold shift showing up on the annual audiogram.

Planning the Audiometric Testing Program

As with the entire hearing conservation program, the audiometric testing program should be an integral part of a company's safety and health program and not a "stand-alone" program. The OHC must operate within a team that may include nurses, industrial hygienists, safety specialists, noise control engineers, and company management and representatives of the financial department, in addition to the audiologist or physician supervisor. In large companies the team may include all of these specialties, and in small ones very few. The OHC will most likely be the focal point of the audiometric program, even though he or she must be supervised by an audiologist or physician. More often than not it will be the OHC who will make sure that things get done and get done right.

The audiometric testing program should comply with the appropriate noise regulation in every respect. The OHC should be prepared to explain the program and reveal all of the audiometric records if a government inspector should request them. It is important, however, to remember that most regulations reflect the minimum "standard of care," and OHCs should be encouraged to improve on them and tailor their programs to their own company's needs and policies, after consulting with their supervising physician or audiologist.

Before undertaking a new audiometric testing program, it is wise to develop and obtain approval of a plan that will include such practical matters as types and costs of equipment needed, methods of recordkeeping, and scheduling practices. This is so that management will know about anticipated expenditures and how much time away from work will be needed to test all of the workers included in the program.

Approaches to the Program

There are two basic approaches to audiometric testing programs: the in-house program and the contracted test service. Most OHCs will probably be involved in in-house programs where the company purchases an audiometer, a sound-booth, and a sound level meter or device to monitor the sound levels in the audiometric booth. Unless there is a physician or audiologist connected to the company, it will be necessary to obtain the services of one of these professionals to interpret audiograms and to provide supervision. It would also be helpful to have the advice of an audiologist, an industrial hygienist, or a noise control engineer to assist in the placement of the booth and to set up the equipment.

An advantage of the in-house program is that the OHC can schedule audiometric tests at the best times—pre-employment or before noise exposure for the baseline, during the shift for the annual audiogram, and at termination of employment. Also, retests may be performed in-house whenever necessary without having to wait until the employee can be scheduled with the contracted test service. Any disadvantages would include the fact that the OHCs bear a great deal of responsibility. They need a close and effective working relationship with their supervising physician or audiologist so that advice and supervision are readily available.

Contracted services may include local physicians or audiology clinics, but they are most often mobile test services. When a company contracts with a mobile service for its audiometric testing program, a van arrives at the plant according to a prearranged schedule; workers are then directed to the van for testing. The technicians employed by mobile test services are usually experienced testers, regularly supervised by an audiologist or physician. These contractors may also provide audiogram review and comparison, employee counseling, and letters to employees when necessary. Many of them have the advantage of testing groups of up to eight employees at a time, enabling the testing process to occur more rapidly. The main disadvantage of this kind of service is that scheduling is less flexible. It is usually necessary to schedule all of the tests at once, and baselines on new employees or retests that must be performed at other times throughout the year, are sent to a local audiologist or otolaryngologist, or performed in-house. An additional disadvantage is that group testing may not afford as much time for training and feedback with individual workers.

Actually, both the OSHA and MSHA regulations give companies that use mobile test services the option of waiting up to a year to complete the baseline audiogram. It is a bad idea, however, to wait that long before the baseline or for appropriate retesting and follow-up. In cases where workers are unavailable for the annual test because of vacation, sick leave, or other reasons, they should be sent to a local audiologist or physician as appropriate, or the company should be prepared to perform the test in-house. Because of this situation, a company should not be completely dependent upon mobile test services.

Equipment Needed

The basic instrumentation in an audiometric testing program consists of an audiometer, a sound-attenuating booth or room, a sound level meter with the ability to measure in octave bands, calibration equipment, and preferably a device to monitor the sound levels in the booth.

Audiometers

Occupational hearing conservation programs should use audiometers and earphones manufactured to meet the requirements of the current ANSI standard. The most recent standard as of this printing is ANSI S3.6-1996, American National Standard Specification for Audiometers. The standard requires Type IV audiometers to have a range of at least -10 dB to 70 dB hearing level (HL) for the frequencies 500, 1000, 2000, 3000, 4000, and 6000 Hz. A footnote to the table listing these requirements states: "The maximum hearing level for Type IV audiometers used for hearing conservation purposes shall be extended to 90 dB HL." (See Table 3 in ANSI, 1996.) There are some audiometers used in occupational hearing conservation that do not test hearing threshold levels below (better than) 0 dB. These audiometers would still comply with the OSHA requirements and with the previous ANSI standard, S3.6-1989, for

Type V audiometers,[25] which were approved for use in industry. Testing below 0 dB, while desirable, may not always be possible in industrial settings because background noise levels can sometimes preclude it.

Audiometer earphones are calibrated to the specific audiometers they accompany and must not be interchanged with another device. The earphones are the most easily damaged part of the system and OHCs must make sure they are not dropped or slapped together.

There are two basic types of audiometers used in industry today: the **manual audiometer** and the **microprocessor**. The **computer-controlled audiometer**, which is widely used today, is a variation of the microprocessor in which the audiometer is used in conjunction with a personal computer.

The Manual Audiometer:

The manual audiometer can be considered the conventional model and has been commercially available since the 1940s. Current models are small, durable, and relatively easy to operate. Figure 7-1 shows an example of a manual audiometer. With this type of audiometer the operator controls the frequency, sound level, and mode of presentation of pure tones. The subject signals that he or she has heard the tone by pressing a switch or raising a hand or finger. The advantages of manual audiometers are that they are the least expensive of all of the types, and that the operator maintains control over the presentation of tones.

The main disadvantage of the manual audiometer is that it is most prone to human error. The number of switches may be confusing and the operator can, for example, forget and test the same ear twice. It is easy for operators to stray from the standard method of tone presentation and to develop a rhythm that is readily anticipated by the person being tested. Also, because the responses must be recorded manually, recordkeeping errors are more likely with manual audiometers than with microprocessors. Without frequent supervision, an OHC may start taking inappropriate short cuts and develop a number of poor habits. These habits are most likely to occur with a manual audiometer.

---

[25] The 1996 revision of ANSI S3.6 has changed the requirements for the various type designations, and the Type V audiometer is now a different instrument, no longer suitable for occupational hearing conservation.

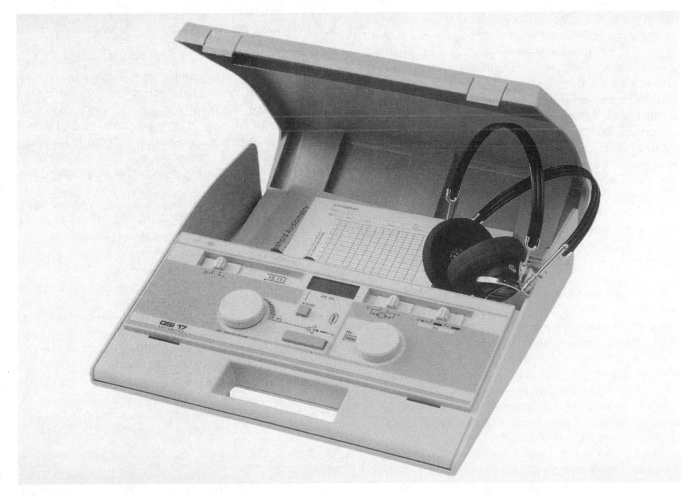

Fig. 7-1. Manual audiometer. (Courtesy of Grason-Stadler, Inc.)

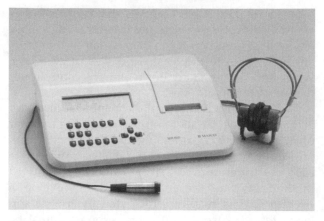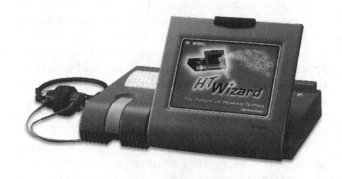

Fig. 7-2. Two examples of microprocessor audiometers. (Left, courtesy of Maico Diagnostics; right, courtesy of Tremetrics)

The Microprocessor Audiometer:

Microprocessor audiometers, sometimes called "automatic audiometers," have become a very popular choice for hearing conservation programs. Figure 7–2 displays two typical microprocessor audiometers. In this type of instrument, a microchip has been programmed to present the test tones, record the subject's responses, and determine the threshold. A printer, either incorporated into the audiometer or as a separate unit, prints the subject's responses and the threshold determination.

The microprocessor uses essentially the same procedure to determine hearing threshold level as the operator of a manual audiometer should use. There may be times when the microprocessor is unable to test an individual whose responses are inconsistent, or when the individual is for some reason difficult to test. In these cases the operator should use a manual override or have a manual audiometer in reserve. Consequently, it is imperative that OHCs develop good skills with a manual audiometer.

Most contemporary models have the capacity of storing a limited number of audiograms or downloading the audiometric data into a personal computer, which can provide for greater data storage and analysis. This system can automatically compare the current test to the baseline, calculate any shifts in hearing that have occurred, especially a standard threshold shift (STS), and even prepare letters to employees. Most modern microprocessor audiometers are programmed for operation independent of a supporting personal computer, while others may include the computer as part of the overall system. Manufacturers typically provide instructions on integrating the audiometer with one's own personal computer system.

Figure 7–3 shows an example of a computer-controlled audiometric system. Audiometer manufacturers will often market software for industrial audiometric programs, or refer the purchaser to a company that sells software for a variety of occupational health programs, including hearing conservation. Some software programs can perform a variety of functions in addition to those mentioned above. These may include identifying both the OSHA/MSHA and NIOSH STS, identifying employees with potentially compensable hearing impairments, and printing out audiograms in graphical form, to name a few. But despite the ability of computers to make calculations and perform all kinds of paperwork, OHCs still need to know what they are doing and supervising professionals are still needed to make many important decisions.

The microprocessor has many advantages. First, it presents the audiometric test in a programmed, consistent sequence, usually more rapidly than an operator can test with a manual audiometer. It avoids most sources of operator error and makes it more difficult to exaggerate a hearing loss. Some models present the user with a hard-copy record, showing every tone presentation and response. Depending on the capabilities of the particular instrument, it can test as many as 16 subjects[26] at a time, and it can do all kinds of useful calculations and recordkeeping. Some models have the capability of giving voice instructions, not only in English but in several other languages.

Among its disadvantages is the lack of a standardized protocol for presenting the pure tones. The resulting variability among different instruments and models can make comparisons difficult. Small differences in hearing threshold levels between different audiometers could affect group STS rates or other measures of program effectiveness. Another disadvantage is the instrument's sensitivity to power surges that can damage equipment and lose records, although surge protectors and built-in

---

[26] Six to eight subjects at a time is usually the maximum number possible without interference caused by the noise of people moving around.

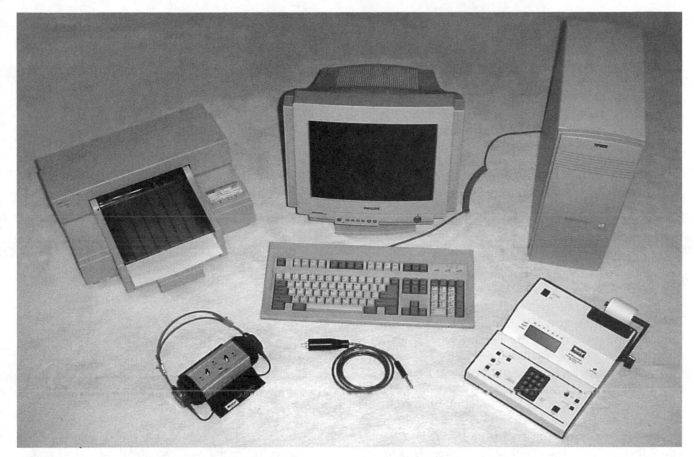

Fig. 7-3. Computer-controlled audiometric system. (Courtesy of Monitor Instruments, Inc.)

power line filters are common in current models. Also, the OHC should be careful not to be lulled into thinking that because a computer "tested" the employee, the test should automatically be considered valid.

Maintaining Consistency in Audiometric Data

Audiometers come in different types and models, and the resulting variety may cause apparent discrepancies in hearing threshold levels in the same individual, in addition to unwanted effects on group data. For this reason it is important that the OHC makes careful selections and continues to use the same type, make, and model of audiometer for as long as is possible. Changing audiometer types or mismatching earphones and audiometers may produce a disruptive effect on the year-to-year sequence of audiograms. Changing to another model, or even adjusting the calibration of an existing audiometer unnecessarily may produce artificial threshold shifts, so it is best to leave the audiometer alone whenever possible. There are times, however, when changes must be made. For example, many companies used to use **"self-recording audiometers,"**[27] which are no longer

being manufactured. After a while it was necessary to discontinue the use of these devices because parts and service were no longer available. When changes such as these do occur it is important to keep careful records of the date of the transition.

Audiometric Test Rooms

Another important area of concern for the OHC is the room in which the audiometric tests are conducted. If the room is too noisy, the employee will be distracted and have difficulty taking the test. Also, the employee's thresholds at 500 Hz and sometimes at 1000 Hz are likely to appear worse than they actually are due to "masking" or interference from the background noise. This can cause problems in comparing the current audiogram with other audiograms at these frequencies.

---

[27] Self-recording audiometers were widely used in occupational hearing conservation programs during the 1970s and 1980s, although they are no longer being manufactured today. They have probably been phased out of virtually all hearing conservation programs, but audiograms produced by these instruments are likely to appear in the files of workers with long-standing tenure in certain jobs. Explanation of these audiograms, along with criteria for reading them and judging their validity will be presented in Chapter VIII.

The OHC should be aware that audiometric rooms are sound-attenuating, but not sound-proof. Even the larger, double-walled type of room will still allow some environmental sounds to come into the room. There are three types of audiometric rooms suitable for testing in the occupational setting: the standard audiometric test enclosure, the "mini-booth" and the sound-treated space in a mobile van. Seen in Figure 7–4 are examples of two mini-booths that have two-inch wall construction and are portable even when assembled. Figure 7–5 shows the larger, "standard" variety, which has four-inch walls and must be disassembled when moved.

The mini-booth is less expensive and has greater portability, but it does not provide as much sound attenuation (reduction) as the standard booth. It may also be very cramped for someone of generous proportions and can induce a feeling of claustrophobia. A recent innovation is the mini-booth with a full-length window to give the person who is being tested a feeling of more space (see Figure 7–4, right). A sensible antidote to claustrophobia practiced by some OHCs is to remind their test subjects that there is no lock on the door and demonstrate before the test begins how easily the door opens.

The sound-treated test enclosure in a mobile van is another type of audiometric test space. This test room is built into the mobile unit and often comes with multiple test spaces separated by curtains or partitions.

Audiometric rooms must be situated (or mobile vans parked) in a location quiet enough to meet OSHA requirements within the room.[28] But the OHC should understand that the OSHA regulation is hardly adequate in this instance and the background sound levels it sanctions will not permit testing to 0 dB hearing threshold level. Therefore, it is advisable to meet the sound pressure levels specified by the American National Standard for Maximum Permissible Ambient Noise Levels for Audiometric Test Rooms (ANSI S3.1-1999). Adhering to the levels of the 1999 ANSI standard for audiometer rooms will ensure that no artificial shifts in hearing level greater than 2 dB will occur due to background noise. Maximum allowable sound pressure levels listed in the OSHA regulation and ANSI standard are given in Table 7.1.

Although it may sometimes be difficult to achieve these criteria at the lower frequencies (500 Hz and below), one should try to come as close as possible. Some people may make excuses for poor testing conditions, saying that this is only "industrial

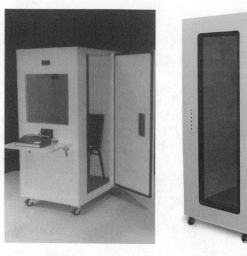

Fig. 7-4. Two examples of audiometric mini-booths. (Left, courtesy of Eckel Industries, Inc.; right, courtesy of Tremetrics.)

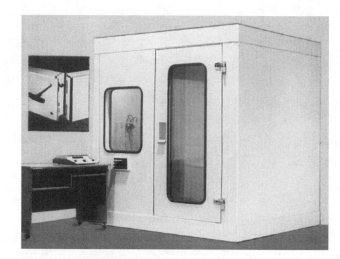

Fig. 7-5. A stationary audiometric booth with 4-inch walls. (Courtesy of Eckel Industries Inc.)

audiometry" and the expectations for quality are therefore reduced. This kind of thinking is counter-productive to a truly effective hearing conservation program, whose purpose is to prevent hearing loss. It is crucial that all changes in hearing threshold level are documented in a program of prevention, particularly when the hearing of young workers with normal hearing is to be conserved.

Measuring the Sound Levels in Audiometer Rooms

It would be wise for the OHC to enlist the help of a noise control engineer or an industrial hygienist in locating the best site for the audiometric test room. To determine how much attenuation is needed, sound pressure levels should be measured in the space where the booth is to be sited before ordering it. It is important to measure the sound levels during a time when audiometric testing is expected to take

---

[28] As mentioned in Chapter VI, MSHA merely requires all audiometric testing to be "conducted in accordance with scientifically validated procedures," and therefore does not specify maximum allowable sound levels in audiometer rooms.

Table 7.1. Maximum allowable sound pressure levels (referenced to 20 μPa) inside audiometer rooms for testing at the frequencies 500-8000 Hz.[29]

Octave-band center frequency	125 Hz	250 Hz	500 Hz	1000 Hz	2000 Hz	4000 Hz	8000 Hz
OSHA Table D-1			40 dB	40 dB	47 dB	57 dB	62 dB
ANSI S3.1	49 dB	35 dB	21 dB	26 dB	34 dB	37 dB	37 dB

place and for the worst case (noisiest) situation. Manufacturers' specified attenuation values can then be subtracted from the environmental sound levels to estimate the sound levels within the room. It is always wise to include a safety factor of 5 to 10 dB in case the background levels turn out to be noisier than expected.

These measurements should be made with a Type I sound level meter and octave-band filter set[30] and they should include the frequencies 125, 250, 500, 1000, 2000, 4000, and 8000 Hz. Particular attention should be given to the sound levels at the lower frequencies (500 Hz and below) since noise at these frequencies is usually the most difficult to control with the use of the sound-attenuating booth.

Once the booth is put into place, the sound levels inside should be checked periodically to make sure that it still meets the desired specifications. NIOSH recommends that the background noise levels in a fixed site be checked at least once a year, and that mobile test areas be checked daily or at each site, whichever is more frequent. During this check all possible sources of noise should be in operation, including the ventilation system and any machines inside or outside of the test room. For future reference, records of the measurements should be maintained so that they can be matched to each person's audiogram.

To make sure that the maximum background levels are acceptable, devices are available that continuously monitor the sound levels in audiometer rooms and indicate whenever a certain level has been exceeded. If these limits are exceeded, the OHC should stop testing until sound levels are again within acceptable levels. In some cases, the monitor is connected to the microprocessor audiometer, which is programmed automatically to make the test procedure pause until background noise levels are adequate for the test to resume. An example of such a device is shown in Figure 7–6. It is especially useful in situations where environmental conditions are marginal for the proper conduct of audiometric testing. Some manufacturers actually combine background noise monitoring instruments with an audiometric calibration device (to be discussed later in this chapter) for their line of audiometers. OHCs

should be aware that the availability of room-noise monitors that can measure sound levels as low as required in the current ANSI standard for background noise (ANSI 3.1-1999) is quite limited.

Noise-Reducing Earphone Enclosures

Noise-reducing earphone enclosures, sometimes referred to as "Audiocups" or "Oto-cups," are occasionally used to supplement the attenuation provided by the audiometric booth. However, the OHC would be well-advised not to rely on them,

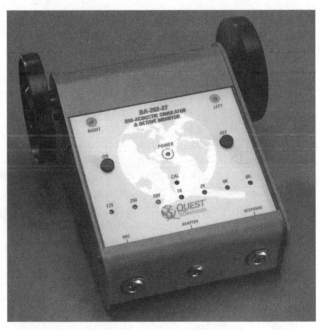

Fig. 7-6. Background noise level monitor for use in an audiometric test space. This device also doubles as a "bioacoustic" simulator. (Courtesy of Quest Technologies)

---

[29] Sound pressure levels in the ANSI S3.1 standard assume that ears will be covered by earphones such as the Telephonic TDH, mounted in MX-41/AR or -51 cushions and connected to a headband with the appropriate force. The reason 125 and 250 Hz are included in the ANSI standard is because high levels of noise at these frequencies can mask thresholds at 500 or even at 1000 Hz.

[30] There will be more information on these instruments in Chapter IX.

and they should never be used in lieu of adequate sound-attenuating audiometric test rooms. These devices consist of standard audiometric earphones built into a solid cup and surrounded by a foam-filled cushion that fits tightly against the head. They are of limited use to the OHC because the attenuation they provide is mainly in the frequencies above 1000 Hz, whereas most room noise problems occur at the frequencies below 1000 Hz. Furthermore, this style of earphones easily causes the external portion of the earcanal to collapse unless they are carefully positioned on the ear. There are no recommended maximum background noise levels for the use of those devices in ANSI S3.1-1999. Although an official interpretation on this issue does not appear on OSHA's website, an OSHA letter dated 6-18-93 states that the use of "circumaural audiometric earphones" violates the noise regulation (OSHA, 1993).

Scheduling

The OHC will probably be the one to develop and coordinate the audiometric testing schedule, and that includes informing management and supervisors about employees' expected time away from work. A schedule that is carefully planned is most likely to be successful.

The Baseline Audiogram

As stated in the previous chapter, it is vitally important that the baseline audiogram be as "pure" as possible, before any noise-induced hearing loss has occurred and without contamination by temporary threshold shift (TTS). Although OSHA and MSHA allow employers to wait up to six months before establishing a baseline audiogram, or even a year if the company uses mobile test services, this is not good practice. Obtaining a baseline before any exposure to noise is in the employee's best interest so that any threshold shifts can be detected as quickly as possible. It is also in the company's best interest to document the employee's hearing status as soon as possible in case hearing loss claims should arise.

The best time to perform a baseline audiogram is before the employee begins to work in a noisy area. If this is not possible, the employee should be tested after at least 14 hours away from workplace noise, preferably at the beginning of the work week. The OSHA/MSHA noise regulations allow employers to use hearing protectors in lieu of the 14-hour quiet period, but because of the many uncertainties regarding hearing protector attenuation, OHCs should avoid this practice whenever possible.

OSHA and MSHA also give employers the responsibility of warning employees to avoid high levels of nonoccupational noise in the 14 hours prior to the baseline audiogram. Of course OHCs cannot control what employees do during their time off, but OHCs have the responsibility to warn against activities like shooting, using power tools, auto racing, and listening to loud music in the hours before the baseline audiogram.

The Annual or Monitoring Audiogram

Although audiometric tests must be given at least once a year to employees exposed above the 85-dBA action level, employers may choose to test some employees more often. For example, workers exposed to time-weighted average levels of 100 dB and above should probably be tested every six months. Perhaps for this reason NIOSH calls the annual (or periodic) audiogram the "monitoring" audiogram. Thresholds obtained on this audiogram should be compared to the baseline audiogram immediately, which is easiest to do with a microprocessor or computer-controlled audiometer. This way the OHC can discuss the results with the employee on the spot, which usually is the best opportunity for counseling. Of course the protocol for discussing the status of the employee's hearing will have been established previously with the OHC's supervising professional.

Unlike the baseline audiogram, the annual (or monitoring) audiogram may be obtained at any time during the work shift. The best time to perform this test is toward the end of the shift so that any TTS can be identified. This procedure may be more time-consuming than testing at the beginning of the work shift if the OHC wishes to perform retests in cases where shifts in hearing have appeared. *Whether or not a retest is performed, testing well into the work shift and identifying TTS is an important precaution that may enable the OHC to prevent the development of permanent hearing loss.* This practice is recommended by knowledgeable hearing conservation professionals, as well as by NIOSH and OSHA (see NIOSH, 1998, p. 49; OSHA, 1981, p. 4144). To conduct the annual audiogram before any noise exposure, and therefore before any TTS appears, is to overlook some vitally important information.

The Retest

If the OHC is unable to obtain a valid audiogram, the employee must be retested by the OHC or referred to an audiology clinic. If the employee demonstrates an STS, then a follow-up retest is advisable. Neither OSHA nor MSHA require a retest when an STS occurs, but if an employee is to be retested, the test must be done within 30 days. As mentioned in Chapter VI, MSHA requires a retest in certain cases when the reviewing professional determines that the initial test was invalid, and this retest must be conducted within 30 days. It is good practice to perform the follow-up retest after at least 14 hours away from noise, although again this requirement is not mandatory. It is always better to administer the retest as soon as possible so that the OHC can counsel the employee and perform other actions as necessary, such as making changes in the use of hearing protectors.

NIOSH recommends that if an STS occurs, the OHC should remove the earphones, reinstruct, reposition the earphones, and retest the worker immediately. By doing an immediate retest a follow-up retest can often be avoided. If on the immediate retest the hearing thresholds return to their original levels, the OHC can be reasonably sure that the employee only needed reinstruction and the shift was not due to TTS. If the STS is still present, the employee should be counseled and scheduled for a retest after 14 hours away from noise.

If on the later retest the STS persists, certain steps need to be taken (discussed in Chapter VIII). If the STS is no longer there, the shift is likely to have been due to TTS. Either way, the retest is an opportune time to counsel the employee and, hopefully, to prevent future TTS that could eventually become a permanent hearing loss.

The Exit Audiogram

OSHA does not require an exit audiogram, but if an employee is leaving the company it is good practice for the OHC to perform an audiometric test after the employee's last exposure to noise. This test may be important in worker compensation cases to see approximately how much hearing loss the company is accountable for. The test results may be especially useful in states where liability may be apportioned to more than one employer.

Taking an Aural History

An aural history should be taken before the baseline audiometric test and updated during annual testing. If there is a significant change in hearing threshold level, the OHC should ask the employee about current auditory complaints, health, and medications and about any changes in workplace noise and noisy non-occupational activities.

The purpose of the aural history is to obtain information that would aid the OHC in administering the audiometric test and to aid the professional reviewer in deciding what kind of follow-up is necessary. For example, the presence of tinnitus (ringing in the ear) may explain why an employee is having difficulty responding reliably to high-frequency pure tones. Or if the employee reports frequent ear infections, the reviewer may have a better idea of how to interpret the audiogram.

Either the OHC may read the questions to the employee and record the responses, or the employee may read the questions and check the conditions that apply. The first method works better if an employee has difficulty reading; and it is convenient if the form is computerized so that the OHC merely enters the responses. The advantage of the second method is that employees can sign their own aural histories in case any controversy arises at a later date.

Table 7.2 lists some of the items that could be included in the aural history. Some supervising professionals may wish to collect more detailed information and others may prefer a more abbreviated history.

Table 7.2. Examples of items that may be included in an aural history.

Hearing loss in the family before age 50	Medical problems	Recreational activities	Additional noise exposure
Self Mother Father Brother Sister Other family	Measles Mumps Diabetes High fever Ear surgery Ear infection Ear ringing Head injury Mycin drugs Hearing aid Chemotherapeutic drugs	Hunting Target practice Auto racing Loud concerts or other music Power tools Motorcycling Hearing protection with any of the above?	Military Noisy past job Noisy second job Noisy farm equipment

Visual Inspection of the Ear

While the OSHA/MSHA noise regulations do not require visual inspection of the ears, it is an essential part of any audiometric testing program. Abnormalities in the earcanal may affect the test results, but more importantly can interfere with the use of hearing protectors. This examination usually involves the use of an **otoscope**, but much information can be gained by simply observing the external ear with the unaided eye and a light source.

The OHC should look at the employee's ears and into the external auditory meatus (the opening to the earcanal), to rule out any obvious dermatitis, drainage, or other medical condition. Pulling the pinna outward and upward will help expose the external auditory meatus. It is important for the pinna pull to be firm and in the correct direction. If there are signs of infection, such as swelling, pain, or discharge, the employee should be referred to a physician. In this case, audiometric testing should be approached cautiously, and the earphone cushions should be thoroughly disinfected afterward. If there is pain when the OHC places the earphones on the employee, the test should not be performed until the condition has been successfully treated.

Additional information may be obtained with an otoscope. Seen in Figure 7–7, the otoscope is a small, hand-held instrument that illuminates the earcanal and tympanic membrane. Before OHCs perform otoscopic inspections they should be well-trained in how to use the otoscope and what to look for. If OHCs are reasonably careful, they do not need to be afraid of causing pain or damage to the ear tissues. Reasonable care means that they should not insert the **speculum** (the otoscope's detachable tip) into an earcanal that is obviously swollen or diseased. When using an otoscope, the ear should be handled gently, and OHCs might consider using specula[31] with soft-flanged tips. For purposes of hygiene, it is best to use a disposable speculum, or else reusable specula must be thoroughly disinfected after each use. Unfortunately, disposable specula do not come in the soft-tipped variety.

The OHC should first visually inspect the ear unaided, then use an otoscope to look more deeply into the earcanal for obvious signs of infection, such as redness or drainage, excessive earwax, foreign bodies (insects, for example), and other obvious abnormalities. Most of these conditions will not actually affect the audiometric test. But, as mentioned above, in cases of painful or discharging ears the otoscopic exam should be discontinued and the employee should receive medical treatment before audiometric testing is conducted.

Most people have some amount of earwax as a normal condition, and even excessive wax does not usually affect the audiogram. It is only when wax completely blocks the earcanal that it can cause a hearing loss. Before fitting insert-type hearing protectors, however, excessive earwax should be removed because an earplug may compress the wax and push it further into the earcanal. This can cause discomfort and irritate the canal walls or pack the wax further into the canal.

Wax removal should only be done by someone who has been technically trained to perform this procedure, such as a physician, audiologist, or nurse. In some cases if a specialist is not available, the OHC may recommend drops that can be obtained over the counter to soften the earwax. However, any history of a perforated eardrum, earaches, or chronic ear infections should be referred to a physician without attempting "self-treatment." Also, the OHC should advise workers not to try to remove earwax with Q-tips® cotton swabs, since this practice can push the wax further into the canal and increase the possibility of discomfort or injury.

The otoscopic procedures should be explained to the employee. Then, when the OHC determines through visual inspection that the external ear and earcanal will permit the exam, the OHC should select the largest speculum that will fit comfortably in the employee's earcanal. The otoscope should be held like a pen between the thumb and the forefinger, as in Figure 7–8, so that the hand can be braced against the cheek for a firm position.

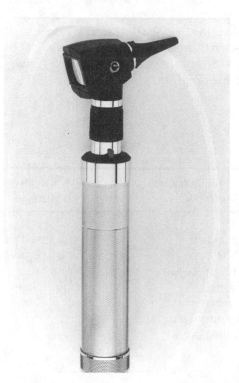

Fig. 7-7. Example of an otoscope. (Courtesy of Welch Allyn Inc.)

---

[31] Specula is the plural of speculum.

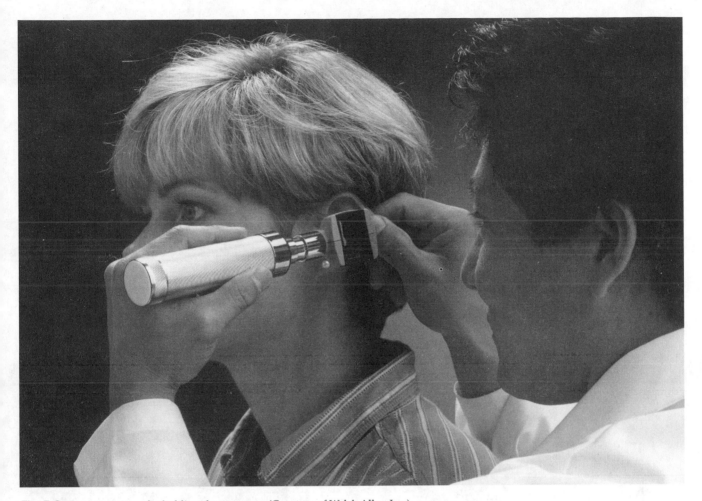

Fig. 7-8. Correct position for holding the otoscope. (Courtesy of Welch Allyn Inc.)

For viewing the right ear, the OHC should brace the right hand firmly against the employee's cheek. When viewing the left ear, the OHC must switch the hand holding the otoscope to the left hand so that once again the fingers are braced against the employee's cheek. The otoscope's speculum is then inserted into the earcanal to view the canal walls and the eardrum. The OHC will need to move the otoscope slightly, as well as his or her eye, to visualize the entire area.

After this procedure, the speculum should be set aside for sterilization, or the disposable speculum discarded, and the results should be recorded. At this point the OHC may want to continue to use the otoscope's light source to check for collapsing earcanals. (The speculum will not be inserted in the earcanal.) The helix (outer edge) of the external ear should be pressed against the head, just as the audiometer earphone would do. If the canal walls close, the employee will probably show an artificial high-frequency hearing loss, as explained in Chapter IV.

If a high-frequency hearing loss occurs in conjunction with collapsing earcanals, the employee may be referred to an audiologist or otolaryngologist for further evaluation. In cases where referral is not convenient, the OHC may attempt to test the employee in either of two ways. A specially designed small plastic nipple may be inserted into the opening of the earcanal, maintaining the earcanal in an open position and allowing the sound to be conducted through. Or the OHC may detach an earphone from the headband and instruct the employee to hold it gently against the ear during the audiometric test. Referral to an audiologist or otolaryngologist is usually preferable.

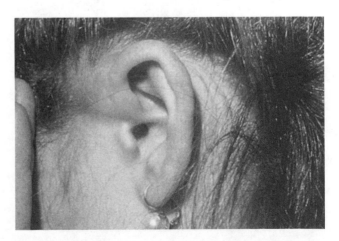

Fig. 7-9a. Normal auricle and earcanal opening. (From Hawke, Keen, and Alberti, 1984)

Figures 7–9 through 7–13 give examples of conditions that can be seen in an examination of the earcanal and eardrum. Figure 7–9a shows a normal auricle and earcanal opening. Figure 7–9b shows an earcanal that has collapsed (vertical slit on right) when pressure has been applied to the pinna. Figure 7–10 is an otoscopic view of a normal eardrum; Figure 7–11 an external otitis (infection of the earcanal); Figure 7–12, a perforated eardrum; Figure 7–13, a thin film of wax almost occluding the entrance of the earcanal.

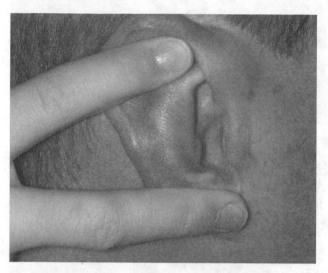

Fig. 7-9b. Collapsed earcanal (vertical slit on right) after applying pressure to the pinna. (Reprinted with permission)

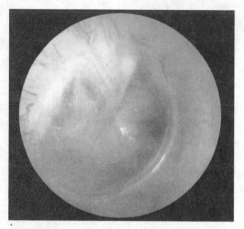

Fig. 7-10. Normal eardrum. (From Hawke, Keen, and Alberti, 1984)

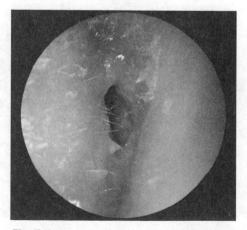

Fig. 7-11. External otitis (infection of the earcanal). (From Hawke, Keen, and Alberti, 1984)

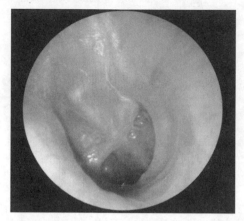

Fig. 7-12. Perforated eardrum: example of a large crescent-shaped perforation in the lower central portion of the eardrum. (From Hawke, Keen, and Alberti, 1984)

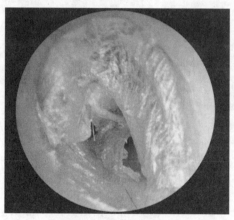

Fig. 7-13. Thin film of wax almost occluding the entrance of the earcanal. (From Hawke, Keen, and Alberti, 1984)

Audiometric Testing Procedures

Seating

During the test, employees should be seated so that they cannot see the audiometer's dials and switches. They should not be able to see the OHC manipulating the switches or the tone-on indicator of the microprocessor audiometer. They should also be positioned so that they do not look directly at the OHC's face or arms. This precaution is taken because individuals can sometimes visually detect the administration of a tone, even subconsciously, just by watching the tester's body motions. But it is important for the OHC to see the employee's face to detect signs of distress or unusual facial expressions. The best way to seat the employee is at a 90-degree angle to the OHC.

Instructions

The OHC's instructions to the employee should be clear, simple, comprehensive, and standard, and they should be given before putting on the earphones. Any employees with hearing aids should keep the aids on during the instructions. It is not a bad idea for the newly trained OHC to write down the instructions and to read them for the first several audiometric tests until he or she is accustomed to giving them in a standard way. The instructions for taking an audiometric test on either a manual or computerized audiometer should be something like this:

✍ *You will hear a series of tones at different pitches through these earphones. Each ear will be tested separately. As soon as you hear a tone, even if it is very faint, press this button [or raise your hand]. Do you have any questions?*

As indicated, the employee's response may also take the form of raising and lowering a finger or a hand, although a hand-switch is a more objective form of response. Smoking and gum chewing can interfere with the employee's ability to listen and should not be permitted during the test.

Placing the Earphones

The OHC should ask the employee to remove eyeglasses, earrings, or anything that might interfere with the proper seating of the earphones. Hair should be pushed away from the external auditory meatus. *Hearing aids should, of course, be removed after the instructions have been given, and beepers and cell phones should be turned off.*

The OHC should then place the earphones directly over the external auditory meatus. If the earphones are not placed correctly, the response to high-frequency tones may be affected. The OHC should adjust the headband to the appropriate height and the employee should be instructed not to reposition the earphones or headband, despite the temptation to do so.

Administering the Pure-Tone Test

Manual Audiometers:

Accepted procedures are spelled out in the American National Standard Method for Manual Pure-Tone Threshold Audiometry, ANSI S3.21-1978 (R1997). The standard is reprinted as Appendix N in the back of this manual. OHCs should reread it periodically to make sure that their testing procedures are in accordance with the standard.

Although it is not essential, it is a good idea to begin the test in the better ear. Rather than look at the previous audiogram, which may bias the results, it is best to ask the employee which is his or her better ear.

The OHC should start by familiarizing the employee with a test tone at 1000 Hz, presented at an easily audible level, such as 30 or 40 dB. If there is no response, the tone should be presented again at 50 dB, and if there still is no response, the hearing level dial should be raised in 10 dB steps until the employee responds.

Once an initial response has been established, the OHC may begin the determination of threshold. The level of the first presentation should be 10 dB below the level of the response during the familiarization procedure. The level of each succeeding presentation depends on whether or not the employee responded to the one before. After a response, the hearing level dial is decreased by 10 dB, and if the employee fails to respond, the level is increased in 5 dB steps until a response occurs. Then move down 10 dB and up 5 dB, "bracketing" the employee's threshold. Give only one presentation of each tone at each level when looking for a response. Hearing threshold level is defined as the lowest hearing level where the subject hears at least 50 percent of the tones, with a minimum of two out of three responses required at a single level.

The duration of each tone presentation should be 1 to 2 seconds, and the interval between tones should never be shorter than the duration of the tone itself. The OHC must be careful to vary the silent interval between tones so that the employee does not pick up a rhythmic pattern and give "false" responses to tones that are not actually perceived. Needless to say, the OHC should never give the employee overt cues during or after presenting the tones.

The sequence of test frequencies is specified in ANSI S3.21. It begins with 1000 Hz, and then proceeds through the high frequencies, including a 1000-Hz retest to confirm test reliability before finishing with 500 Hz. The standard also specifies that if the 1000-Hz retest shows a difference of more than 5 dB, the lower threshold may be accepted and at least one other test frequency should be retested. However, most professionals now recommend that if the difference at 1000 Hz is greater than 5 dB, the OHC should remove the earphones and reinstruct the employee, and the entire audiogram should be repeated.

Many hearing conservation professionals advocate (and many manufacturers of computerized audiometers use) a slightly different testing order: 1000, 500, 1000 Hz, followed by the higher frequencies. This order enables the tester to quickly detect potential test reliability issues such as excessive ambient noise or employee misunderstanding of test instructions. The extent to which the OHC departs from the ANSI standard's recommended procedure and arbitrary order of test frequencies, should be the decision of the OHC's professional supervisor.

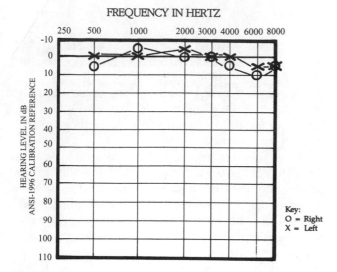

Fig. 7-14. Example of an audiogram showing normal hearing in both ears.

Each time a threshold is determined, the OHC should record it on an audiogram form. If symbols are used, an "X" represents the left ear's threshold and an "O" represents the right ear.[32] Figure 7–14 shows an audiogram of a subject with normal hearing in both ears.

Table 7.3 displays the same audiogram, using numbers for hearing threshold levels instead of symbols. The retest results for 1000 Hz have been recorded to the right of the original threshold levels. It is always a good idea to record the retested thresholds, even if they agree very well with the original results.

Microprocessor Audiometers:

The initial procedures for operating a microprocessor or computer-controlled audiometer will be much the same as for the manual audiometer. Seating the employee, giving the instructions, and placing the earphones will be the same. The actual test (and sometimes the instructions too, as described earlier) will then be administered by the microprocessor according to procedures similar to those outlined above. But the OHC must stand by in case the employee needs further instruction or the audiometer stops testing because its reliability or validity criteria have been exceeded. The OHC will then need to use the audiometer's manual override feature to test certain frequencies, or possibly have to repeat the entire test in the manual mode.

Different microprocessors use different criteria for accepting or rejecting a response. Also, the method of tone presentation may not be uniform among these instruments, so comparisons between tests performed on different instruments may not be consistent. These are good reasons for becoming thoroughly familiar with the instruction manual and for staying with one instrument once it has been purchased.

As mentioned in Chapter VI, the OSHA noise regulation states: "A technician who operates microprocessor audiometers does not need to be certified."[33] This is a misleading statement; first because it ignores the multitude of other duties that the OHC will have, but also because handling a microprocessor is not something to do in one's sleep. Besides, the microprocessor will stop testing an employee from time to time, and the OHC must know how to perform the test manually. OHCs need to be sure to back up their data from microprocessors every day, to enter or transcribe the data accurately, and to maintain the security of all passwords.

Audiometer Calibration

The validity of audiometric testing depends on a number of factors, but one of the basic essentials is that the frequency and level of the tones produced by the audiometer are in fact what they are supposed to be. In other words, the audiometer needs to be in calibration. There are three types of calibration that the OHC needs to know about: the **daily calibration check**, the **acoustic calibration**, and the **exhaustive calibration**. Both the first and second types are really **calibration checks**, and only

---

[32] Because most audiometric data are computerized, the use of numbers is preferable for recordkeeping purposes. The traditional audiogram, however, with the "X" and "O" symbols may be quite helpful in discussing the hearing loss with the employee and demonstrating changes in hearing threshold levels. Some software programs offer the graphic form as an additional option.

[33] The reader should be reminded that the MSHA regulation does not carry this statement, and the states of Oregon and Washington require CAOHC certification.

Table 7.3. Hearing threshold levels in dB (audiogram in tabular form).

Frequency, Hz	500	1000	2000	3000	4000	6000	8000
Left ear	0	0/0	-5	0	0	5	5
Right ear	5	0/-5	0	0	5	10	5

in the third type, the exhaustive calibration, are adjustments actually made to the audiometer. The phrase "in calibration" means that you should be able to compare the sound level output of the audiometer on the day it is being used to the numbers from the exhaustive calibration and they should be the same. If not, there are steps that must be taken.

For the sake of consistency in the audiometric testing program, it is preferable to adjust the audiometer's output (in the exhaustive calibration) as little as possible. Whenever the actual output of the audiometer is changed there is the possibility of "false" threshold shifts that are unrelated to the actual hearing of those being tested. These shifts may occur in individuals or even in large groups of employees. A stable audiometer that is properly cared for is always the best answer.

The Daily Calibration Check

OSHA requires that the operation of the audiometer be checked before each day's use. There are two parts to this procedure. First, the audiometer's sound level output must be verified using an electronic device or a subject with known, stable hearing threshold levels. This test is sometimes called the **biological check**. To accomplish the biological check an electronic device is preferable because it is usually more stable than a human subject. It can be performed by an instrument sometimes called a **"bio-acoustic simulator"** or an **"electro-acoustic ear,"** pictured in Figure 7–15. The audiometer's earphones are placed on the instrument, and the OHC tests the instrument as though it were a person. If a microprocessor audiometer is used, the test runs automatically. Several companies manufacture these devices specifically intended for use with the company's own audiometers, so the OHC should make sure that the audiometer and simulator will be compatible before purchasing them.

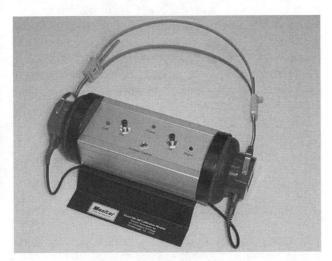

Fig. 7-15. Simulator used to perform the daily check of an audiometer's calibration. (Courtesy of Monitor Instruments, Inc.)

Lacking an electronic simulator, the biological check may be carried out using a person with known, stable hearing threshold levels. This person need not have normal hearing, but his or her hearing threshold levels must not fluctuate. Therefore it is safer to use someone whose hearing is normal. There may be cases where the OHC is alone and without an electronic simulator. In these instances the OHC may use herself/himself as the subject for the biological check, but this is not the most efficient and reliable approach. In any case, the subject is tested to make sure that the audiometer's output is within at least 10 dB of its specified level. Deviations of 10 dB or greater require the next level of calibration, the acoustic calibration.

The other aspect of the daily calibration check is called the **"functional"** or **listening check**. This check involves listening to and inspecting the audiometer for any malfunctions. For example, the OHC should check the earphones at a hearing level of about 50 or 60 dB to make sure that the test signal is not "leaking" to the non-test earphone. This is done by listening for the test tone in the non-test earphone. The switches should be checked to make sure that the signal is pure and not distorted or accompanied by any unwanted static or hum. These kinds of checks should be carried out at each test frequency.

Because the earphone cords may become brittle and worn, it is a good idea to manipulate them while listening through the earphones to make sure the signals are not broken or intermittent. The earphone cushions, which should be cleaned periodically, will eventually become stiff and pitted and will require periodic replacement. The OHC should be aware of these kinds of maintenance needs in case they are not attended to during the exhaustive calibration. The OHC should keep a record every time the daily calibration checks are performed. The records should include the hearing levels of the simulator or individual with stable hearing and a checklist for the various items comprising the audiometer inspection.

The Acoustic Calibration

The acoustic calibration is actually another form of calibration check, and is accomplished with an **audiometer calibration system**. An example of such a system is shown in Figure 7–16. It consists of a sound level meter, an octave-band filter set, and a special coupler — **the NBS 9A coupler** — with weights that exert a standard amount of pressure on the earphone to ensure an adequate seal with the sound level meter's microphone.[34]

---

[34] NBS stands for the National Bureau of Standards, which is now the National Institute of Standards and Technology. These calibration methods are spelled out in more detail in American National Standard Method for Coupler Calibration of Earphones, ANSI S3.7-1995 (R1999).

OSHA requires the acoustic calibration to be performed at least once a year or whenever the results of the functional (or daily biological) check indicate a deviation of 10 dB or more between the audiometer's dial setting and its output. OSHA spells out these requirements in Appendix E of the noise regulation (see Appendix C of this manual). The basic components of the acoustic calibration are checks on the **sound pressure output** and the **linearity** of the attenuator (the hearing level dial). To check the output, the hearing level dial is set at 70 dB and each frequency is checked to make sure that the output is correct. The linearity of the attenuator is checked at 1000 Hz to make sure that each increase and decrease of 10 dB is really 10 dB, and not substantially greater or less.

Tables E–1 and E–2 of the OSHA regulation give the expected sound level meter reading when the audiometer's hearing level dial is set at 70 dB for two common types of earphones. The regulation advises an exhaustive calibration when the measured sound levels deviate by plus or minus 3 dB for the frequencies 500 Hz through 3000 Hz, 4 dB at 4000 Hz, and 5 dB at 6000 Hz. An exhaustive calibration is *required* when the deviations are greater than 10 dB or at any test frequency.[35]

The deviations allowed by the OSHA regulation are quite high, so the OHC may wish to post any changes of 10 dB on the audiometer and apply them as corrections to the audiogram, or, preferably, have an exhaustive calibration at an earlier time. Either

way, there are likely to be disruptions to the consistency of the audiometric testing. It is always better to avoid making these changes, if possible. But if an exhaustive calibration is necessary, the OHC should be careful to record exactly when it was done so that any widespread changes in audiometric thresholds may be explained.

OHCs who perform acoustic calibration should be technically trained in the procedures and should be thoroughly familiar with the audiometer, the calibration equipment, the instruments' specifications, the OSHA noise regulation's requirements, and the relevant paragraphs of ANSI S3.6-1996, American National Standard Method Specification for Audiometers.[36] Because the audiometer can lose its calibration in the shipping process, it is preferable to perform the acoustic calibration on-site, rather than sending it out.

The Exhaustive Calibration

OSHA requires the audiometer to be calibrated "exhaustively" every two years or earlier if needed as a result of the acoustic calibration. NIOSH recommends that the exhaustive calibration be performed annually. In this type of calibration the audiometer may actually be adjusted, if needed, to conform with certain sections of ANSI S3.6-1996. This process may be done on-site by a specialist, such as a staff member of the audiometer distributor, or it can be carried out in a laboratory or by the audiometer's manufacturer. It is important to request special handling of the audiometer when it is shipped, and to check it acoustically or with a thorough "daily" check when it returns.

An interesting recent development is the establishment of a manufacturer's trade association called the National Association of Special Equipment Distributors (NASED). Companies that are members of this association employ trained staff who can service and calibrate audiometric instruments and certify that they meet relevant government standards, such as those of the National Institute of Standards and Technology (NIST), formerly the National Bureau of Standards. A list of member companies and their addresses is available on the NASED website, **www.nased.com**.

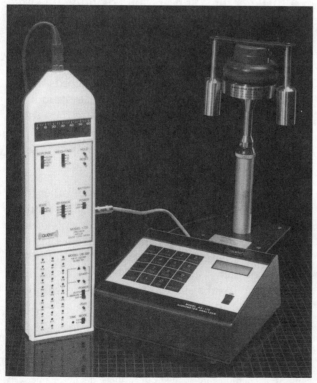

Fig. 7-16. A calibration system used for the acoustic calibration of audiometers. (Courtesy of Quest Technologies)

---

[35] Section (h)(5)(ii) of the OSHA regulation states that "deviations of 15 dB or greater" require an exhaustive calibration, while the regulation's Appendix E specifies deviations "greater than 10 dB." These values are actually the same because nowadays all of the audiometers that will be used in industry measure in 5-dB increments.

[36] The OSHA regulation refers to an earlier ANSI standard, S3.6-1969. Although the ANSI standard was updated in 1989 and again in 1996, the more recent version's Table 6 gives the same information contained in OSHA's tables E-1 and E-2.

References

ANSI (1996). American National Standard Method Specification for Audiometers. ANSI S3.6-1996, Acoustical Society of America, Melville, NY.

ANSI (1997). American National Standard Method of Manual Pure-Tone Audiometry. ANSI S3.21-1978 (R1997), Acoustical Society of America, Melville, NY.

ANSI (1999). American National Standard Method for Coupler Calibration of Earphones. ANSI S3.7-1995 (R1999), Acoustical Society of America, Melville, NY.

ANSI (1999). American National Standard for Maximum Permissible Ambient Noise Levels for Audiometric Test Rooms, ANSI S3.1-1999, Acoustical Society of America, Melville, NY.

Hawke, M., Keene, M., and Alberti, P.W. (1984). *Clinical Otoscopy.* Churchill Livingstone, New York. [Photos reprinted by permission of publisher, pages 33,42,59,69,71.]

NIOSH (1998). "Criteria for a recommended standard: Occupational noise exposure: Revised criteria, 1998." DHHS (NIOSH) 98–126. Dept. Health and Human Services, Public Health Service, Cincinnati, OH.

OSHA (1981). "Occupational noise exposure: Hearing conservation amendment." U.S. Dept. Labor, Occupational Safety and Health Admin., 46 *Fed. Reg.*, 4078–4179.

OSHA (1993). Letter to Deanna Meinke dated 6-18-93 from Edward Kaggak, Assistant Regional Administrator, Federal State Operations, OSHA, Denver, CO.

Quiz

1. Which is the most delicate part of the audiometric test system?

2. What are the two main advantages of manual audiometers? What is the main disadvantage?

3. Why is it important for OHCs to develop skills with a manual audiometer, since microprocessor audiometers are so widely used today?

4. Why are comparisons between audiograms from different makes of computerized audiometers sometimes difficult?

5. Why is it important that the audiometric test room be sufficiently quiet?

6. What is the maximum allowable sound level in audiometer rooms at 500 Hz according to OSHA? According to ANSI S3.1? (You may need to refer to Table 7.1.)

7. According to OSHA policy, noise-reducing earphone enclosures may be used instead of sound-attenuating audiometric test rooms. (True or False)

8. What is the best time to schedule the baseline audiogram? Why?

9. What is the best time to schedule the annual audiogram? Why?

10. OSHA requires employers to warn employees to avoid high levels of non-occupational noise for at least _____ hours prior to the baseline audiogram.

11. When is a retest mandatory?

12. How can the OHC avoid causing pain or discomfort to the employee when performing an otoscopic inspection?

13. Earwax usually interferes with the audiogram and should be removed before audiometric testing. (True or False)

14. The best way to seat an employee for audiometric testing is at a _____ degree angle to the operator.

15. The audiometric test should be initiated in the _____ ear. (better or worse)

16. Accepted procedures for administering pure-tone audiometric tests with a manual audiometer are spelled out in what standard?

17. Hearing threshold level is defined as the lowest hearing level where the subject hears at least 50 percent of the tones. (True or False)

18. The duration of each tone presentation should be _____ seconds.

19. An OHC who has a microprocessor audiometer does not need to know how to conduct a manual audiometric test. (True or False)

20. What are the three types of audiometer calibration required by OSHA? In which types is the audiometer actually adjusted?

21. List at least three actions that should be performed during the daily calibration check in addition to testing using an electronic simulator or a person with stable hearing threshold levels.

Abbreviations Used in Chapter VII

ANSI	American National Standards Institute
dB	Decibels
dBA	Decibels measured on the A scale of the sound level meter
HL	Hearing Level
Hz	Hertz
NASED	National Association of Special Equipment Distributors
NBS	National Bureau of Standards (now the National Institute of Standards and Technology)
NIOSH	National Institute for Occupational Safety and Health
NIST	National Institute of Standards and Technology
OHC	Occupational Hearing Conservationist
OSHA	Occupational Safety and Health Administration
STS	Standard Threshold Shift
TTS	Temporary Threshold Shift

Recommended Reading

American Academy of Otolaryngology—Head and Neck Surgery. *Doctor, explain earwax.* (Free pamphlet) AAO-HNS Inc., 1 Prince St., Alexandria, VA, 22314–3357.

Franks, J.R., Stephenson, M.R., and Merry, C.J. (1996). *Preventing occupational hearing loss—A practical guide.* DHHS (NIOSH) 96–110. Department of Health and Human Services, Public Health Service, National Institute for Occupational Safety and Health, Cincinnati, OH.

NIOSH (1998). "Hearing loss prevention programs (HLPPs)." Chapter 5 in *Criteria for a recommended standard: Occupational noise exposure: Revised criteria.* DHHS (NIOSH) 98–126. Dept. Health and Human Services, Public Health Service, Cincinnati, OH.

Royster, J.D. (2000). "Audiometric monitoring phase of the hearing conservation program." Chapter 5 in E.H. Berger, L.H. Royster, J.D. Royster, D.P. Driscoll, and M. Layne, (Eds.), *The Noise Manual, Fifth Edition.* American Industrial Hygiene Assoc., Fairfax, VA.

Tufts, J., and Frank, T. (Spring 2000). "Permissible noise levels in audiometric test rooms." CAOHC *Update, 11*(1) 1.

Websites

http://asa.aip.org
Acoustical Society of America (for information on ANSI standards)

www.nased.com
National Association of Special Equipment Distributors

www.hearingconservation.org
National Hearing Conservation Association (NHCA)

www.cdc.gov/niosh
National Institute for Occupational Safety and Health (NIOSH)

www.osha.gov
Occupational Safety and Health Administration (OSHA)

Chapter VIII

Understanding the Audiogram and Follow-up Procedures

The OHC's Role in Audiogram Review

An effective audiometric testing program involves much more than testing hearing and filing the audiograms. It is usually the OHC's responsibility, after coordinating with the professional supervisor, to determine the basic validity of the audiogram. Although the OSHA regulation has no specific requirement on this subject, the preamble to the 1983 version states that technicians are permitted a preliminary review of audiograms and that they must refer "problem audiograms or audiograms of questionable validity" to a professional reviewer for further evaluation (OSHA, 1983, pp. 9758–9759). The MSHA regulation clearly states that the determination of audiogram validity is the responsibility of a physician, audiologist, *or* a qualified technician under the direction or supervision of a physician or audiologist (see MSHA regulation, Section 62.172, in Appendix F of the manual).

According to OSHA and MSHA, each audiogram must be compared to the employee's baseline audiogram to determine if a standard threshold shift has occurred. The regulations state explicitly that the comparison may be done by a technician. OSHA goes on to state that the audiologist, otolaryngologist, or physician must review "problem" audiograms and determine whether there is a need for further evaluation. OSHA does not define the words "problem audiogram." This means that the OHC and the supervising professional need to come to an understanding about the characteristics of valid audiograms and problem audiograms, as well as the role that each person will play in reviewing the audiograms and coordinating the follow-up.

The purpose of this chapter is to acquaint the OHC with a variety of audiogram types and to suggest examples of problem audiograms. It will not be an exhaustive analysis of audiometric patterns, nor is it meant to be a training course in audiology. As OHCs become experienced and as they work with their supervising professionals they will gain confidence in their abilities to review audiograms and coordinate follow-up procedures within the framework of their roles.

About the Audiogram

"Normal Hearing"

One should remember that a 0-dB hearing threshold level (HTL) on the audiometer is not the same as a 0-dB sound pressure level (SPL) on the sound level meter, but it has been adjusted to reflect the softest sound that normal-hearing listeners could hear at each frequency. (See Fig. 5-5 and the discussion of this topic in Chapter V.) Some individuals tested by the OHC will hear better than 0-dB HTL and quite a few will hear somewhat worse. Needless to say, as people's hearing becomes worse, it takes greater levels of sound pressure to reach their thresholds and this is reflected by a progression toward the lower portion of the graph.

There has been controversy in the professional community about the definition of normal hearing. Some would say that it depends upon a person's age since normal hearing for an 80-year-old would not be considered normal for a 15-year-old. In general, thresholds better than 20–25 dB are considered to be within normal limits, although some would say that the limit of normal hearing would be more like 0–15 dB, especially for the low and middle frequencies.

It is safe to say that the definition of normal hearing and, by default, the definition of impaired hearing, is dependent on both age and frequency. For example, a 60-year-old worker with a hearing threshold level of 30-dB at 4000 Hz would be considered within the range of normal, while a 20-year-old worker with the same hearing might not be. Likewise, a 30-dB hearing threshold level at 500 Hz would not be considered normal for any age group.

Relating the Audiogram to Hearing Handicap

Interestingly, the correlation between hearing threshold level on the audiometer and the problems experienced in daily life as measured by hearing handicap questionnaires is not strong. One reason is that the pure-tone audiogram does not always reflect a person's ability (or disability) to understand speech, especially in less-than-ideal conditions. Another is that different individuals will have different communication needs and preferences. While some people may not be overly concerned about a mild or even a moderate hearing loss, others may consider themselves significantly handicapped from the same pure-tone loss.

Most individuals with hearing losses will have difficulty understanding speech in a noisy background, especially if it is a reverberant room. The exception is people with conductive hearing losses due to outer or middle ear problems. But people with the sloping losses typical of noise-induced hearing loss will have particular trouble understanding speech in unfavorable listening conditions. Whenever people speak softly or indistinctly, when they attempt to communicate at a distance, or when there is noise in the background, people with sensorineural hearing losses are likely to have much more difficulty than in ideal face-to-face communication situations. Examples of challenging listening conditions include most social gatherings (like in the church foyer), conversations in a group, in the restaurant environment, driving or riding in a car, walking down a noisy city street, and communicating when the TV is on.

Characteristics of Audiograms

Examples of the two principal types of audiometers were presented in Chapter VII. The conventional audiogram chart was pictured, which is often used with the manual audiometer. Because this type of audiogram gives a comprehensible, graphic picture of hearing loss it will be used here to display various hearing loss patterns. Possible causes or etiologies will be given for each type of audiogram.

These possible causes are given only to provide some background for the different types of hearing impairment and to assist the OHC in determining the proper follow-up procedure. The OHC must remember never to speculate on the medical cause of a hearing loss with the employee, but only to observe the pattern of the loss and to refer the employee for additional testing, counseling, or medical treatment as necessary.

Hearing Within Normal Limits

Figure 8-1 shows an audiogram of an individual whose hearing is within normal limits. As explained previously, the O symbolizes the right ear's response and the X symbolizes the left's response. Note that the hearing threshold level (HTL) is somewhat greater (worse) than 0 dB in all frequencies, but it is not considered impaired. These HTLs are probably worse than one would expect from an 18-year-old, but better than one would expect from most 60-year-olds.

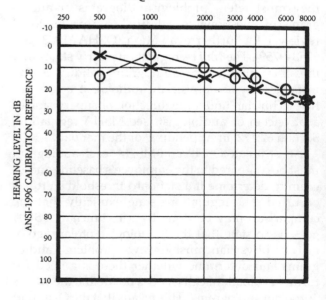

Fig. 8-1. Audiogram of a person whose hearing is within normal limits.

Most OHCs will prefer to keep audiograms in tabular form for easier recordkeeping and ready access to previous audiograms. This is how Figure 8-1 looks as a table:

Table 8.1. Figure 8-1 in tabular form

Freq. Hz	500	1000	2000	3000	4000	6000	8000
Left	5	10	15	10	20	25	25
Right	15	5	10	15	15	20	25

Unilateral Loss

Sometimes an employee will have normal or near-normal hearing in one ear and some degree of hearing loss in the other. This is called a **unilateral** hearing loss. If the hearing in neither ear is normal, but one ear is considerably better than the other, this condition is usually referred to as an **asymmetric** hearing loss. If the HTLs in the better ear are within normal limits, this person will usually not have difficulty understanding speech in good listening conditions, even if the loss in the poorer ear is substantial. But problems may occur in unfavorable listening conditions, such as the ones mentioned above, especially in a noisy or reverberant environment or if the speech is coming from the side of the poorer ear. People with unilateral or asymmetrical hearing losses will often have trouble identifying the direction a sound is coming from.

Unilateral hearing losses are not usually caused by noise exposure, although it is possible to sustain a sudden hearing loss in one ear from an extremely intense sound, such as an explosion or a firecracker (resulting in acoustic trauma). Actually, most cases of sudden hearing loss are not due to acoustic trauma but to viral, vascular, or other medical causes. More commonly, unilateral hearing losses are caused by a childhood disease, such as mumps, or by an outer or middle ear pathology. One very serious condition that can present as a unilateral or asymmetric hearing loss is a tumor of the auditory nerve, an acoustic neuroma. When the OHC encounters a unilateral or asymmetric hearing loss with a large difference between ears, this person should be promptly referred to an otologist or otolaryngologist unless another cause has already been established.

Figure 8-2 shows an example of a unilateral hearing loss in the right ear that is quite severe in the high frequencies. There is also some hearing loss in the left ear, so the loss could also be categorized as asymmetric, and there are substantial differences between the thresholds of the two ears. There is actually no response in the right ear at 6000 and 8000 Hz; this is symbolized by the little arrow extending downward at an angle from the O representing the right ear. The arrow on the right ear's symbol points downward and left and, if there was no response on the left ear, the left ear's symbol would point downward and right (see page 5 of the ANSI standard S3.21 in Appendix N of this manual). Note that the no-response symbols are placed at 90 dB at 6000 Hz and 80 dB at 8000 Hz because these are the upper limits for these two frequencies in this particular audiometer. Some audiometers, particularly those used in audiology clinics, will be able to test to 100 and 90 dB (Type 2) or even 110 and 100 dB (Type 1) respectively at these frequencies. OHCs should be familiar with the upper limits of their own instruments.

This is how Figure 8-2 would appear in tabular form:

Table 8.2. Figure 8-2 in tabular form

Freq. Hz	500	1000	2000	3000	4000	6000	8000
Left	0	10	15	20	35	30	30
Right	40	60	70	75	90	90+	80+

Flat Audiogram

In some cases the audiometric pattern may be relatively flat across all frequencies. This is often characteristic of outer or middle ear involvement, due to causes such as middle ear infections, chronic allergies, or abnormalities of the tympanic membrane. In such cases the loss would probably be conductive and amenable to medical treatment. Occasionally flat losses may be sensorineural. Possible causes could be Meniere's disease, or a severe case of the

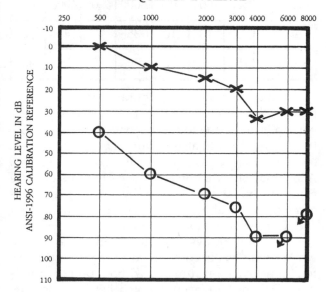

FREQUENCY IN HERTZ

Fig. 8-2. A unilateral hearing loss in the right ear. Since there is some loss in the left ear, this could be considered a severely asymmetric hearing loss.

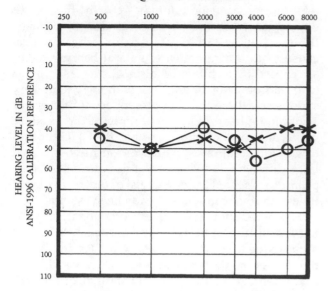

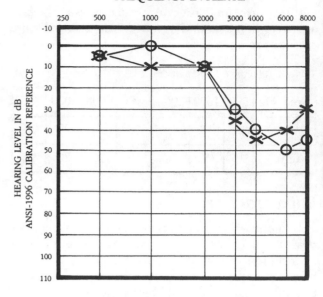

FREQUENCY IN HERTZ

Fig. 8-3. An example of a flat audiometric configuration.

Fig. 8-4. Sloping audiogram with a "notch" configuration.

measles, or the loss could be congenital due to a problem during pregnancy. Also, it is not uncommon for flat audiograms to result from equipment malfunctions or from pseudohypacusis (functional hearing losses); if suspected, both of these possibilities would need to be investigated. The first encounter of a flat loss in a worker should be discussed with one's supervising professional or referred promptly for medical or audiological follow-up.

Figure 8-3 gives an example of a flat threshold pattern. Note that the hearing loss is not absolutely flat, and that the HTLs are slightly different for the two ears. In fact, HTLs are only rarely identical in both ears.

This is the flat loss pictured in Figure 8-3, now in the form of a table:

Table 8.3. Figure 8-3 in tabular form

Freq. Hz	500	1000	2000	3000	4000	6000	8000
Left	40	50	45	50	45	40	40
Right	45	50	40	45	55	50	45

Sloping Configuration

Probably the most common audiometric pattern, especially in people in noisy occupations, is the hearing loss that slopes toward the high frequencies. Sometimes the HTLs improve in the audiogram's highest frequencies, which forms a "notch" configuration. The notch from occupational noise exposure most often occurs at 4000 Hz, but it can frequently occur at 3000 or 6000 Hz. The exact location of the notch depends on many factors, including the

frequency spectrum of the noise, the size and shape of the individual's earcanal, and the sensitivity of the individual's cochlea. It is not unusual to see notches at different frequencies in each ear for the same individual. Also, notches may be caused by factors other than noise, such as viral infections.

Figure 8-4 shows a sloping audiogram with the notch configuration. Note that the notch occurs at 4000 Hz in the left ear and 6000 Hz in the right ear.

Here is the tabular form of the loss depicted in Figure 8-4:

Table 8.4. Figure 8-4 in tabular form

Freq. Hz	500	1000	2000	3000	4000	6000	8000
Left	5	10	10	35	45	40	30
Right	5	0	10	30	40	50	45

Another common configuration is the high-frequency drop-off with no notch. Although this pattern is often due to presbycusis, the hearing loss from aging, it could also be caused by noise, disease, ototoxic drugs, or any combination of these factors. A loss may show a notch in the early years of noise exposure, but as the years go by, the noise-induced component combines with the aging component and the notch is no longer evident.

Figure 8-5 shows an audiogram typical of a worker who has been exposed to high noise levels for many years, presumably without proper protection. If there had been a notch before, it is now obscured by presbycusis. Note also that there is now some loss in the mid-frequencies, which also can be characteristic of long-term noise exposure.

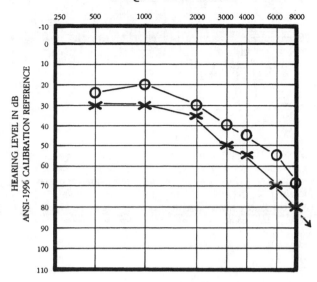

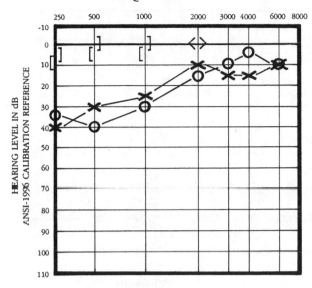

Fig. 8-5. Typical audiogram of a worker who has been exposed to noise for many years.

Fig. 8-6. Example of an audiogram with a rising configuration, and including bone conduction thresholds.

This is the tabular form of Figure 8-5:

Table 8.5. Figure 8-5 in tabular form

Freq. Hz	500	1000	2000	3000	4000	6000	8000
Left	30	30	35	50	55	70	80↑
Right	25	20	30	40	45	55	70

Rising Configuration

The type of audiogram where hearing threshold levels improve in the high frequencies is rather unusual. These losses are rarely caused by noise exposure, although a traumatic loss from a low-frequency or mid-frequency noise source could conceivably cause this kind of pattern. More typically these losses are conductive or occasionally sensorineural due to some form of pathology, such as Meniere's disease. An example of this type of configuration is shown in Figure 8-6.

Bone Conduction and Masking

In Figure 8-6 the familiar **air conduction** symbols are accompanied by **bone conduction** symbols in the form of hatch-marks. Although the OHC will not be performing bone conduction testing (unless trained as an audiologist), she or he might encounter audiograms with bone conduction symbols coming from an audiology clinic or physician's office. Basically, bone conduction testing bypasses the outer and

middle ears and stimulates the inner ear directly by setting the bones of the skull into vibration at the frequencies selected. The bone conduction symbols, represented by > for the left ear and < for the right, indicate that the loss in Figure 8-6 is a conductive one because the bone conduction symbols show hearing threshold levels considerably better than the hearing threshold levels by air conduction. Thresholds for the 250-Hz frequency are also included because they will be a part of the clinical audiogram although once again, the OHC will not be testing this frequency.

Sometimes the clinical audiogram will contain a different type of symbol for bone conduction threshold, which is in the shape of a bracket. The right ear is represented by [and the left by]. These symbols signify that the audiologist has used a procedure called **"masking."** Briefly, this means that the audiologist has introduced a noise into the non-test earphone to keep that ear busy while the other ear is being tested. Masking prevents the tone from crossing over to the non-test ear. Because the tone crosses over easily by bone conduction, masking is very often used with bone conduction testing. But it is also used with air conduction testing when there is a significant difference in HTL between the two ears. The symbol for the right ear when the left is masked is a square □ and the symbol for the left ear when the right is masked is a triangle ∆. In Figure 8-6, note that masking has been used to arrive at the bone conduction HTLs at 250, 500, and 1000 Hz.

The tabular form of Figure 8-6 includes bone conduction as well as air conduction thresholds:

Table 8.6. Figure 8-6 in tabular form

Freq. Hz	250	500	1000	2000	3000	4000	6000
Left (air)	40	30	25	10	15	15	10
Right (air)	35	40	30	15	10	5	10
Left (bone)	5	0	0	0			
Right (bone)	10	5	5	0			

It is not unusual for hearing loss to be partly conductive and partly sensorineural, in which case it is called a **mixed** loss. The audiogram will be characterized by bone conduction thresholds that are better than air conduction thresholds, but not all within normal limits. Once again, the OHC will not be testing with bone conduction, but it is useful to know that these types of hearing losses exist.

Other Types of Audiograms

In addition to the graph and table forms demonstrated above, there are two other types of audiograms that the OHC may encounter: the audiogram produced by the self-recording audiometer and that produced by the computerized audiometer.

Audiogram from the Self-Recording Audiometer

As explained in the preceding chapter, the self-recording audiometer is virtually obsolete at this time, but the audiograms may very well persist in the records of a company's hearing conservation program. Examples of these audiograms are shown in Figures 8-7 and 8-8 below.

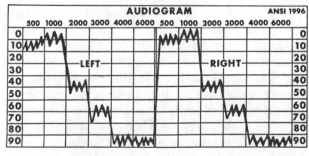

Fig. 8-7. Audiogram from a self-recording audiometer showing a moderate-to-severe hearing loss in the frequencies above 1000 Hz. If a line were drawn horizontal to the time axis, there would be at least six crossings at each frequency, so the audiogram is acceptable.

One of the problems with self-recording audiometry has been that the OHC must be able to know when an audiogram is acceptable or unacceptable and how to score it. Appendix C of the OSHA noise

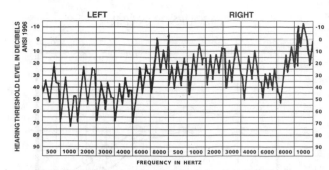

Fig. 8-8. Audiogram from a self-recording audiometer showing excursions that are too wide at nearly every frequency for the mandatory six crossings to be achieved. This audiogram is, therefore, unacceptable. Note that the retest at 1000 Hz in the right ear shows nearly normal hearing, whereas the audiogram shows a loss of about 25 dB at the same frequency (same ear) earlier in the test.

regulation (found in Appendix C of this manual) gives specific mandatory instructions for self-recording audiometry. First, there are specifications for the audiometer and the chart that actually concern the manufacturer rather than the OHC. The important instruction to the OHC is found in section (E):

> *It must be possible at each test frequency to place a horizontal line segment parallel to the time axis on the audiogram, such that the audiometric tracing crosses the line segment at least six times at that test frequency. At each test frequency the threshold shall be the average of the midpoints of the tracing excursions.*

This statement means that an audiogram such as the one seen in Figure 8-7 would be acceptable, but the one in Figure 8-8 would not. It also tells the OHC that threshold is determined by averaging the midpoints of the pen's up and down excursions. If this process is done carefully, it is possible to determine thresholds for increments smaller than 5 dB. If the audiogram contains the necessary six crossings for each frequency, threshold determination is not difficult. Many of these audiograms will meet the OSHA criteria. However, quite a few will not, either because the subjects have not been adequately instructed or because, for a number of reasons, they found the task too difficult. Such audiograms would be of limited use to the hearing conservation program.

Sometimes these audiograms are more easily interpreted once they have been converted to tables like the ones described above. The OHC may be tempted to round the threshold values to the nearest 5-dB increment to make them comparable to the results of manual or computerized audiometers. It is better, however, to leave the threshold values exactly as read from the audiogram since it is easy to make errors in doing the rounding.[37] In other words, if the

---

[37] Because translating from the tracings to numerical values is somewhat subjective, it is all too easy to make errors during this procedure. The process of rounding is then likely to compound the errors.

threshold at 1000 Hz is 7 dB and the threshold at 2000 Hz is 23 dB, it is better to leave them that way than to round them to 5 dB and 25 dB respectively. If, however, the data will be entered into a computer and the program will not accept thresholds that do not end in "0" or "5," then rounding will be necessary.

Audiogram from the Microprocessor Audiometer

Figure 8-9 gives an example of the detailed data that some models of microprocessor audiometers can produce. In the upper portion of the left strip, below the employee's identifying information, audiometric thresholds are displayed vertically. Thresholds for each ear are stated as current (CT) and baseline (BL) values, and the amount of shift for each frequency is given. Below each column of numbers is the average hearing threshold level at 2000, 3000, and 4000 Hz and the average shift from baseline at these frequencies. The next line displays the average shift, after being adjusted for presbycusis according to the method in OSHA's Appendix F and MSHA's Tables 62-3 and 62-4. Further down the strip are hearing handicap calculations (percent binaural impairment—PBI) according to the AAO formula, classification codes, such as the ones used by the DoD, information on certain calibration checks, and employee demographics.

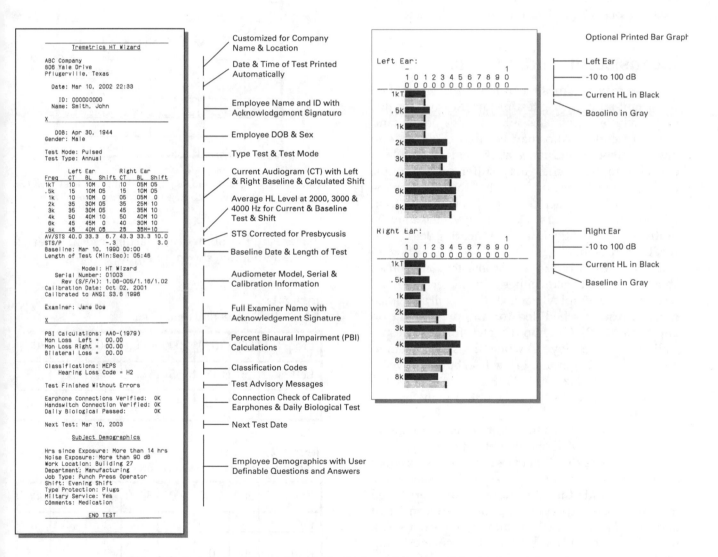

Fig. 8-9. Detailed audiometric and identifying data produced by a microprocessor audiometer. (Courtesy of Tremetrics)

The strip displayed on the right shows a bar graph of the current audiogram's thresholds (in black) compared to those of the baseline (in grey), which provides a quick and easy means of visualizing any changes.

Not shown in Fig. 8-9 are certain codes that the audiometer may use to indicate errors in testing or other reasons for failing to achieve threshold. Two examples of these codes are: "UN" (unknown), meaning that the threshold level is unknown because the maximum number of presentations has been exceeded without a reliable response; and "NR" (no response), meaning that the audiometer's upper limit has been reached. Each manufacturer of microprocessor audiometers has its own set of codes and OHCs need to be thoroughly familiar with the meaning of each code used by their audiometer.

Inconsistent Audiometric Tests

There may be times when it is difficult to obtain consistent audiometric test results. Reasons for this may include employees who do not understand the instructions, who may be tired or ill, or who have engaged in substance abuse and are unable to concentrate. Also, they may suffer from tinnitus, causing them to respond to what they think is the test tone when, in fact, the stimulus is coming from within their own ears. Occasionally they may be motivated to exaggerate their hearing losses for whatever reason.

Employees who give inconsistent responses should be tested again, either immediately or after a few hours. An employee who is tired or ill should be given a rest or scheduled for an appointment on another day. OHCs should watch for cases, especially in new employees, where thresholds seem to be poor at the beginning of the test, but improve by the time 3000 Hz or 4000 Hz is tested, as the employee begins to get acquainted with the test procedure.

If an employee is confused or possibly exaggerating the loss, the OHC should patiently reinstruct the person, encouraging him or her to listen as carefully as possible. Often the responses will become more consistent and the thresholds may very well improve. If the responses continue to be inconsistent and the OHC feels that the audiogram is not valid, these cases should be referred to the supervising professional or to an audiology clinic for further evaluation. Both OSHA and MSHA require that the employer obtain a valid audiogram, and if this cannot be done on-site, then the employee must be referred to a specialist at the company's expense.

Figure 8-10 shows a hypothetical case where the subject gave somewhat inconsistent responses, was reinstructed to listen very carefully and to respond even if the tone is very soft, and then was tested again. Note that in the first test the hearing loss was rather flat, with slightly worse hearing in the high frequencies. Upon retesting, the thresholds are within normal limits, except for a slight loss in the high frequencies. This pattern could be encountered in an employee who has a slight noise-induced loss but who is exaggerating a greater one.

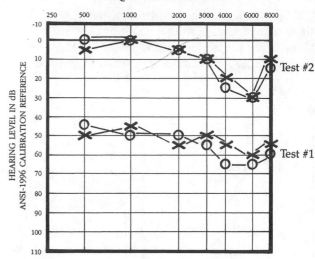

Fig. 8-10. Audiogram showing marked improvement (Test #2) after reinstruction and encouragement to listen carefully.

Here are the numerical hearing threshold levels for the audiogram shown in Figure 8-10:

Test #1:
Table 8.10. Figure 8-10 in tabular form

Freq. Hz	500	1000	2000	3000	4000	6000	8000
Left	50	45	55	50	55	60	55
Right	45	50	50	55	65	65	60

Test #2:
Table 8.11. Figure 8-10 in tabular form

Freq. Hz	500	1000	2000	3000	4000	6000	8000
Left	5	0	5	10	20	30	10
Right	0	0	5	10	25	30	15

Once again, it is very important for the OHC to realize that there may be several reasons for inconsistent audiograms and that the exaggeration of HTLs is only one of them. OHCs should never accuse employees of deliberately misleading them.

Even if the OHC is reasonably certain that this is taking place, the best course is to let the individual save face by attributing the inconsistencies to the uncertainties involved in taking the test. In any case, it is a good idea for the OHC to document any impressions about the employee's ability to communicate and possible inconsistencies during the testing, without making any judgments about his or her behavior.

Reprinted in Appendix J are some tips on dealing with hard-to-test workers from an article by Linda Frye in the CAOHC *UPDATE*. These include switching from a microprocessor to manual testing, the use of a "pulsed" tone if the employee is bothered by tinnitus,[38] and the importance of giving employees a break after they have been in the test booth for more than 10 minutes at a time. Perhaps the person has had a hard day, or perhaps he or she is self-conscious or worried about having a hearing loss. Patience on the part of the OHC will often make the test go more smoothly.

Problem Audiograms

OSHA requires that an audiologist or physician review **"problem audiograms"** and determine whether there is a need for further evaluation, but the agency provides no definition of a problem audiogram. This is something that the OHC needs to work out with the professional supervisor before embarking on an audiometric testing program. At this time, a committee of the National Hearing Conservation Association (NHCA) is drafting guidelines, and OHCs should check the NHCA website to see if they have been made final (**www.hearingconservation.org**). NHCA's draft recommendations include the following:

1. OSHA-defined STS (DoD-defined STS for military facilities) on annual audiogram.

2. Change of +15 dB or more at any frequency either ear on annual audiogram, compared to the baseline audiogram.

3. Improvement of −15 dB or more at any frequency either ear on annual audiogram, compared to the baseline audiogram.

4. Asymmetry
   a. Difference of 40 dB or more between ears at any frequency on baseline.
   b. Difference of 25 dB or more between ears at two consecutive frequencies on annual audiogram.

5. Unreliable audiograms: inconsistent/unreliable thresholds— differences of 10 dB or more between annual and follow-up audiograms, or compared to the previous year's test(s), at the same frequency(ies) in the same ear.

6. Low-frequency hearing loss
   a. Average hearing level greater than 25 dB at 500, 1000, and 2000 Hz on the baseline audiogram.
   b. Shift of 10 dB average at 500, 1000, and 2000 Hz on annual audiogram.

7. Technician unable to obtain audiogram using standard procedures.

Although these recommendations may be slightly changed in their final form, they reflect a cautious, common-sense approach that OHCs would do well to follow. With regard to recommendation A, it is important that OHCs understand that the existence of an STS does not mandate referral to an audiologist or physician. While it is necessary for supervising professionals to review the audiometric history of an employee who incurs an STS, this does not automatically require medical or audiological follow-up unless the supervisor advises it.

Standard Threshold Shift (STS)

For many years STS stood for "significant threshold shift," which conveys the meaning of this occurrence somewhat more appropriately than "standard threshold shift." The word "significant" was changed to "standard" when OSHA's hearing conservation amendment was revised in 1983. The OHC should be aware that some programs still use the word "significant." Both NIOSH (1998) and the Department of Defense (DoD, 1996) use the term "significant," and even OSHA may return to it at some time in the future.

Calculating STS

All OHCs ought to know how to calculate STS, even those with computerized audiometric systems. As explained in Chapter VI, the definition of STS used by OSHA and MSHA is an average shift from baseline of 10 dB or more in the frequencies 2000, 3000, and 4000 Hz in either ear. Because noise tends to affect the higher frequencies earlier and more severely than the lower or middle frequencies, it is not unusual for a shift to be as much as 20 or even 25 dB at 4000 Hz, with little or no shift at the others; and the loss still would not be considered an STS.

Some programs have used a different definition of STS, either instead of or in addition to the OSHA/MSHA definition. For example, the DoD

---

[38] Many audiologists prefer to use a pulsed tone for all pure-tone audiometric tests.

currently uses the OSHA/MSHA definition plus a change of 15 dB or greater at any of the frequencies 1000, 2000, 3000, or 4000 Hz in either ear. In its Criteria for a Recommended Standard, NIOSH uses a shift in either ear of 15 dB or more in any of the test frequencies, 500–6000 Hz, which persists on a retest within 30 days. In fact, NIOSH recommends an immediate retest, and if a shift of 15 dB or more is not evident, then further testing is unnecessary until the next annual test. Neither the DoD nor the NIOSH criteria allow adjustments for presbycusis in the calculation of STS. If a company wishes to use another definition in addition to the OSHA/MSHA definition, it is, of course, free to do so.

To calculate an OSHA/MSHA STS, take the average hearing threshold level at 2000, 3000, and 4000 Hz in each ear for the current audiogram, and compare it to the average for these three frequencies in the baseline audiogram. If the current average is 10 dB or greater than the baseline in either ear, an STS has occurred. Here is an example of an STS calculation for a man who received his baseline audiogram in 1987 at the age of 28 and his most recent audiogram in 2001 at the age of 42:

Current audiogram (2001)

Freq. Hz	500	1000	2000	3000	4000	6000	avg. 2,3,4k
Left	15	10	20	25	40	45	28
Right	10	15	15	30	45	40	30

Baseline audiogram (1987)

Freq. Hz	500	1000	2000	3000	4000	6000	avg. 2,3,4k
Left	0	0	15	10	20	15	15
Right	5	0	10	20	25	10	18

This man would have developed an STS in both ears because the difference between the current audiogram and the baseline exceeds the 10 dB average at 2000, 3000, and 4000 Hz. (Left ear 28-15=13; right ear 30-18=12.)

The OSHA and MSHA regulations allow the use of presbycusis tables to adjust the current audiogram when calculating STS. This practice is not mandatory, but many employers want to use this adjustment since it takes the natural aging process into account and reduces the apparent differences between the baseline and current audiograms. Some professional supervisors will prefer not to use these adjustments because they are based on average (median) data for groups of people and it may not seem appropriate to apply them to individuals

since one never knows exactly how much loss an individual would have had from aging. Two state OSHA programs, Oregon and Washington, do not allow an adjustment for presbycusis when calculating STS.

Appendix F of the OSHA regulation lists median hearing threshold levels according to age, with separate tables for men and women. To adjust the audiogram for presbycusis, locate the presbycusis levels at 2000, 3000, and 4000 Hz for the age of the employee at the time of the baseline audiogram and subtract those levels from the presbycusis levels corresponding to the age of the employee at the time of the current audiogram. These difference values are then subtracted from the HTLs of the current audiogram. The current audiogram is then compared to the baseline to see whether or not an STS has occurred.

According to the presbycusis table for men in the OSHA regulation's Appendix F:

	2000	3000	4000 Hz
age 42	7	11	16 dB
age 28	4	6	8
difference	3	5	8

Subtracting the difference values from the current audiogram's HTLs:

Left ear	20	25	40 dB
	3	5	8
Adjusted threshold	17	20	32
Right ear	15	30	45 dB
	3	5	8
Adjusted threshold	12	25	37

Now comparing the current adjusted audiogram with the baseline:

Current audiogram (adjusted for presbycusis):

Freq. Hz	500	1000	2000	3000	4000	6000	avg. 2,3,4k
Left			17	20	32		23
Right			12	25	37		25

Baseline audiogram:

Freq. Hz	500	1000	2000	3000	4000	6000	avg. 2,3,4k
Left			15	10	20		15
Right			10	20	25		18

At this point there is no longer an STS in either ear. (Right ear 25–18=7; left ear 23–15=8.)

In cases like this it is tempting to believe that there is no problem. But the employee's hearing does appear to be growing worse, so it would be a good idea to retest him (if this has not been done already), to counsel him, and to take steps to prevent further deterioration, even though his threshold shift may not be "official" as far as OSHA and MSHA are concerned.

Retesting

When an STS occurs, the best practice is to retest the worker right away, and it will often happen that the shift will disappear and further retesting will be unnecessary. If the STS persists (or if immediate retesting is not possible), OSHA and MSHA state that the employer *may* perform a retest within 30 days.[39] Although it is not mandatory, workers should be retested, whenever possible, and it is important to make sure that retesting is done after at least 14 hours away from noise, under the same conditions that the baseline was performed. Performing the retest under quiet conditions can expose the occurrence of TTS on the annual test, and the OHC can take steps to prevent the temporary loss from becoming permanent.

Baseline Revision

A paragraph in Chapter VI described OSHA's provisions for revising the baseline audiogram. According to OSHA, an annual audiogram *may* be substituted for the baseline when the reviewing professional determines that an STS is persistent. If, after retesting, an STS persists, then the retest audiogram may become the new baseline. Also mentioned in Chapter VI is the case where hearing in both ears has deteriorated, and yet only one ear exhibits an STS. OSHA *allows* employers to revise the baseline in both ears in these cases, but recommends that the thresholds for each ear be assessed and revised independently, since this method is more protective (see the interpretation on the OSHA website, McCully, 1996). OHCs should follow OSHA's recommended practice and always treat the audiometric results for the two ears separately when it comes to revision.

Interestingly, while OSHA *allows* the annual audiogram to be revised when the professional reviewer determines that an STS is permanent, MSHA actually *requires* it. (Appendix F, this manual, section 62.170(c)(1).)

Another aspect of STS needs to be mentioned—the occurrence of improved HTLs. It is not unusual for an employee's hearing to improve from year to year, especially during the first few years of testing. Improvements may result from better use of hearing protectors; or the employee may have had a cold or allergy at the time of the baseline and has subsequently recovered. Also, it appears that people become more skilled at taking the audiometric test (the "learning" or "improvement" effect), causing HTLs to improve between the baseline and subsequent tests. OSHA recommends revising the baseline when another audiogram shows better HTLs, then comparing future audiograms to the new baseline, but the agency gives no guidance on exactly when to revise the baseline in cases of improved hearing. Again, MSHA *requires* the baseline audiogram to be revised when the annual audiogram indicates "significant improvement" over the baseline, but does not define the word "significant."

In the absence of regulatory guidance, NHCA has issued a professional guide for audiometric baseline revision (NHCA, 2001). This useful guide discusses revisions for both improved hearing and for persistent STS. It has also been reprinted in an issue of the CAOHC *UPDATE*, and is reproduced as Appendix K in this manual. Although these guidelines are to be implemented by the supervising professional, it is useful for OHCs to be familiar with them, and CAOHC has urged OHCs to share them with the supervisors of their audiometric testing programs.

According to the NHCA criteria, if the average hearing threshold level for 2000, 3000, and 4000 Hz in either ear shows an improvement of 5 dB or more and the improvement persists on the next test (either retest or annual), the worker's audiometric record should be flagged for review by an audiologist or physician for potential baseline revision. Age corrections are not to be applied in cases where baselines are revised for improved hearing.

Sometimes a periodic audiogram will show improved thresholds at certain frequencies and worse thresholds at others. OSHA has given no recommendations about what to do in such a case. Some professionals advocate making a composite audiogram that includes the best thresholds at each frequency. This procedure is risky, however, because it reflects a departure from the actual test results. It is probably safer just to use one or the other of the two best audiograms. When in doubt, the supervising professional should be consulted.

Follow-up Procedures

The fact of audiometric testing does nothing to save hearing unless it is followed with an effective intervention. This is why the actions resulting from the test are so important.

---

[39] The MSHA regulation stipulates that only one retest may be performed after an STS has been identified.

First, OHCs should be thoroughly familiar with the requirements for follow-up found in section (g)(8) of OSHA's noise regulation and sections 62.173–175 of the MSHA regulation. These requirements are paraphrased below and they are printed in boldface so the reader can differentiate between requirements and commentary.

Time Limits

OSHA:

If there is an STS, the employee should be informed of this fact in writing within 21 days of the time the STS is determined. When using a computerized audiometric system the determination usually will occur right away, so the clock starts ticking at the time of the test. If the professional reviewer needs to see all audiograms, then the 21 days would start when the reviewer informs the employer of the STS.

MSHA:

The mine operator must notify the miner in writing within 10 days of receiving the results of an audiogram or a follow-up evaluation. The MSHA requirement covers any audiogram or follow-up exam, not just STS. The mine operator has other duties to be performed within 30 days of the occurrence of an STS, unless the STS is not work-related (see below).

Duties

OSHA:

When an STS occurs the employer must take certain steps unless a physician determines that the STS is not work-related or aggravated by occupational noise. These steps are:

1. Employees who are not using hearing protectors must be fitted with them, required to use them, and trained in their use and care. This refers to employees exposed to TWAs between 85 and 90 dBA since those exposed to TWAs above 90 dBA are already required to wear hearing protectors.

2. Employees already using hearing protectors must be refitted and retrained. Also, they must be provided with protectors that afford greater attenuation if necessary. Most employees will not need hearing protectors with greater attenuation, but will need to wear their current protectors more effectively.

3. If additional testing is necessary or if the employer suspects that a medical problem is caused or aggravated by the use of hearing protectors, the employee must be referred to an audiologist or otolaryngologist as appropriate. As mentioned earlier, the employer is responsible for obtaining a valid audiogram and if the OHC is unable to do this, then referral is necessary. Also, if the noise conditions necessitate the use of hearing protection devices, the employer is responsible should these devices cause or aggravate a medical problem. OSHA has interpreted this section to mean that the employer must bear the expense of medical treatment or audiological evaluation in these cases.

The OSHA regulation is not completely clear on two points. First, this requirement is part of a section on what to do about employees who develop an STS. But if the OHC is unable to obtain a valid audiogram, how do we know that an STS has occurred? Obviously, the employer must refer the worker for further testing regardless of whether an STS has been demonstrated.

The second case also involves an employee who has not yet experienced an STS and who may not even have had a baseline audiogram. What should the OHC do about an employee who must wear hearing protectors but who comes to the hearing conservation program with an infection of the outer ear? In this case the problem is not caused or aggravated by the protectors, but it clearly would be if the individual used an earplug or possibly a muff as well. Another example would be the employee with excessive earwax, which could cause a medical problem if it were repeatedly packed in by an earplug. Both of these conditions could take place without the occurrence of an STS. OSHA does, however, make the employer responsible for protecting the employee from noise hazards, and if the employee needs to wear hearing protectors to be adequately protected, it is clearly the employer's duty to have these conditions treated.

4. If there is a medical problem of the ear that is not related to the wearing of hearing protectors, the employee must be informed of the need for an otological examination. Examples of this kind of problem might be a persistent cold or allergy, or a one-sided hearing loss that has not been previously checked. In this case the company is not obligated to bear the expense, but the chances of follow-up would be improved if it did.

If after an employee has been retested there is no longer an STS and if the employee's TWA is less than 90 dBA, the employee may discontinue wearing hearing protectors. In this case the employee must be informed of the new audiometric interpretation. Despite the regulation's allowances, it is not good practice to discontinue the use of hearing protection if the OHC is reasonably sure that some temporary loss has been caused by workplace noise. If this is the case, the company may require the employee to keep on wearing the hearing protection and he or she should definitely be counseled. If there is some noise exposure during recreational activities, the employee should be advised to use hearing protection away from work as well.

Many people are under the impression that OSHA requires any employee who experiences an STS to be referred to a physician or audiologist. This is not true. Probably the majority of STS cases will be caused by noise exposure, and medical treatment will not be of help. The course of action for these cases is thoughtful and persistent counseling by the OHC or the professional supervisor, working with employees to improve the effectiveness of their hearing protection, motivating them to wear it faithfully, replacing the devices when necessary, and advising employees about protecting their hearing off the job. If indeed occupational noise exposure is causing the STS, management should be encouraged to control the noise at the source.

MSHA:

1. In case a valid audiogram cannot be obtained due to a medical condition that the physician or audiologist believes to be aggravated by occupational noise or by hearing protectors, the miner must be referred for a clinical-audiological evaluation at no cost to the miner. If the condition preventing a valid audiogram is unrelated to occupational noise or hearing protectors, the miner must be referred, but the mine operator does not bear the cost. These requirements are not contingent upon an STS, but on obtaining a valid audiogram. MSHA seems to be clearer than OSHA, that if the OHC cannot obtain a valid audiogram for anything other than medical reasons, the employer's duties stop there. Even so, the recommended practice would be for the mine operator to take all necessary steps to obtain a valid audiogram, since audiometric testing is a critical element of the hearing conservation program.

> **2. When an STS occurs, within 30 days the mine operator must:**
> **a. Retrain the miner according to the requirements in section 62.180,**
> **b. Provide the miner with the opportunity to select new or different hearing protectors,**
> **c. Review the effectiveness of any engineering or administrative controls to identify and correct deficiencies.**

The above requirements are similar to OSHA's except for the addition of #3 concerning engineering or administrative controls.

AAO-HNS Referral Criteria

In addition to the OSHA/MSHA requirements, there is another set of follow-up procedures that the OHC should know about. It is the Otological Referral Criteria for Occupational Hearing Conservation Programs developed by the American Academy of Otolaryngology—Head and Neck Surgery (AAO-HNS, 1997).[40] The purpose of these criteria is to identify larger changes in hearing that are likely to be significant, both medically and in terms of communication difficulties. *For these criteria, the original baseline should always be kept and used to compare with the current audiogram.*

The AAO-HNS recommends medical referral on the basis of the baseline as well as the periodic audiogram. Referral should be made under the following circumstances:

1. Baseline Audiogram
   a. Average hearing level at 500, 1000, 2000, and 3000 Hz greater than 25 dB in either ear.
   b. Difference in average hearing level between the better and poorer ears of more than 15 dB at 500, 1000, and 2000 Hz or more than 30 dB at 3000, 4000, and 6000 Hz.

2. Periodic Audiograms
   a. Change for the worse in average hearing level in either ear compared to the baseline audiogram of more than 15 dB at 500, 1000, and 2000 Hz or more than 20 dB at 3000, 4000, and 6000 Hz.

The AAO-HNS also recommends the following medical criteria for referral:

1. History of ear pain; drainage; dizziness; severe, persistent tinnitus; sudden, fluctuating, or rapidly progressive hearing loss; or a feeling of fullness or discomfort in one or both ears within the preceding 12 months.

2. Cerumen accumulation sufficient to completely obstruct the earcanal.

The AAO-HNS emphasizes the importance of communication between the referring individual and the otolaryngologist.

These referral criteria are not mandatory, unlike the OSHA/MSHA follow-up procedures, but they are recommended as an important part of a hearing health program. The extent to which employees need follow-up examinations and treatment in addition to that specified by federal regulations should be a topic of discussion between the OHC and the supervising professional.

---

[40] A free copy of the AAO-HNS leaflet may be ordered by e-mail: **orders@entnet.org** or by calling the AAO-HNS headquarters at (703) 299-1121. It is also available on the organization's website, **www.aaohns.org.**

References

AAO-HNS (1997). *Otologic Referral Criteria for Occupational Hearing Conservation Programs.* American Academy of Otolaryngology–Head and Neck Surgery Foundation, Inc., Alexandria, VA.

DoD (April 22, 1996). Department of Defense Instruction No. 6055.12.

McCully, R. (1996). "Baseline audiograms." OSHA Standards Interpretations and Compliance Letters, 2-23-96.

NHCA (January 2001). "Professional guide for audiometric baseline revision." *Spectrum, 1,* suppl. 2.

NIOSH (1998). "Criteria for a recommended standard: Occupational noise exposure: Revised criteria, 1998." DHHS (NIOSH) 98-126. Dept. Health and Human Services, Public Health Service, Cincinnati, OH.

OSHA. (March 8, 1983). "Summary and explanation of actions taken." Occupational Noise Exposure; Hearing Conservation Amendment; Final rule, 48 *Fed. Reg.*, 9742–9772.

Quiz

1. The pure-tone audiogram is always a good predictor of how people understand speech in everyday living conditions. (True or False)

2. Under what conditions will people with sloping sensorineural hearing losses have the most difficulty understanding speech?

3 What are the air conduction and bone conduction symbols for left and right ears?

4. The technical term for a one-sided hearing loss is a _____ loss. When both ears show a hearing loss but one ear is considerably better than the other, it is referred to as an _____ loss.

5. A hearing loss that is relatively flat across frequencies is often characteristic of a _____ hearing loss.

6. What is the most common audiometric configuration for people who work in noisy environments?

7. A hearing loss that is partly conductive and partly sensorineural is called a _____ loss.

8. Tinnitus may be the cause of inconsistent audiometric responses. (True or False)

9. What should the OHC do if she or he feels that an employee is exaggerating the hearing threshold levels?

10. Is the definition of STS used by OSHA and MSHA an average shift greater than 10 dB at 2000, 3000, and 4000 Hz or an average shift of 10 dB or greater at 2000, 3000, and 4000 Hz?

11. In adjusting for presbycusis the appropriate amount is subtracted from the (baseline or current) _____ audiogram.

12. Besides the occurrence of a persistent STS, when should the baseline audiogram be revised?

13. OSHA requires all employees with a persistent STS to be referred to an audiologist or otolaryngologist. (True or False) Does MSHA?

14. Who should bear the responsibility for medical referral if an employee is unable to wear hearing protection because of a pre-existing external otitis?

15. The AAO-HNS referral procedures are not mandatory, but are a helpful adjunct to a hearing health program. (True or False)

Abbreviations Used in Chapter VIII

AAO-HNS	American Academy of Otolaryngology—Head and Neck Surgery
dB	Decibels
dBA	Decibels on the A scale of the sound level meter
DoD	Department of Defense
HTL	Hearing threshold level
Hz	Hertz
MSHA	Mine Safety and Health Administration
NHCA	National Hearing Conservation Association
NIOSH	National Institute for Occupational Safety and Health
OHC	Occupational Hearing Conservationist
OSHA	Occupational Safety and Health Administration
SPL	Sound pressure level
STS	Standard threshold shift
TTS	Temporary threshold shift
TWA	Time-weighted average exposure level

Recommended Reading

American Academy of Otolaryngology—Head and Neck Surgery Foundation, Inc. (1997). *Otologic Referral Criteria for Occupational Hearing Conservation Programs*. One Prince St., Alexandria, VA, 22314-3357.

NIOSH (1998). "Hearing loss prevention programs, (HLPPs)." Chapter 5 in *Criteria for a Recommended Standard: Occupational Noise Exposure: Revised Criteria, 1998*. DHHS (NIOSH) 98-126. Dept. Health and Human Services, Public Health Service.

Royster, J.D. (2000). "Audiometric monitoring phase of the hearing conservation program." Chapter 5 in E.H. Berger, L.H. Royster, J.D. Royster, D.P. Driscoll, and M. Layne, (Eds.), *The Noise Manual, Fifth Edition*. American Industrial Hygiene Assoc., Fairfax, VA.

Websites

www.aaohns.org
American Academy of Otolaryngology—Head and Neck Surgery

www.msha.gov
Mine Safety and Health Administration

www.hearingconservation.org
National Hearing Conservation Association (NHCA)

www.cdc.gov/niosh
National Institute for Occupational Safety and Health (NIOSH)

www.osha.gov
Occupational Safety and Health Administration (OSHA)

Chapter IX

Noise Measurement and Control

Introduction

The OHC is not expected to become an instant expert on noise measurement and control. In fact, most OHCs will probably not make any noise measurements, let alone decisions about controlling noise. Those who usually measure noise are noise control engineers and industrial hygienists, although a variety of personnel may perform this function if they have been sufficiently trained. They include various types of engineers, audiologists, and safety specialists.

But it is always a good idea for the OHC to have a rudimentary knowledge about noise measurement and control. Since the OHC is often the key person around whom the hearing conservation program revolves, she or he may need to coordinate the activities of others in this area and may even need to ensure that the OSHA and MSHA requirements are being met.

Purposes of Noise Measurement

There are three main purposes of noise measurement in industry: (1) to identify overexposed workers and quantify their exposures, (2) to assess the noise situation for potential engineering and administrative controls, and (3) to assess the background levels in audiometric test rooms.

Identifying and Quantifying Workers' Noise Exposures

Workers who are exposed to noise at or above the action level, an 8-hour TWA of 85 dBA, need to be included in a hearing conservation program; workers whose exposures exceed the 90-dBA TWA must wear hearing protectors.[41] MSHA requires miners exposed above a TWA of 105 dBA to wear dual hearing protectors (plug and muff concurrently). Workers' noise exposures must be measured to determine if they fall into either of these categories. In addition, noise exposures must be measured from time to time to make sure that they have not changed. Changes in equipment, work process, or scheduling may shift a worker from below the action level to above it, or even above the 90 dBA permissible exposure level (PEL), where hearing protection becomes mandatory. Likewise, changes may shift workers into lower exposure categories, where hearing protection may no longer be mandatory or even where a hearing conservation program is no longer required.

In addition, workers' noise exposures must be quantified to know how much attenuation is required from hearing protection devices. For example, if an employee's TWA is over 105 dBA, the OHC will know that a hearing protector with substantial attenuation is required (or dual protectors), as well as

---

[41] Workers in Washington state must wear hearing protectors when exposed at or above a TWA of 85 dBA.

close supervision of the use of that protector. If, however, the TWA is more like 92 dBA, it would be a mistake to select a protector with too much attenuation.

Noise measurements may also be used for educational and motivational purposes. Workers are often interested in the details of their exposures, especially when noise levels can be related to specific equipment. Software is now available that can link employees' TWAs not only to their job, but also to their audiometric test results. With this kind of knowledge they may be more willing to respect the integrity of noise control devices, wear their hearing protectors, and participate more fully in the hearing conservation program.

Finally, noise measurements may be useful if worker compensation claims are filed, since some jurisdictions give definitions of "hazardous noise levels" (see Appendix I). In addition, they are useful in the process of hearing conservation program evaluation in that they provide information about what may be expected from a certain work area. For example, an employee's deteriorating hearing levels are unlikely to be caused by workplace noise if the TWAs are consistently less than 85 dBA. He or she may have a medical problem or may be receiving considerable off-the-job noise exposure.

Assessing the Potential for Engineering Controls

Noise control engineers need to assess the levels and spectral qualities (frequencies) of the noise emitted by various machines and work processes. By doing so they can determine exactly which part of the process or machine is the major source of noise, in what order the noise problems should be tackled, and what type of noise control treatment will be the most effective and economical. These measurements need to be done with knowledge and precision so that funds are not wasted on ineffective or inappropriate controls.

Measuring the Background Levels in Audiometer Rooms

As explained in Chapter VII, it is important to keep the background noise levels to within specified limits for the audiometric test to be valid. To make sure that these levels are not exceeded, they must be measured regularly with a sound level meter (including an octave-band filter set) or a specially designed background noise monitor (see discussion in Chapter VII).

Instruments for Measuring Noise

The basic instruments for measuring industrial noise are the sound level meter, the noise dosimeter, and their calibrators. Noise control engineers often use additional equipment, such as tape recorders, sophisticated frequency analyzers, and vibration analyzers, but the OHC does not need to be concerned with these particular instruments.

Sound measuring equipment has been available for more than 60 years, although in recent decades it has become much more flexible and precise. The introduction of microcomputers has greatly expanded the range of possible noise measurements and the ease with which they can be made.

All instruments used for noise measurement should conform to the appropriate ANSI standards: American National Standard Specification for Sound Level Meters (ANSI S1.4-1983), American National Standard for Personal Noise Dosimeters (ANSI S1.25-1991), and American National Standard Specification for Acoustical Calibrators (ANSI S1.40-1984).

The Sound Level Meter

Use of the Sound Level Meter:

Sound level meters are often used in industry for conducting **area noise measurements**. This is to determine the noise levels near particular machines, in the aisles between machines, or in certain noisy locations that may be posted as "high noise areas." A **noise map** of an industrial plant, similar to a topographic map, may be constructed using area noise measurements. These measurements do not necessarily reflect individual employee's noise exposure measurements unless the noise is continuous, as in a textile weaving plant.

Sound level meters can be used to assess employees' noise exposures, even when the noise levels vary somewhat, but it is usually a complicated and time-consuming project to use them. Before the advent of noise dosimeters, the engineer or industrial hygienist would follow the worker with a sound level meter and stopwatch, recording the noise levels and the amount of time the worker was exposed to each level. Today this is almost always done automatically with a dosimeter.

Measuring the background levels in audiometer rooms, calibrating audiometers, and assessing the need for engineering controls are other important uses for sound level meters, as stated previously. For many of these purposes the sound level meter must include attachments or possess more sophisticated capabilities than the simple, general purpose model.

Important Features of Sound Level Meters:

Type: The two types of sound level meters most often used in industry are the **general purpose** meter (**Type 2**) and the **precision** sound level meter (**Type 1**). Figure 9-1 shows an example of both the Type 1 (left) and Type 2 (right) sound level meters.[42] There is also a Type S, which stands for "special purpose" that is not usually used in industry because it tends to have limited capabilities, such as a limited dynamic range or only one weighting network (the A scale). The general purpose sound level meter should be adequate for virtually all the measurements taken for the hearing conservation program. According to the American Standard Specification for Sound Level Meters (ANSI S1.4), the allowable **tolerances** (accuracy limits) for Type 2 are ± 1.5 dB in the mid-frequency range (100 Hz–1250 Hz), and somewhat greater for the lower and higher frequencies.[43] OSHA requires the use of a sound level meter that meets or exceeds the Type 2 specifications, although MSHA makes no specific requirements.

Another type of sound level meter that deserves mention is the **integrating/averaging** sound level meter (usually just referred to as the "integrating" sound level meter), which is especially useful when noise levels fluctuate considerably. It contains the same basic functions of Type 1 or 2 meters, but it samples the sound level according to a predetermined schedule and averages the responses logarithmically over a prescribed period of time.

Basic sound level meter characteristics: There are certain characteristics of the basic sound level meter that OHCs should be familiar with. Most of these instruments show the sound level output with a liquid crystal display (LCD) in tenths of a decibel. The **dynamic range**, (usually referred to as just the "range"), is often selectable for low (e.g., 30–100 dB) or high (e.g., 70–140 dB) settings. You can also choose between the **A-** and **C-**weighting networks, using the A network for most occupational noise measurements, and the C network when the contribution of low-frequency noise is of interest or when you want to assess the effectiveness of hearing protector attenuation (more on this in Chapter X).

Basic sound level meters also have a switch to

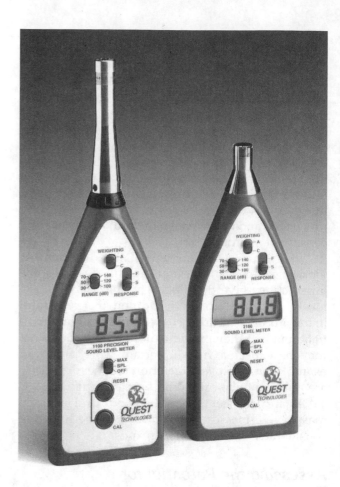

Fig. 9-1 A Type 1 precision sound level meter (left) and a Type 2 general purpose sound level meter (right). (Courtesy of Quest Technologies, Inc.)

choose between **"slow"** and **"fast" meter response**. The term "meter response" refers to the time the meter takes to reach its final reading. The concept was initiated to "slow the meter down" sufficiently to make it easier to read the values consistently. The slow meter response is standardized at 1 second and the fast response at 0.125 second. For most purposes, OSHA requires the use of the slow meter response.

If there is some concern that an impulse noise may have exceeded the 140-dB level, the meter's **"peak"** or **"instantaneous"** setting should be used.[44] In the peak mode, the meter is required to measure an impulse as short as 100 microseconds. Some meters also offer an **"impulse"** mode but, ironically, this setting should not be used for measuring industrial impulses (or impacts) because it does not measure the true *peak* sound pressure level.

---

[42]Although these two meters look much the same, there are internal differences.

[43] Some may wish to use a precision sound level meter to measure the background levels in audiometer rooms because measurements are required up to 8000 Hz. The Type 2 tolerance at this frequency is ±5 dB, whereas the Type 1 tolerance is tighter, +1.5 and −3 dB. Unless there is an unusual problem with high-frequency background noise, however, this should not be necessary, and there are Type 2 sound level meters, when coupled with octave band filter sets, that can do the job.

[44] While most Type 2 sound level meters have the capability of measuring peak sound pressure levels, there are a few that do not. If there are high levels of impulse noise in the work environment, the user should make sure to select a meter that has this feature.

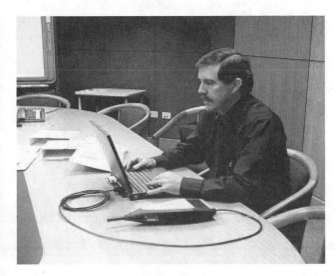

Fig. 9-2. Downloading data from a sound level meter to a lap-top. (Courtesy of Brüel & Kjær)

Special sound level meter characteristics: Not only Type 1 sound level meters, but also many Type 2 meters offer a variety of special characteristics. The OHC who wants only to take "spot checks" will not need these special features, but most sound level meters can perform a large variety of functions for those who want to take advantage of them. Many will measure according to the 3-dB exchange rate as well as the OSHA/MSHA 5-dB rule, and some offer 4 dB (for certain DoD agencies) or even 6 dB as well. Some have extended dynamic ranges (e.g., 30–140 dBA), and quite a few are capable of integrating and logging data and creating files. The files may be stored within the sound level meter and later transferred to a computer and printed out. Figure 9–2 shows the process of downloading data from a sound level meter to a laptop computer.

Microphones: Even though microphones for industrial use have increasingly been manufactured to be rugged, the microphone is still the most fragile part of the sound level meter, and it is one of many reasons why the meter should not be dropped. Most Type 2 instruments will be accompanied either by a ceramic or a condenser microphone. The ceramic microphone is fairly resistant to wear and tear, but tends to be susceptible to temperature changes. The condenser, or "condenser electret," is usually more expensive, tends to be more accurate in the high frequencies, and is somewhat more fragile. Type 1 sound level meters will almost always use a condenser microphone. Both types of microphones should be stored away from high levels of humidity.

Most microphones manufactured in the U.S. will be calibrated to be "**random-incidence**" microphones that should be held at a slight angle (70 to 80 degrees) to a direct sound source. European microphones are usually calibrated to be "**free-field**" microphones and should be pointed directly at the

sound source. To be on the safe side, the manufacturer's instructions on microphone placement should *always* be followed.

Attachments: Whenever sound levels at specific frequencies are to be measured, some sort of frequency analyzer must be used. The most practical way to do this in the occupational setting is to attach an **octave band filter set** to the sound level meter, as seen in Figure 9-3.[45] This enables a person to measure the sound energy in each octave band, for purposes of assessing the background levels in audiometer rooms or to identify the noisiest frequencies emitted by a particular machine.

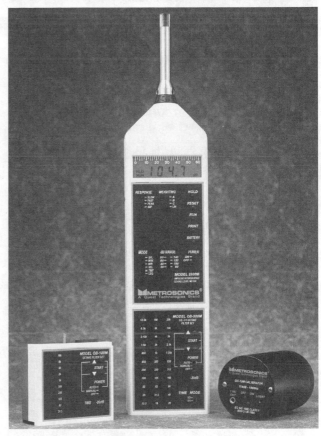

Fig. 9-3. Type 2 sound level meter with octave-band filter set (left), ⅓ octave band filter set (attached to meter) and calibrator (right). (Courtesy of Metrosonics)

Another useful attachment is the **windscreen**, which fits snugly over the microphone. Seen in Figure 9-4, it reduces the effects of air movement on sound level measurements. Even when there is relatively little perceptible wind, it is a good idea to use a windscreen, not only outdoors but also in large indoor spaces.

---

[45] Some sound level meters contain built-in frequency analyzers, so it is not always necessary to attach them or have them attached.

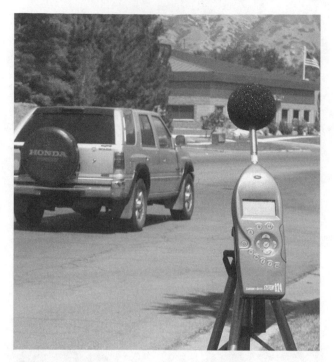

Fig. 9-4. A windscreen should be used indoors as well as outdoors whenever there is some movement of air. (Courtesy of Larson-Davis Laboratories)

The Noise Dosimeter

The noise dosimeter is a small, integrating sound level meter that calculates the noise dose automatically. It is worn clipped to the belt or to a shirt pocket with the microphone placed in the vicinity of the ear, preferably attached to the clothing at the top of the

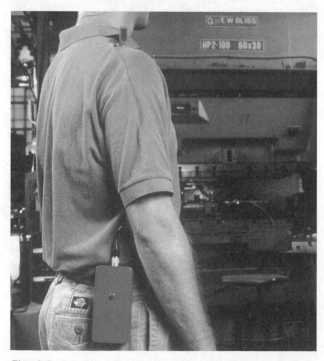

Fig. 9-5. A noise dosimeter as worn on the job. (Courtesy of Quest Technologies)

shoulder. Figure 9-5 displays a dosimeter as it is worn by a worker and Figure 9-6 shows the instrument at close range.

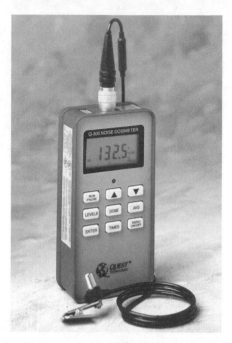

Fig. 9-6. Example of a noise dosimeter. (Courtesy of Quest Technologies)

Dosimeters can perform a great variety of functions, many of them simultaneously. All of the major manufacturers of acoustical equipment make noise dosimeters that can "profile" or "log" a worker's noise exposure. They measure, store, and analyze the data; and when connected to a printer or computer they will produce hard-copy printouts of a worker's noise exposure history. The history may include a number of pertinent statistics, such as the time (by the minute) of the noise exposure, the noise level and dose at specific times, the dose at the end of a period, the maximum and minimum noise levels, and noise level histograms, etc.

Many of these instruments allow the user to set the exchange rate (3, 4, or 5 dB) and the lower threshold, the level in dBA below which the instrument does not measure. OSHA and MSHA specify a lower threshold of 80 dBA or below for compliance with the action level, and many dosimeters will begin measuring at 70 dBA or below. Some people prefer to set the lower threshold at 90 dBA to assess compliance with OSHA/MSHA requirements for engineering controls, but this practice is not recommended because the dosimeter will fail to integrate all sound levels below this point, treating them as if they are completely harmless. The ear does not conform to such abrupt demarcations. Those who use this lower cutoff are probably complying with the letter of the noise regulations, but certainly not with the spirit.

Most dosimeters can compute doses using either the A- or C-weighting networks, and some instruments will measure A and C noise doses simultaneously. This function may be helpful for making calculations of hearing protector attenuation using the NRR. Today's dosimeters can also give measurements based on fast, slow, and instantaneous response, as well as other meter dynamics, and some will measure and store the dose using both the 3-dB and 5-dB exchange rates, which can be helpful if you want to compare the results using the OSHA/MSHA method with results using the NIOSH/ACGIH/international method. Most of them have very large dynamic ranges over which they can measure accurately, some as large as 110 dB. In addition they have the capacity to measure accurately short-duration, high-level impulses. These instruments can also be used as sound level meters as well as dosimeters.

Government agency inspectors usually rely on dosimeters to assess compliance with noise regulations, using the sound level meter mainly as a back-up instrument. All dosimeters should, of course, comply with the specifications of the American National Standard for Personal Noise Dosimeters (ANSI S1.25-1991).

Calibrators

Calibration is a necessary part of any noise measurement. Most professionals advocate checking the calibration of the instrument before and after each period of use. A typical calibrator is shown in Figure 9-7, and Figure 9-8 shows a calibrator being applied to the microphone of a sound level meter. Calibrators should be purchased at the time of purchase of the sound level meter or dosimeter and must be compatible with the instrument with which they will be used. Their performance should meet the requirements of American National Standard Specification for Acoustical Calibrators (ANSI S1.40-1984), and they should be returned to the factory or laboratory for periodic calibration.

It is also good practice to send sound measuring equipment back to the manufacturer periodically for a thorough calibration, since the calibrator will not be able to detect all problems. A two-year interval is considered appropriate for this level of calibration, although meters that are heavily used should be sent back more often.

Regulatory Requirements for Noise Measurement

Although most of the requirements for noise-exposure monitoring have been discussed in Chapter VI, they will be summarized again below

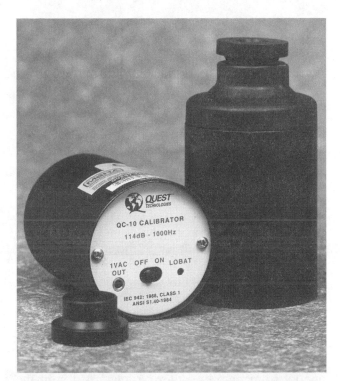

Fig. 9-7. A sound level calibrator with adaptor rings for different-sized microphones. (Courtesy of Quest Technologies)

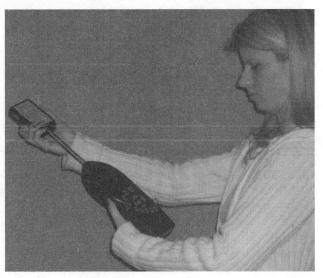

Fig. 9-8. A sound level meter's calibration is being checked. (Courtesy of Larson-Davis Laboratories)

and supplemented with a discussion of OSHA's mandatory Appendix A and the comparable appendix in the MSHA regulation. Readers are urged to study the exact wording of the OSHA and MSHA requirements in Appendices C and G of this manual.

The OSHA requirement for noise measurement should be considered a performance regulation as opposed to a specification regulation, leaving most of the details of noise measurement procedures, instruments, and calibration up to the employer or the professional who performs the measurements.

MSHA's requirements are even less specific, basically that the mine operator must establish a monitoring system that is sufficient to determine compliance with the regulation (see Section 62.110 in Appendix G of the manual).

The OSHA regulation calls for the monitoring of all employees exposed to TWAs of 85 dBA and above, and for feasible engineering controls to be instituted at TWAs of 90 dBA and above. Area monitoring is permitted, but "representative personal sampling"[46] must be performed when there is a high degree of worker mobility, significant variations in sound level, or a significant component of impulse noise present in the work environment. What is meant by "significant" is not defined, but left to the employer (or the professional making the measurements).

Both OSHA and MSHA require the integration of all sound levels between 80 dBA and at least 130 dBA to comply with the 85-dBA action level. OSHA specifically requires all continuous, intermittent, and impulsive noise to be included in the assessment of noise exposure, which means that the sound energy from impulses *must* be integrated with the other types of noise. (This is only possible with a dosimeter or integrating sound level meter.) A footnote to the regulation's Table G–16 states that exposure to impulsive or impact noise should not exceed a peak sound pressure level of 140 dB and, as mentioned above, the possibility of this occurrence should be measured with the "peak" setting on the sound level meter. These two measurement procedures are not incompatible; they merely give different types of information. MSHA requires the integration of all sound levels from 90 dBA to at least 140 dBA for measuring compliance with the PEL.

Both OSHA and MSHA specify that employees or their representatives must be given the opportunity to observe the monitoring and *they must be notified of the results* (a requirement that companies often seem to miss). MSHA requires that miners be notified in writing within 15 days of the exposure determination.

Compliance with OSHA's Appendix A is mandatory, as is MSHA's Appendix to Part 62, so these materials should not be overlooked. The OSHA appendix gives examples for computing noise dose from sound levels in the worker's environment and the durations of exposure at each level. These computations will not usually be necessary because most employers will choose to use dosimeters for this purpose. It is interesting to note, however, that Table G-16a gives a range of reference durations from 32 hours for a level of 80 dBA to 0.031 hour at a level of 130 dBA.[47] This not only means that all of these levels must be included in the measurements, but that durations longer than 8 hours must be assessed as well. Flexible work plans that include 10- and 12-hour work shifts are increasingly common. Some occupations, such as long-distance truck driving, may entail noise exposures during "rest" periods as well as work hours. If these long durations are an integral part of the employee's job, the noise exposures should be included in the assessment of dose.

As mentioned earlier, both OSHA and MSHA consider a TWA of 90 dBA to be 100 percent dose. This TWA is based on an 8-hour exposure duration. If the duration is shorter, higher noise levels are permitted. Likewise, if the duration is longer than 8 hours, the permissible average level is lower than 90 dBA. According to OSHA's Table G-16a and MSHA's Table 62-1, the "reference" or allowable duration for a 12-hour shift is 87 dBA; for a 16-hour shift it is 85 dBA and for a 20-hour shift it would be about 83.5 dBA.

An employee's noise dose, which is read from the dosimeter in terms of percentages, may be converted to the equivalent 8-hour TWA by using OSHA's Table A-1 or MSHA's Table 62-2. By reading these tables you can see that a dose of 87 percent is equivalent to an 8-hour TWA of 89 dBA, 150 percent is equivalent to an 8-hour TWA of about 93 dBA, 300 percent is equivalent to about 98 dBA, and so forth.

Some Tips on Making Noise Measurements

It is not enough to have good equipment, well-cared-for and calibrated. Those who make noise measurements must know when and what to measure, how to do it, and how to make sure they have taken sufficient measurements. While this chapter does not constitute an instruction manual, there are certain practical matters that the OHC should at least be aware of.

Know when and whom to measure: Not all employees who work in noisy environments need noise monitoring. Strictly speaking, those whose

---

[46] OSHA does not require the monitoring of every single noise-exposed worker if all the workers in a certain group appear to be similarly exposed. In this case the employer may select one worker for monitoring. If there is any difference in their exposures, the employer should select the worker whom he/she believes has the highest noise exposure to represent the group.

[47] The inclusion of levels above 115 dBA does not mean that exposure to these levels is permitted for continuous noise or even intermittent noise. (See discussion of this topic in Chapter VI.) A logical question would be: Why did OSHA stop at 130 dBA when noise above this level is even more hazardous? The answer is that at the time the hearing conservation amendment was drafted the range from 80 to 130 dBA represented the limits of dosimeter technology. Today's dosimeters have much broader dynamic ranges, so it would make no sense to ignore any sound levels above 130 dBA should these high levels occur. MSHA's Table 62-1 stops at 115 dBA for a period of 15 minutes, and carries a requirement that "at no time shall any excursion exceed 115 dBA." Again, this does not mean to ignore sound levels above 115 dBA, but those who measure them should know that such levels are in violation of MSHA's regulation.

TWAs are below 85 dBA do not need to be monitored. But how are you to know who falls above and who falls below this criterion? The rule of thumb is that when employees have difficulty communicating at a distance of about 3 feet, the noise levels are above 85 dBA. Other signs of excessive noise levels are the occurrence of tinnitus or a "dullness" of hearing (or TTS) at the end of the work shift. When in doubt, it is always wise to go ahead and make noise measurements. Moreover, documentation of TWAs below 85 dBA may be useful for legal and administrative purposes.

Plan ahead: Arrangements should be made ahead of time to secure the cooperation of management, supervisors, union health and safety representatives, and other key personnel. Then, it is always a good idea to walk through the area or plant to be measured, assessing the situation with nature's built-in sound measuring system—the ears. This will help with decisions regarding the most appropriate type of equipment, whether to use area or personal monitoring (or possibly both), and where to concentrate your efforts.

Familiarize yourself with the equipment: Presumably those who perform the noise monitoring will be thoroughly familiar with their equipment, will have studied the manufacturer's instructions, will know the type of microphone and therefore the correct microphone incidence, will have checked the instrument's calibration before taking the measurements, and will check it again afterward.

In addition to holding the sound level meter at the correct incidence with respect to the sound source, it is important to hold it away from the body to minimize the reflections and shielding that the body may cause.

When taking measurements of background levels in audiometric test rooms it is important to make sure that the sound level meter is capable of measuring sound levels low enough to comply with the appropriate criteria (preferably the ANSI S3.1-1999 standard). In other words, it makes no sense to use a meter whose "**noise floor**" (lower limit of measurement) at 500 Hz is at 30 dB when you want to measure down to 21 dB. Also, the OHC must remember that a sound level meter with only the A-weighting, or A- and C-weighting networks, is not sufficient for measuring background levels in audiometric booths. A meter that can measure octave-band noise levels is required. These kinds of problems should be addressed before purchasing the instrument.

Be mindful of wind and weather: It is good policy to use the microphone's windscreen whenever measurements are taken out-of-doors, or even when there is some air movement indoors. (When in doubt, use the windscreen.) Dosimeters also have small windscreens that fit snugly over their microphones. Outdoor noise monitoring in rainy weather

should not be performed; even monitoring in high humidity should be limited depending on the manufacturer's suggestions. Temperature extremes may cause problems for certain microphones, in which case the manufacturer's instructions should be followed.

Take sufficient measurements: If a sound level meter is used exclusively, it is important to make sure that enough measurements are made to describe an employee's noise exposure adequately. In most cases employers will choose to use dosimeters for this purpose, but in the event that a dosimeter is not available, the person who makes the measurements needs some guidance as to the number of samples (measurements) that are needed. The correct number is contingent upon the amount of fluctuation in the noise level. Sampling guidelines are available in the textbook chapter by Royster, Berger, and Royster listed at the end of this chapter.

Measure impulse noise correctly: Some years ago one school of thought advocated measuring impulse noise separately from other types of noise, such as continuous and intermittent noise. The theory was that the original OSHA regulation was unclear on how to measure impulse noise. When OSHA issued the hearing conservation amendment, the agency clarified the issue by stating explicitly that all types of noise should be added into the assessment of dose—including impulse noise—for compliance with all parts of the OSHA noise regulation. MSHA's requirement is similar: to integrate all sound levels over the appropriate range. The only practical way to do this assessment is to use a dosimeter or an integrating sound level meter. This does not preclude taking measurements of the peak sound pressure level, as stated above, which should be done using the "peak" or "instantaneous" settings on the sound level meter or dosimeter (not the "impulse" setting), to see if the 140-dB peak has been exceeded.

ANSI guidelines for noise measurement: There is an ANSI standard for measuring occupational noise exposure, ANSI S12.19-1996 (R2001), which includes topics such as calibration, measurement conditions, microphone placement, and many other practical matters. The standard's Annex A contains methods for calculating employee noise exposures using a sound level meter and timing device. The standard allows the use of a basic sound level meter to assess worker exposure when the sound level of an activity is steady, which is defined as varying no more than ±2.5 dB. When the levels vary more than that amount, a dosimeter or integrating sound level meter must be used.

The scope of the standard applies to users who are proficient, or under the direction of a person who is proficient in noise measurement. This statement could well apply to the whole topic of noise measurement.

Noise Control

Those responsible for developing and implementing noise control solutions will usually be trained as engineers, industrial hygienists, or safety specialists. In most cases, the professional of choice will be the noise control engineer since this person's training and expertise enables her or him to do the job the most effectively. In the absence of a noise control specialist, the OHC may need to be the one who identifies noise problems that would be candidates for noise control, and he or she may have to advocate for the funds to perform the work. In addition, the input of workers should always be sought since they are often the ones who have the most intimate knowledge of their machines. Their participation in the fact-finding process and their support of the noise control treatments increase the chances for a successful project. The OHC may be the one who acts as liaison between workers and noise control professionals.

Sometimes engineering controls are thought of in a separate category from hearing conservation programs. Actually, they should be considered an integral part of an effective hearing conservation program. Of all the program's elements, noise control is the best long-term solution to the prevention of noise-induced hearing loss. In some cases these controls may be extremely expensive and hearing protectors are needed to do the job indefinitely. But noise control may be accomplished quite reasonably in many other situations, and it can often be cost effective. This is where the ingenuity of those who have a thorough knowledge of the machines and work processes plays a part.

Some practical advice on noise control in articles written by noise control engineer and CAOHC member Beth Cooper, has appeared in issues of the *UPDATE*. They are reprinted as Appendix M of this manual. Cooper points out several advantages of noise control; among them are:

- Reduction in the time and expense of other hearing conservation measures such as audiometric testing and hearing protectors for employees whose exposures no longer exceed a TWA of 85 dBA.
- Prevention of noise-induced hearing loss—eliminating the noise problem is the most effective way.
- Improvements in safety, productivity, and communication. For example, noise reduction can make it easier for employees to hear radio communication as well as important sounds like paging and warning signals.
- Noise control may also eliminate an adverse effect on the neighboring community (which especially applies to construction noise).

Briefly, noise control is accomplished in three ways: by controlling the **source**, the **path**, and the **receiver**.

Source: The most effective way to control the noise source is to design a quieter method of carrying out an industrial process or to purchase a quieter piece of equipment. Managers may accomplish this by including requirements for noise limits when specifying new machines or building new plants. But existing machinery can also be quieted in a variety of ways. These include isolating a vibrating machine to cut down on the noise radiating from it, reducing the speed of a particular machine, or reducing the pressure of a compressed air device. For example, noise can be controlled by decreasing the velocity of air flow or by substituting mechanical ejection for compressed air. Existing noise sources may also be retrofitted with quieter parts. Damping material can be applied to the sides and bottom of bins in which parts are dropped. Sometimes simple maintenance procedures, such as replacing worn bearings, can lower noise levels considerably. These changes can lead to increased efficiency or a reduction in energy expended, and consequently improve cost-effectiveness. In other cases the cost of controlling noise may be excessive and treatments to the path or receiver may be preferable.

Path: Reducing the noise along its path may involve building an enclosure around a noisy machine or tool. Enclosures should be carefully designed so that the worker's ability to control or repair the machine is not adversely affected. If the noise control treatment is the type that must be removed for maintenance of the machinery, the employer may need to monitor its use to make sure that employees put it back on afterward. This is particularly true if the maintenance employees did not participate in the final design of the treatment. Other treatments to impede the transmission of noise along its path include the use of sound-absorbing materials on walls and ceilings to reduce the reflection of sound waves indoors and fixing noise "leaks" by repairing or replacing parts. Also, barriers or large curtains—made of loaded vinyl or other heavy materials—may be erected or hung around noisy areas. These methods are mainly effective at controlling high-frequency noise.

Receiver: Finally, noise can be controlled in the receiver's immediate environment by constructing a booth or control room around the worker. That way the worker may do the job with only occasional excursions into the noisy environment. While this method may work quite well, it can cause a feeling of isolation. A booth that is big enough for two or more people to communicate may be helpful. Controlling the noise at the receiver's end of course includes the use of hearing protection devices.

Administrative Controls

One more approach to noise control that deserves mention is the use of administrative controls—the policy of rotating workers out of noisy jobs to prevent them from exceeding the action level or the PEL. Presumably, non-noise-exposed workers would then take their places. In actuality, this kind of administrative control is not used very often because it tends to disrupt established work practices and interfere with union contracts. Besides, even though individuals' exposures are somewhat reduced, this practice can spread the risk to a greater number of workers.

This use of administrative controls should not be confused with the practice of providing workers with quiet rest areas and cafeterias, which can facilitate recovery from TTS, even though they do not necessarily reduce the hazardous dose. Average sound levels in these areas should be kept below 70 dBA to the extent possible.

Feasibility

Both the OSHA and MSHA regulations give priority to the use of feasible engineering and administrative controls. Strictly speaking, employers are to require the use of hearing protectors above the PEL (a TWA of 90 dBA) only in circumstances where engineering controls are not feasible or while they are in the process of being installed. There has been a great deal of controversy about the concept of feasibility, however, and in recent years the courts have interpreted it, at least in OSHA cases, as including economic as well as technological feasibility. Unfortunately, while there is quite a bit of information about the technological feasibility of noise control, there is relatively little information available about its economic feasibility.

Another disincentive for the use of engineering noise control is OSHA's current policy, discussed in Chapter VI, which allows employers to substitute "effective" hearing conservation programs for engineering controls between TWAs of 90–100 dBA. Several of the larger companies, however, have not adopted this approach, but prefer to use engineering controls above 90 dBA or even 85 dBA whenever feasible. As stated previously, OSHA's policy could be withdrawn at any time, and MSHA enforces the use of engineering controls above the PEL. Engineering noise control should always be the goal for long-term solutions to the adverse effects of noise.

References

ANSI (1983). American National Standard Specification for Sound Level Meters. ANSI S1.4-1983 (R2001). Acoustical Society of America, Melville, NY.

ANSI (1984). American National Standard Specification for Acoustical Calibrators. ANSI S1.40-1984 (R2001). Acoustical Society of America, Melville, NY.

ANSI (1991). American National Standard Specification for Personal Noise Dosimeters. ANSI S1.25-1991 (R1997). Acoustical Society of America. Melville, NY.

ANSI (1996). American National Standard Measurement of Occupational Noise Exposure. ANSI S12.19-1996 (R2001). Acoustical Society of America. Melville, NY.

Quiz

1. What are the three main purposes of noise measurement in the occupational setting?

2. The Type _____ sound level meter is adequately precise for most occupational noise measurement conditions.

3. The integrating sound level meter and noise dosimeter average sound levels _____ (arithmetically or logarithmically).

4. For most purposes OSHA requires the _____ (fast or slow) meter response.

5. When measuring the peak sound pressure level of an industrial impulse, one should use the sound level meter's "impulse" setting. (True or False)

6. The main reason why the sound level meter (or dosimeter) should not be dropped is so that the _____ will not be damaged.

7. What is the purpose of the octave band filter set?

8. Many dosimeters can _____ a worker's noise exposure, in that they can keep a time history of the noise exposure throughout the work shift that may be converted into hard copy.

9. Government agency inspectors rely primarily on _____ (sound level meters or dosimeters) to enforce the noise regulation.

10. When should the calibration of sound measuring equipment be checked?

11. OSHA requires the integration of impulse noise into the assessment of worker noise dose. (True or False)

12. Both OSHA and MSHA require the integration of all sound levels between _____ dBA and _____ dBA to comply with the action level.

13. How would you find out the allowable TWA for a 12-hour work shift? What is this level?

14. Before taking any measurements, what are three indications that noise levels in the work environment exceed 85 dBA?

15. It is good practice always to use a _____ when taking measurements outdoors or indoors in large spaces.

16. The three basic types of engineering controls are to control noise at the _____, _____, and _____.

17. Name at least three advantages to performing noise control in the occupational setting.

Abbreviations Used in Chapter IX

ACGIH	American Conference of Governmental Industrial Hygienists
ANSI	American National Standards Institute
CAOHC	Council for Accreditation in Occupational Hearing Conservation
dB	Decibels
dBA	Decibels measured on the A scale of the sound level meter (or dosimeter)
DoD	Department of Defense
Hz	Hertz
LCD	Liquid crystal display
MSHA	Mine Safety and Health Administration
NIOSH	National Institute for Occupational Safety and Health
NRR	Noise Reduction Rating
OHC	Occupational Hearing Conservationist
OSHA	Occupational Safety and Health Administration
PEL	Permissible exposure level
TTS	Temporary threshold shift
TWA	Time-weighted average exposure level

Recommended Reading

ANSI (1996). R2001 (1996). American National Standard Measurement of Occupational Noise Exposure. ANSI S12.19-1996 (R2001). Acoustical Society of America, Melville, NY.

Cooper, B.A. Reprints from *UPDATE* (see Appendix M).

Driscoll, D.P., and Royster, L.H. (2000). "Noise control engineering." Chapter 9 in E.H. Berger, L.H. Royster, J.D. Royster, D.P. Driscoll, and M. Layne, (Eds.), *The Noise Manual, Fifth Edition*. American Industrial Hygiene Assoc., Fairfax, VA.

Earshen, J.J. (2000). "Sound measurement: Instrumentation and noise descriptors." Chapter 3 in E.H. Berger, L.H. Royster, J.D. Royster, D.P. Driscoll, and M. Layne, (Eds.), *The Noise Manual, Fifth Edition*. American Industrial Hygiene Assoc., Fairfax, VA.

Measuring Sound. Booklet produced by Brüel & Kjær, 2850 Naerum, Denmark, 1984.

OSHA (1980). *Noise Control: A Guide for Workers and Employers*, available on the Noise Pollution Clearinghouse website; **www.nonoise.org**.

Royster, L.H., Berger, E.H., and Royster, J.D. (2000). "Noise surveys and data analysis." Chapter 7 in E.H. Berger, L.H. Royster, J.D. Royster, D.P. Driscoll, and M. Layne, (Eds.), *The Noise Manual, Fifth Edition*. American Industrial Hygiene Assoc., Fairfax, VA.

Website

www.nonoise.org
Noise Pollution Clearinghouse

Chapter X

Hearing Protectors

Worker Acceptance

There used to be a saying among industrial hygienists and safety specialists that if hearing protectors didn't hurt they were not doing the job. Fortunately that is no longer true, if indeed it ever was. It is true that hearing protection is not everybody's favorite thing and, as with many types of safety equipment, workers would much prefer not having to bother with it. But by interacting with employees in a persistent and sensitive manner, the OHC can play a critical role in the extent to which they will accept hearing protection devices. Workers are more apt to wear hearing protectors if they are encouraged to participate actively in the hearing conservation program, if they fully understand the need for protectors, and if they are given a choice of types and brands. Acceptance is also more likely to occur if employees are convinced that hearing protectors are an interim solution; in other words, if the workers understand that the company has an engineering control plan and can see that the plan is being implemented.

The NIOSH Criteria Document lists several important factors that determine the extent to which workers will accept hearing protectors and wear them consistently (NIOSH, 1998, p. 64):

- Convenience and availability
- Belief that the device can be worn correctly
- Belief that the device will prevent hearing loss
- Belief that the device will not impair the ability to hear important sounds
- Comfort
- Adequate noise reduction
- Ease of fit
- Compatibility with other personal protective equipment

These factors don't just happen; the OHC needs to train and work with employees to convince them of the advantages of hearing protectors and ensure that the right device is selected.

Success of the program also depends on the tone that management sets. If upper management supports the hearing conservation program, the company should have a policy that everyone—from the corporate CEO to the foreman to occasional visitors—should wear hearing protectors in noisy areas. If the hearing protectors are earplugs, even visiting dignitaries should make sure that they are properly inserted, and not treated merely as a formality.

If OHCs are to be effective in this area, they must be well informed about hearing protectors. This involves doing some outside reading, being familiar with the pertinent regulatory requirements, and talking with distributors and others who are familiar with the various products. OHCs should make sure that the employer offers a variety of appropriate types of protectors, not just the one plug and one muff required by OSHA or, in the case of miners, the two of each type required by MSHA. It is always good practice for OHCs themselves to try out every type of protector the company offers and, if possible, to wear each protector for an extended period of time. By doing this they will develop first-hand knowledge of the fitting, insertion, attenuation, comfort, and other qualities of the protectors.

Types of Hearing Protectors

The three basic types of hearing protection devices are earplugs, earmuffs, and semi-inserts. A fourth category, that of special protectors, will also be discussed.

Earplugs

A properly selected, fitted, and inserted earplug can provide considerable attenuation (noise reduction) and can be worn comfortably for many hours at a time. These devices come in many shapes, sizes, and materials.

User-Molded Earplugs:

Probably the most popular plug at present is the **user-molded** or **formable** plug, manufactured out of soft polymer foam. The foam plug is sometimes referred to as the "roll-down" plug, since it needs to be compressed before it is inserted. Other user-molded plugs include the "glass down," silicone putty, and the wax-impregnated cotton varieties. Figure 10-1 shows a collection of these types of earplugs.

Figure 10-2 gives an example of a popular foam earplug. This particular one comes in two sizes and may be attached by a cord.

Premolded Earplugs:

Another common type is the **premolded** earplug, as seen in Figure 10-3. These devices are formed from flexible materials like foam, vinyl, silicone, or similar materials, and may include one or more flanges or sealing rings. They are flexible and durable, usually come in a range of sizes, and they have a stem or tab for ease of insertion and removal. Correct sizing and fitting are particularly important with this type of plug. Ear gauges are available from some manufacturers to aid in this process, but they cannot substitute for careful fitting with the actual plug. Whenever a multi-sized plug is used, the OHC should be sure to order the full range of sizes.

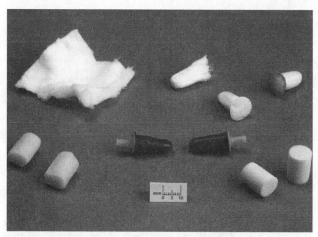

Fig. 10-1 A group of user-molded ear plugs. (Courtesy of E·A·R/Aearo Company)

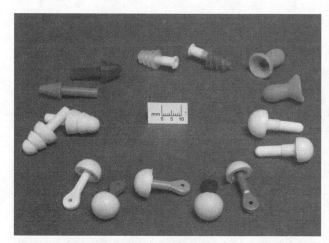

Fig. 10-3. Medley of premolded earplugs. (Courtesy of E·A·R/Aearo Company)

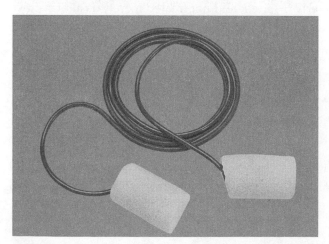

Fig. 10-2. Pair of corded foam plugs. (Courtesy of E·A·R/Aearo Company)

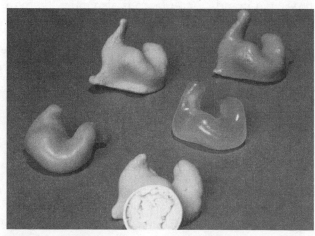

Fig. 10-4. Examples of custom-molded earplugs. (Courtesy of E·A·R/Aearo Company)

Custom-Molded Earplugs:

A third type, seen in Figure 10-4, is the **custom-molded** earplug, which is made from a mold of the individual employee's earcanal and concha. While somewhat more expensive than the other types, it may give workers added satisfaction because it is custom-made for each person. Also, because it follows the individual ear's contours, it may be easier to insert correctly. OHCs should be aware, however, that the earcanal impression for a custom-molded earplug must be made by an individual with considerable skill, otherwise the plug will not fit well or attenuate effectively.

Earmuffs

The use of earmuffs has been evident to air travelers for decades because they are often worn by airline mechanics and baggage handlers. They are also common in other occupational situations, but are not as widely used as earplugs.

Earmuffs consist of plastic cups attached by an adjustable headband. The earcups fit snugly against the head by means of cushions that are filled with foam or liquid. Some earmuffs are meant to be worn with the band only over the head, while with others the band may be worn behind the head or under the chin if they are to be used in conjunction with a hard hat or other safety equipment. They do not come in various sizes, although some types and brands of muffs are smaller or larger than others. In other words, they have to be individually fitted, not just handed out.

An example of a large-volume earmuff is shown in Figure 10-5. These muffs usually provide more attenuation than the smaller-volume devices, especially in the low and middle frequencies.

The small-volume muff, seen in Figure 10-6, can be useful for work in confined spaces and when conditions allow somewhat lower levels of attenuation.

Figure 10-7 shows an earmuff–hard hat combination. The muffs are fitted into a slot on the hard hat

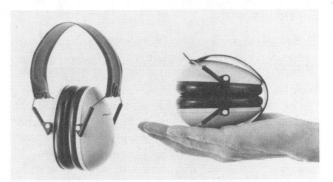

Fig. 10-6. A small-volume, folding earmuff. (Courtesy of Peltor)

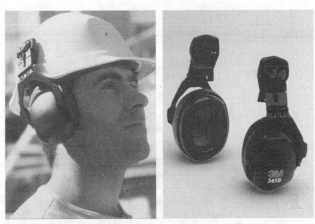

Fig. 10-7. Earmuff attached to a safety helmet (left); earmuffs detached (right). (Courtesy 3M Occupational Safety and Environmental Health Division)

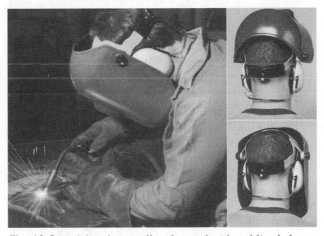

Fig. 10-8. Back-band earmuffs to be used with welding helmets or other types of hoods and safety gear. (Courtesy of Peltor)

and they can be turned out and away from the helmet when not in use. The necessary tension is provided by a spring-loaded device.

Earmuffs can also be an integral part of other safety equipment. Figure 10-8 displays a back-band set of muffs that can be used with welding helmets or other types of hoods and face shields. Manufacturers often sell muffs that can be used with or attached to a variety of safety gear in addition to hard hats, such as rain shields, safety glasses, and visors with various kinds of face shields.

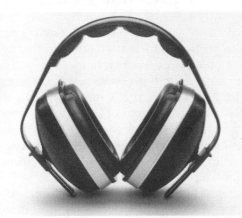

Fig. 10-5. A large-volume earmuff. (Courtesy of Bilsom, a Bacou-Dalloz Company)

Semi-Inserts

Semi-inserts, sometimes referred to as **canal caps** or **banded earplugs**, are pictured in Figure 10-9. They consist of earplug-like tips connected by a lightweight headband. The semi-insert devices having pod-type tips, which actually extend into the ear-canal, are likely to provide slightly greater attenuation than the cap-type models. Semi-inserts are usually intended for short-duration, on-and-off wearing, since they are sometimes uncomfortable if worn for extended periods of time. They should not be worn in very high levels of noise because their attenuation may not be sufficient.

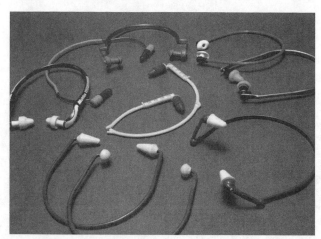

Fig. 10-9. Medley of semi-insert hearing protectors. (Courtesy of E·A·R/Aearo Company)

Dual Protection

"**Dual protection**," sometimes referred to as "**double protection**," is the condition where earplugs are worn in combination with earmuffs. Dual protection can be helpful in very high noise levels or when levels of about 105 dBA are experienced over long periods of time. The OHC should note that the resulting attenuation rating is *not* doubled. OSHA presumes an increase of about 5 dB over the attenuation of the better device alone. The increase is somewhat larger in the low frequencies when an earmuff is worn over a properly inserted foam plug, and this can be useful in high levels of industrial noise.

According to an OSHA interpretation letter, employers can require the use of dual protection, especially if an employee demonstrates progressive noise-induced hearing loss (Miles, 1994). The MSHA regulation actually requires dual protection at TWAs above 105 dBA. The NIOSH criteria document recommends dual protection at exposures greater than 100 dBA. OHCs need to be careful, however, to require or recommend dual protection only during high noise level exposures to prevent problems with overprotection (to be discussed at more length later in the chapter).

Special Protectors

There are some useful devices designed to improve the ability to communicate and hear warning signals in situations where hearing protection must be worn. These devices include **level-dependent** protectors, **noise-cancelling** protectors, and **communication headsets**. Hearing protectors with "**uniform attenuation**" (meaning similar amounts of attenuation across the frequency spectrum) are also helpful when communication is important, and although they are categorized here as special protectors, they will be discussed, later in this chapter, in the section on hearing protectors and communication.

Level-Dependent Protectors:

Level-dependent hearing protectors, sometimes called **amplitude-sensitive** or **nonlinear** protectors, provide different amounts of attenuation, depending on the sound level in the employee's environment. They can be particularly useful during the quiet periods of intermittent noise exposure. They are intended to allow low and moderate levels of sound to enter the ear naturally, while attenuating high-level sounds. This way they should enable the wearer to hear speech and warning sounds while providing protection against noise at hazardous levels. Some protectors accomplish their intended purpose more successfully than others, so OHCs should obtain as much information as possible before making a selection. These devices may be divided into the categories of "**active**" and "**passive**."

Active hearing protectors use electronic circuitry to accomplish the level-dependence. One type, called **sound transmission** earmuffs, uses an amplifier to permit the passage of low and moderate level sound; then at a level of 85 or 90 dB, the amplification stops and the muffs attenuate like ordinary earmuffs.

Passive level-dependent hearing protectors may take the form of earplugs or earmuffs. Passive earplugs attempt to attenuate high-level sounds by means of small holes or valves, while allowing low-level sounds to enter. The effectiveness of these plugs is limited since most of these devices provide the major portion of their attenuation in the high frequencies, and the level dependency is activated only at very high sound pressure levels. However, a recent military design, the "Combat Arms" earplug, provides a greater degree of level-dependence in a color-coded, dual-ended earplug. Worn with one end in, it provides a passive level-dependency, but turned around with the other end in it performs as a conventional earplug.

Passive level-dependent attenuation is more promising with earmuffs. For example, there is a commercially available passive earmuff that uses a valve system to accomplish the level-dependence.

This muff also gives significant attenuation in the low and mid frequencies as well as the high frequencies at high sound levels. This relatively "flat" attenuation across frequencies can be beneficial to speech communication. But because most of these devices don't start to increase their attenuation until levels of at least 110 dB, their best use is to protect the wearer from impulse noise, mainly from gunfire.

Noise-Cancelling Hearing Protectors:

Noise-cancelling hearing protectors, often referred to as **active noise-reduction** devices, generate a signal within the protector itself that cancels certain incoming sounds. Noise-cancelling protectors are most effective at reducing low-frequency noise. The extra low-frequency protection can be helpful in environments that are dominated by low-frequency noise, such as locomotive cabs, military vehicles, and certain industrial settings. Although they are expensive, noise-cancelling protectors can be effective, and in some situations, worth the added cost.

Communication Headsets:

When communication is a necessary part of the job, some companies may choose to purchase communication headsets for their employees. An example of such a device is shown in Figure 10-10. The receiver is built into the earmuff, providing radio communication (FM, infrared, or wired systems) and the muff attenuates the noise in the worker's environment. The microphone is often of the "noise-canceling" type, which allows better communication. Some of these headsets have limiting devices to prevent the radio signal from attaining hazardous levels. A recent development is a commercially available

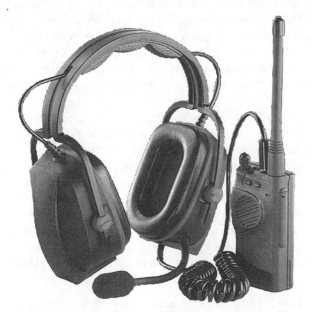

Fig. 10-10. An earmuff communication headset. (Courtesy of Bilsom, a Bacou-Dalloz Company)

communication system that is connected to an earplug so that an earmuff may be worn over it for protection in very high noise levels. Although they can be expensive, noise-attenuating communicating systems may prove to be invaluable when safety and efficiency are important factors.

Recreational Headsets:

Ordinary radio earphones provide little useful attenuation and are not recommended for use by personnel in a hearing conservation program. The foam earphones that often accompany portable radios and CD players provide virtually no attenuation. Moreover, if an employee listens to music through headsets, there is the temptation to turn the volume high enough to override the background noise, which can lead to temporary or permanent hearing loss as well as reduce the ability to hear necessary communication and warning sounds.

An OSHA interpretation memo discourages the use of recreational headsets in occupational noise environments and cites situations where typical headset outputs were 99–100 dBA (Anku, 1987). The memo states that headsets that limit music sound levels to 90 dBA would be permitted by OSHA, but management should be aware that these devices may pose a hazard to hearing.

Advantages and Disadvantages of the Different Types

Earplugs—Pros and Cons

If they are fitted and worn correctly, earplugs are often more comfortable than earmuffs for long wearing periods. They are cooler in hot weather, easier to wear in confined spaces, and more comfortable because of the lack of headband pressure. They are generally cheaper than muffs (except for the "disposable" earplugs) and are compatible with hard hats and other safety gear.

On the other hand, the attenuation of earplugs is more variable than that of earmuffs because they are more dependent on proper fitting and insertion practices. Their use is more difficult to monitor by a supervisor because they are not as obvious, and they are easier for the worker to lose. Earplugs may be difficult to use in an intermittent noise environment, especially when communication is required during quiet periods, because they may need to be taken in and out. (The premolded plugs attached by a long cord, however, may be as satisfactory as earmuffs in intermittent noise.) Also, some types of plugs tend to work loose simply from chewing or talking and need to be reinserted.

Frequent reinsertion may be a particular problem in environments where there is a lot of dust, dirt, or metal shavings, especially with user-molded plugs. Employees should roll down and insert user-molded plugs with clean hands only, and this is often inconvenient. Custom-molded plugs may receive better acceptance than other varieties, although they are not a panacea. Their effectiveness may be compromised unless the individual who makes the earcanal impression (mold) is very skillful.

Earmuffs—Pros and Cons

Earmuffs are easier to fit to most individual head shapes and sizes, and their attenuation is less variable in actual use than earplugs. Their use is generally easier to enforce because they are so visible, although the supervisor is not always able to identify muffs that have become worn out, cracked, or "modified" to cover transistor radios. Earmuffs are comfortable in cold environments, and they tend to have slightly greater attenuation than most plugs at 500 Hz and 1000 Hz. They are particularly suited for intermittent or occasional use because they are not subject to many of the reinsertion problems described above.

Certain disadvantages to earmuffs are that the headband pressure can become quite uncomfortable for extended wearing periods; and in hot weather, perspiration can collect under the earcup, causing discomfort and annoying sounds in the earcanal and concha. Compatibility with other safety gear can be a problem, especially when worn in conjunction with safety glasses. The muff's cushion will tend to press against the temple bars, particularly when the temple bars are thick, causing discomfort as well as a leak in the muff's attenuation. A small pad that fits around the temple bar can relieve the discomfort, but it is usually accompanied by some loss of attenuation. If it means that both pieces of safety equipment will be worn, however, the trade-off may be worthwhile.

Semi-Inserts—Pros and Cons

The most important advantage of semi-insert protectors is that they can be put on and taken off quickly and easily, making them very convenient for short-duration intermittent exposures. But their attenuation tends to be less than that offered by other types of protectors, particularly in the low frequencies. As mentioned above, some of these protectors may be uncomfortable if worn for extended periods, but others can be fairly comfortable, so OHCs should try a variety of devices, preferably on themselves first.

An additional drawback to semi-insert protectors is that the **occlusion effect** is most noticeable with these devices. This is the term used to describe the low-pitched, hollow sound of one's own voice when the earcanal is covered at its entrance.[48] The occlusion effect also occurs to a lesser degree when earplugs are inserted only minimally and with small-volume earmuffs. Semi-inserts with tips that are inserted in the canals, like earplugs, produce less occlusion effect than those that merely cap the earcanals.

Another common complaint with semi-inserts is that hitting or bumping the headband can produce a sound that is annoying to the wearer. This is less likely to occur when the band is worn over the head than when it is worn under the chin.

Hearing Protection and Communication

A Justified Complaint

Employees frequently complain that hearing protectors interfere with the ability to hear certain crucial communications, including instructions or warnings from other workers, audible alarms, and the sounds of their machinery malfunctioning. These problems may be compounded by the tendency of well-meaning safety and health professionals to provide as much attenuation as possible by selecting the protector with the highest **Noise Reduction Rating** (**NRR**).

In the past, audiologists and industrial hygienists have told workers that hearing protectors would actually enhance their abilities to hear speech and warning signals because the protector would attenuate the desired signal and the noise by the same amount. The sound levels of both the signal and noise would be reduced to a more comfortable listening level with less distortion. There is some truth to this argument, especially for communication in very high noise levels. But evidence is now available that shows instances where hearing protectors can be a communication problem (e.g., Hörmann et al., 1984; Lazarus, 1983; Suter, 1992). For example, one communication problem arises from the fact that people who wear hearing protectors tend unconsciously to reduce their voice levels because the occlusion effect makes them think their voices are louder than they really are (Tufts, 2002).

In intermittent noise conditions, hearing protection users typically have increased difficulty hearing speech and warning signals when the noise level drops below about 85 dBA. This is why there is a tendency to remove the protectors during intermittencies (the relatively "quiet" periods). But even in much

---

[48] Readers can experience the occlusion effect simply by covering their ears with the palms of their hands and noticing the change in their vocal quality.

higher noise levels, hearing protectors can interfere with the perception of speech or warning signals when workers already have some hearing loss.

Additional Problems of the Hearing-Impaired

Workers with existing hearing losses will often resist wearing hearing protectors because they have trouble hearing important sounds of their machines, speech communication, or warning sounds. These claims can be quite valid.

For these reasons, some workers will want to wear their hearing aids in the workplace. Although this desire is understandable, the hearing aid can create additional problems by amplifying noise to unsafe levels. For example, one study found that even a mild-gain (low power) hearing aid increased exposures from 83 dBA to nearly 92 dBA (Dolan and Maurer, 2000). Moreover, hearing aid earmolds, even with the aid turned off, do not usually offer as much attenuation as a properly worn plug or muff (Berger, 1987).

OHCs should therefore discourage the use of hearing aids in noisy areas, but they must also be sensitive to the problems of hearing-impaired workers and seek the safest possible solution, whether it is controlling the noise in some way or providing specialized hearing protectors.

Most hearing protectors attenuate the high frequencies quite a bit more than the lower frequencies. Sensorineural hearing loss, which is the most common type of hearing loss among adults, also affects the high frequencies more than the lower frequencies. The combination of these characteristics causes many of the consonant sounds, whose energy is mainly in the high frequencies, to be inaudible. Speech to the hearing-impaired person wearing a high-frequency attenuating hearing protector can sound like a muffled, incomprehensible blur.

There is also a potential safety hazard when hearing protectors, added to hearing impairment, make warning sounds inaudible. Accidents and fatalities have occurred when high levels of noise have drowned out warning signals (Laroche et al., 1995), and the use of hearing protectors may, in some situations, compound the problem (Suter, 1992).

Localization

Another problem, more characteristic of muffs than plugs, is interference with the ability to localize a sound—to identify the direction that a sound is coming from. The ability to localize in the vertical plane is particularly impaired by earmuffs. This could have serious implications for construction workers or other employees who need to be able to identify the sources of sounds above and below their positions (Suter, 1992).

Solutions

The dilemma the OHC faces is that hearing protectors can interfere with speech and warning signals on the one hand, but on the other hand the absence of protection can lead to hearing loss. There is no easy solution to this dilemma. Eliminating the noise hazard is the most obvious one, but that is not always possible. In addition, there are certain kinds of hearing protectors that can be helpful. Today both plugs and muffs are commercially available with attenuation fairly evenly spread across the frequency spectrum, which are referred to as protectors with **uniform** or **flat** attenuation (Berg and Hiselius, 2000). The advantage of these protectors is that they reduce the low-frequency noise as, or nearly as, effectively as they do for high-frequency noise. This way they avoid the pitch "imbalance" that often occurs with conventional protectors. By attenuating the high frequencies only moderately, they allow better speech perception than protectors that attenuate heavily in the high frequencies. OHCs should be aware that most of these protectors provide the benefits of flat attenuation only as long as they are inserted or worn properly.

These hearing protectors generally provide more moderate attenuation with a lower NRR than many others. This is actually a beneficial characteristic because high levels of attenuation are not necessary in most industrial environments. For noise exposures between 85 dBA and 90 dBA, which are typical of most industries, an NRR of 29 is unnecessary. In fact, it may be overkill and encourage non-use of the protectors.

In addition to hearing protectors with uniform attenuation, other types of protectors, like the level-dependent protectors and communication headsets described above, can often be beneficial. Employers should also give consideration to other safety features, such as visual warning signals, vibrating beepers, or more efficient auditory signals. For these solutions the OHC may want to consult a noise control engineer or industrial hygienist.

OHCs need to remember the old adage that the only effective hearing protector is the one that is worn, and they must educate those in charge of purchasing equipment that **overprotection is not a good idea**. Most hearing protectors with uniform attenuation are somewhat more expensive than conventional protectors because special design features may be required to effect the desired response (although some are quite reasonably priced). There may be situations where communication headsets or active attenuators are the best solution, which would be an added expense. However, the benefits in terms of successful communication, hearing saved, and accidents avoided are likely to be well worth the expense.

Use and Care of Hearing Protectors

Regulatory Requirements

Sections (i), (j), and (k) of OSHA's noise regulation and Section 62.160 of the MSHA regulation outline the employer's responsibilities for hearing protectors. OHCs should be thoroughly familiar with these requirements, which are found in Appendices C and F of the manual. They state that employees must be given the opportunity to select their hearing protectors from a variety of suitable hearing protectors. This requirement has been interpreted to mean that employers should offer at least a plug and a muff, and preferably three or more devices. An OSHA interpretation memo states that the term "suitable" means "comfortable to wear and that offer sufficient attenuation to prevent hearing loss" (Miles, 1983). The MSHA regulation requires that employees be able to choose from a selection that includes at least two plugs and two muffs, and when dual hearing protectors are required, to choose one of each type.

Both regulations state explicitly that employees must be trained in the fitting, care, and use of hearing protectors. Workers must be trained in the purpose of hearing protectors, the advantages, disadvantages, and attenuation of various types, and be given instruction on their selection, fitting, use, and care. Moreover, the employer is responsible for ensuring that hearing protectors are worn, and worn correctly.

Fitting and Insertion

By now the OHC knows that no hearing protector should be merely handed out without fitting it individually. This applies to muffs and semi-inserts as well as plugs. Heads come in different sizes and shapes, and what is a perfect muff for one person may not do at all for another. Figure 10-11 illustrates that point very well. Also, some muffs are designed with left and right ears specified, while others may be worn in either orientation.

Before fitting any hearing protector the OHC should visually inspect the ear. When fitting earplugs, the inspection should be done with an earlight or an otoscope. Any signs of infection should rule out the use of plugs until the infection has been successfully treated. If there is a minor infection it may be permissible for the employee to wear an earmuff, but if there is any pain or drainage, no hearing protection should be worn. A small amount of cerumen is normal and should not interfere with the wearing of an earplug. But if there is excessive cerumen, it can become impacted and possibly cause problems. When in doubt, it is best to have the employee examined by a health professional.

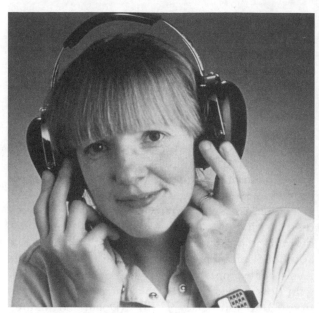

Fig. 10-11. Earmuffs do not fit all head sizes. (Courtesy of E·A·R/Aearo Company)

If the employee's condition prohibits the use of either plugs or muffs, the employee should not be exposed to high levels of noise. This may mean that the employee is not able to work in his or her regular job until medical clearance is obtained. Because it is the employer's responsibility to provide a safe and healthful workplace, the employee must not be penalized for any temporary layoff due to the inability to wear hearing protection.

When dealing with a multi-sized plug, the OHC should select the plug that feels reasonably comfortable, but fits snugly. Inexperienced fitters tend to select plugs that fit too loosely; this can cause the wearer discomfort because to achieve the desired attenuation the plug must be pushed in too far. Also, the OHC should keep in mind that individuals will often wear different sizes in each ear.

A useful technique for inserting any kind of earplug is illustrated in Figure 10-12, where the subject reaches around his head with the opposite hand, grasps the pinna, and pulls it gently up and out. This helps to straighten out the earcanal.

When inserting the foam plug, the plug should be rolled tightly between the thumb and forefinger[49] (with clean hands), inserted while still compressed well into the earcanal, and held for a few moments until it has expanded to fill the canal and its entrance.

A properly inserted plug can be seen to block the earcanal, and the user will say that it muffles the noise. Depending on the degree of occlusion effect, the user may report that his or her own voice sounds somewhat louder and lower in pitch. If the fitting is

---

[49] When rolling down foam earplugs, regardless of their initial shape, they should be rolled into a tight crease-free cylinder before insertion.

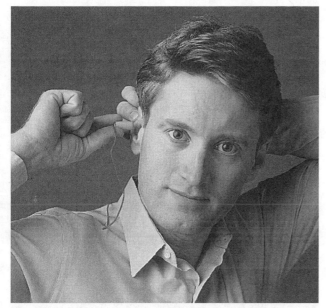

Fig. 10-12. Reaching in back of the head to grasp the pinna and pulling it slightly up and out makes it easier to insert an ear plug. (Courtesy of 3M Occupational Safety and Environmental Health Division)

done in a quiet place the OHC may want to turn on a radio or some other sound source to help the user decide when the optimum attenuation has been achieved. When a premolded plug with a stem has been correctly inserted, there should be some tension on the stem when trying to remove it.

The drawing in Figure 10-13 demonstrates a properly (left) and improperly (right) inserted foam

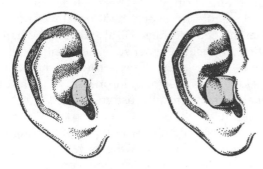

Fig. 10-13. Properly (left) and improperly (right) inserted foam plugs. (Courtesy of E·A·R/Aearo Company)

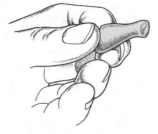

Fig. 10-14. Example of a foam earplug after removal from an earcanal in which it has been allowed to expand for about a minute. (Courtesy of E·A·R/Aearo Company)

earplug. The drawing in Figure 10-14 shows what a foam earplug should look like after it has been allowed to expand in the earcanal for about a minute before removal. Note that about half of the plug is compressed into the shape of the earcanal, with no creases or folds.

The next set of photographs shows the contrast between properly and improperly inserted hearing protectors: glass down in Figure 10-15; premolded plugs in Figure 10-16; and semi-inserts in Figure 10-17.

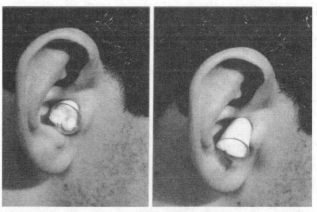

Fig. 10-15. Properly (left) and improperly (right) inserted glass down earplug. (Courtesy of E·A·R/Aearo Company)

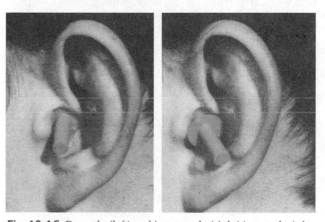

Fig. 10-16. Properly (left) and improperly (right) inserted triple-flanged premolded plug. (Courtesy of E·A·R/Aearo Company)

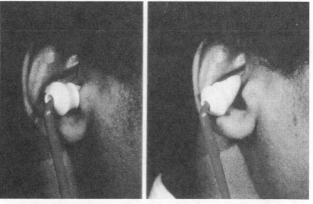

Fig. 10-17. Properly (left) and improperly (right) inserted pod-type semi-inserts. (Courtesy of E·A·R/Aearo Company)

The OHC should be aware that the premolded plug should be removed slowly. If there is an effective seal and it is removed too rapidly, the eardrum can be painfully distorted and, in rare cases, even damaged. This is not true of the foam or fiberglass varieties.

One method to test the effectiveness of the fit of earplugs is to cup both hands and place them over the ears while listening in a background of noise. If the earplugs are fitting properly there will be little perceptible difference in the noise level between the hands-cupped and hands-away positions.

Some of the same hints for fitting earplugs apply to the fitting of the insert type of semi-inserts. Also, it may help to wiggle the pods or canal caps back and forth to make sure that the best seal is obtained.

When fitting earmuffs the OHC should make sure that the flexible cushions completely surround the pinna and when it is properly adjusted that the headband rests on the top of the head. Each earcup should be checked to make sure that it seals tightly against the head and that the seal is not interrupted by an individual's facial contours or by excessive hair. Hats or other headgear should not interrupt the seal of the muffs, and the temple bars of eyeglasses should be as thin as possible. The OHC should also remember that comfort is always important, and that headband pressure that is too great will result in unused earmuffs. If a particular muff does not provide a good seal or if it is not comfortable, the OHC should try another type or brand.

For additional tips on fitting hearing protectors, see Appendix L.

Hygiene

Premolded earplugs should be washed and earmuff cushions should be wiped off regularly. Although some prefer to dispose of them after every use, foam plugs can also be washed and reused several times.[50] Some OHCs tell employees to save up a number of used foam plugs, tie them into an old piece of pantyhose, and throw them into the washing machine with other clothes. This practical bit of advice seems to work very nicely. Employees should be discouraged from sharing hearing protectors.

Replacement

No hearing protector lasts forever, not even heavy-duty earmuffs. The covering on the muff's cushions will eventually harden and fail to provide an adequate seal. The cushions should be checked every six months and replaced as necessary. In addition, the headband tends to loosen with age or it can

become sprung (sometimes deliberately to make it more comfortable) and fail to provide the necessary pressure to hold the ear cups tightly against the ears. Figure 10-18 shows two pairs of earmuffs, one with the headband distorted to the point that its attenuation would be significantly reduced.

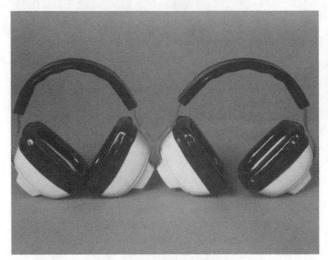

Fig. 10-18. The headband of the earmuff on the right has been distorted so that it will not fit tightly against the head and provide the intended attenuation. (Courtesy of E·A·R/Aearo Company)

Foam earplugs should be discarded if they fail to recover their original shape when they are taken out of the ear. Premolded plugs may last for months, or they may shrink and harden within a matter of weeks depending upon the characteristics of the wearer's cerumen and skin oils. These plugs should be checked regularly every two or three months. Custom-molded earplugs will also shrink and harden with time, reducing their effectiveness, and should be checked periodically. Even routine anatomical changes, such as weight gain or loss, can affect the earcanal, and, as a result, custom-molded plugs may no longer fit snugly.

The OHC should check all types of hearing protectors for modifications by the user. Such modifications can make the protector more comfortable, but significantly degrade its attenuation. Examples would be springing the muff's headband or drilling holes in the earcups. With plugs, the flanges may be cut off or the whole plug can be cut in half. These modifications may not always be visible from the outside, but they will sabotage the protector's intent. A good time to check protectors for wear and tear or any kind of modification is during the audiometric test, although all hearing protectors should be checked more often than once a year.

Wearing Time

Most workers probably don't realize that if they remove their hearing protectors in high levels of

---

[50] Foam plugs cost only a few cents apiece when they are purchased in bulk. However, they are among the most expensive protectors if they are thrown away after each use.

noise, even if only for a few minutes, the protection offered will be substantially reduced. The higher the NRR (and the higher the noise level) the greater will be the reduction in effectiveness. If workers have a tendency to remove protectors because of discomfort, the OHC should fit them with a more comfortable model, even if the NRR is lower. If workers tend to remove protectors when they need to communicate, the OHC should try to fit them with a protector offering uniform attenuation, or perhaps another special protector or communication system. OHCs should also train workers to put protectors on before entering noisy areas. A protector with only moderate attenuation can be more effective than a heavy-duty protector if it is the one that is worn continuously in hazardous noise levels.

Wearing Protectors Away From Work

Figure 10-19 shows good use of hearing protectors off the job. Because non-occupational noise exposure can be a significant contributor to noise-induced hearing loss, employees should be encouraged to use hearing protection when engaging in activities such as target shooting, hunting, attending concerts with loud music, using woodworking tools, or even mowing the lawn. The best way to promote these practices is to allow, or better yet to encourage, workers to take their protectors home. If this means purchasing an extra pair of muffs for certain workers, the company needs to understand that this kind of generosity is in everyone's best interest.

Hearing Protector Attenuation

The NRR

Hearing protector attenuation is measured in the

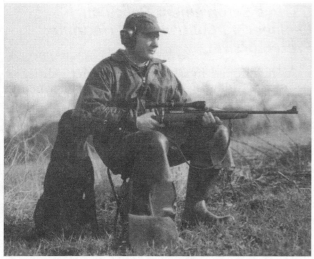

Fig. 10-19. Hearing protectors should be used off the job as well. (Courtesy of Bilsom, a Bacou-Dalloz Company)

laboratory with a standardized procedure called **"real-ear attenuation at threshold."** Noise signals at a variety of frequencies are presented to trained listeners with and without hearing protectors, and the difference between the two conditions reflects the protector's attenuation. The examiner then combines the attenuation values for the frequencies tested over a series of tests and makes some adjustments to the data. The resulting number is the Noise Reduction Rating or NRR. The U.S. Environmental Protection Agency (EPA) requires hearing protector manufacturers to print the NRR on the protector's package. The main purpose of the NRR is not to predict exactly what the worker will or will not hear with the protector in place, but to enable the purchaser to choose from among a variety of protectors.

Regulatory Requirements

OSHA:

Section (j) of the OSHA regulation gives the requirements for evaluating the attenuation of hearing protectors as they are to be used on the job. Hearing protectors must attenuate most employees' exposures at least to a TWA of 90 dBA, but if an employee has experienced a standard threshold shift the protector must attenuate at least to a TWA of 85 dBA. To be on the safe side, many employers will choose a protector whose NRR will reduce the exposure to 85 dBA, regardless of the occurrence of an STS.

The regulation also states that the protector's attenuation should be evaluated (with respect to the employee's noise exposure measurement results) to see if the protector is providing sufficient attenuation. The employer[51] must provide more effective hearing protectors when necessary. Although the regulation does not specify how often the employer should perform this evaluation, it should be done on a regular basis, at least once a year.

Employers are given a choice of methods by which to estimate the adequacy of hearing protector attenuation. These methods are given in the regulation's (mandatory) Appendix B. Employers *may* use any one of three methods developed by NIOSH and described in its "List of Personal Hearing Protectors and Attenuation Data" (NIOSH, 1975), but the simplest and by far the most commonly used is the NRR.

When using the NRR, the employer should subtract the protector's NRR from the C-weighted noise-exposure level (TWA) in the worker's environment. This is the way the EPA designed the NRR to be used.

---

[51] The regulation actually uses the word "employee" when it should say "employer." One can see by the context that this is a typographical error.

The most convenient way to obtain the C-weighted TWA is with a dosimeter that uses the C- as well as the A-weighting networks. Lacking that, the employer may use a sound level meter set on the C-weighting network and take enough measurements to estimate the TWA.

Employers who are unable to make C-weighted measurements may use the A-weighting network, but first they must subtract 7 dB from the protector's NRR to account for the lack of spectral information incurred by not having C-weighted measurements. The OHC should note that the 7 dB adjustment is *not* meant to account for the difference between laboratory and "real-world" use. Instead it accounts for the absence of a proper assessment of the contribution of low-frequency noise, which the C network supplies.

MSHA:

MSHA's noise regulation does not require any particular method for evaluating the attenuation of hearing protectors for the work environment in which they are to be used. The Program Policy Letter merely states that a hearing protector must have an NRR or some other "scientifically accepted indicator of noise reduction" (Nichols and Teaster, 2000).

Field Attenuation

Not long after OSHA's hearing conservation amendment was promulgated, the professional community became aware that the performance of hearing protectors in the field (in actual use) was not nearly as favorable as the NRR would indicate. Hearing conservation professionals, including NIOSH contractors, used special equipment to assess the attenuation that workers received from hearing protectors on the job. A series of studies using a variety of hearing protectors showed that the actual field attenuation that workers received was only about one-third to one-half the attenuation they received in the laboratory. In addition, the variability among wearers, as shown by the standard deviation, was two to three times greater than in the laboratory.

The graph in Figure 10-20 shows the difference between real-world results, averaged over 22 field studies, compared to laboratory data. You can see that the "NRR" derived from the field studies is significantly lower than the laboratory-based NRR. In fact, some earplugs show attenuation values that are only a small fraction of what would be predicted by the NRR. In general, earmuffs and foam earplugs seem to perform better in actual use than the other earplugs, since most of them offer an on-the-job attenuation of at least 10 dB. Some plugs, however, show field NRRs of only 2 or 3 dB.

The attenuation values portrayed in Figure 10-20 are not conventional averages (means or medians), but are calculated the same way the NRR is calculated. Amounts representing the variance (standard deviations) have been subtracted from the mean attenuation, which reduces the final value. For illustrative purposes, the author of this graph, Elliott Berger, has subtracted only one standard deviation from his "field NRR," instead of the usual two standard deviations that are subtracted in calculating the laboratory NRR. If he had subtracted two standard deviations from the field data averages, some protectors would yield an NRR of 0 dB. In fact, some wearers of hearing protectors actually receive no attenuation at all, but most will receive at least a few decibels.

There are many reasons why workers do not receive as much attenuation from hearing protectors as laboratory subjects. First of all, in the conventional laboratory procedure, subjects are usually highly trained listeners and the experimenter selects and inserts the earplugs in the subjects' ears or places the muffs. The protectors are sized carefully and plugs are usually inserted very tightly. After all, these subjects can put up with discomfort for the duration of the test, but workers can hardly be expected to tolerate these conditions for long periods of time.

Most people who are occupational users of hearing protectors, on the other hand, have had little training in the proper insertion of hearing protectors. They tend to fit these devices fairly loosely, for reasons of comfort or the need to communicate, or simply because they do not know how to insert them correctly. In addition, the protectors will attenuate less efficiently as they age, as mentioned above, and may loosen from chewing or talking. All of these factors indicate a need for vigilance on the part of the OHC and the entire hearing conservation team.

OSHA's Enforcement Policy on Engineering Controls and Hearing Protectors

As mentioned in Chapter VI, OSHA's Office of Health Compliance Assistance issued Instruction CPL 2-2.35 in 1983, guidelines to its inspectors for enforcing the noise regulation. While the guidelines applied only to federal OSHA inspectors, every state OSHA program except North Carolina has adopted them.

Briefly, the guidelines instructed inspectors not to cite a company for failing to use feasible engineering or administrative controls between TWAs of 90 and 100 dBA unless the company did not have "an effective hearing conservation program." Unfortunately, OSHA never gave an explanation of exactly what constituted an effective hearing conservation

Labeled vs. Field Attenuation

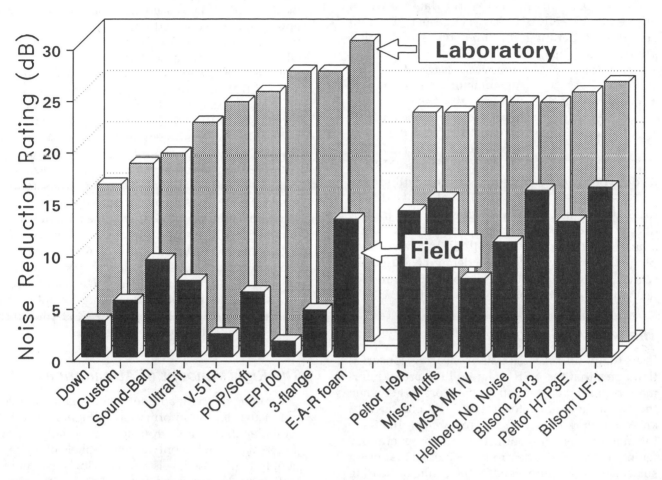

Fig. 10-20. This graph contrasts the attenuation received in actual use with that found in laboratory evaluations. The laboratory NRRs are calculated in the conventional manner using a two-standard deviation subtraction. The field "NRRs" are calculated using a one-standard deviation subtraction. These data were analyzed and combined by Elliott Berger from the results of 22 field studies. (Courtesy of E·A·R/Aearo Company)

program. OSHA did, however, instruct its inspectors to derate the hearing protector's expected attenuation by 50 percent when assessing the relative effectiveness of hearing protectors and engineering controls according to these enforcement guidelines.

For example, an employee in a textile weaving plant could have had an A-weighted TWA of 98 dBA, and the company did not intend to reduce the exposure through engineering controls. Her employer did not have access to a dosimeter with a C-weighting network and did not wish to estimate the C-weighted TWA with a sound level meter. The hearing protector she used had an NRR of 24 dB. The OSHA inspector would, therefore, subtract 7 dB from the NRR, which would give 17 dB. Derating the NRR by 50 percent would give 8.5 dB, and subtracting that from her TWA of 98 dBA would yield 89.5 dBA. According to OSHA's enforcement policy, this worker's employer would just barely be in compliance with the regulation. If, however, she had previously experienced an STS or not yet received a baseline audiogram, the company would not be in compliance because, in that case, the derated NRR must attenuate to at least 85 dBA.

No doubt, the motivation for this enforcement policy was economic and political, an attempt to relieve employers of any potential burdens from costly engineering controls. But the OSHA staff was aware of the field studies on hearing protector attenuation and the dangers of relying on the NRR.

The reader must bear in mind that this enforcement policy is not a regulation. OSHA did not go through the procedural requirements, including public involvement, necessary in the making of a regulation. Therefore this policy does not have the power of law and it could be withdrawn by the agency at a moment's notice. On the other hand, it may be the agency's practice for some years to come and it is useful information for the OHC. It is also important to remember that MSHA has no equivalent policy and requires engineering controls for compliance with its PEL.

The NIOSH Recommendations for Derating

On the basis of the real-world data shown in Figure 10-20, NIOSH has suggested different amounts of derating for three types of hearing protectors (NIOSH, 1998):

- Earmuffs — Subtract 25% from the manufacturer's labeled NRR
- Foam earplugs[52] — Subtract 50% from the manufacturer's labeled NRR
- All other earplugs — Subtract 70% from the manufacturer's labeled NRR

For example, with an earmuff whose NRR is 24 dB, you would reduce its NRR to 18 dB for use with C-weighted TWAs (a 25% derating of 6 dB), or to 11 dB for use with A-weighted TWAs (a 25% derating of 6 dB, plus a 7-dB spectral uncertainty adjustment because of use with dBA). With a foam plug whose NRR is 29 dB, the derated NRR for use with dBC measurements would be 14.5 dB, and for use with dBA measurements it would be 7.5 dB.

The New ANSI Standard

Virtually all professionals in hearing conservation agree that the NRR provides little useful information about the attenuation that workers get when they wear these protectors on the job. Consequently, an ANSI working group has researched this issue for many years and conducted tests in several different laboratories. The group concluded that using subjects who are untrained in the fitting of hearing protection and who put on the protectors themselves gives a better estimate of on-the-job attenuation than the traditional method for making attenuation estimates, which uses highly trained subjects and experimenter fit. The result of the group's efforts has been a revision of the ANSI hearing protector standard (ANSI S12.6-1997), reprinted as Appendix O in this manual. The new standard's "Method B" provides attenuation estimates based on the responses of subjects who are given the manufacturer's directions and are told to fit the device themselves as best they can.[53] The NRR derived from Method B more closely resembles the real-world performance of hearing protectors, and would be especially useful for OHCs who want to rank-order several different protectors.

The problem with the new ANSI standard is that the EPA closed its Office of Noise Abatement many years ago and is not currently in a position to change the old NRR. Some hearing protector manufacturers, however, have collected data using Method B and the new results would be available on request. If OHCs wish to see these data, they should ask the manufacturer's representative specifically for the Method B NRR. If the EPA should reopen its office, or if another agency would take on the task of revising the NRR, OHCs can be sure that they will be notified of this event in future issues of the CAOHC *UPDATE*.

Interestingly, several professional organizations, including the National Hearing Conservation Association (NHCA), have endorsed the new ANSI standard's Method B. Moreover, the current version of the OSHA Technical Manual refers to a task force of organizations created by the NHCA to tackle the problem of the NRR's inadequacy. OSHA mentions the advantages of Method B, not to actually require its use, but to provide information to interested readers. (See Appendix III.5 of the OSHA Technical Manual, available on OSHA's website.)

The Right Amount of Attenuation

Gauging the right amount of attenuation is a delicate balance. The information in Figure 10-20 is a reminder that many protectors, especially certain plugs, may provide only a few decibels of attenuation. In high noise levels a few decibels may not be sufficient. But the need for communication, especially in highly intermittent noise environments, must be taken seriously. Requiring a large-volume earmuff in only moderate noise levels would be a mistake.

Too much attenuation not only interferes with communication, but can cause a feeling of isolation that separates workers from the world around them. The result of over-attenuation may be that the protector is worn only in the supervisor's presence, and the majority of the time is not worn at all. Hearing loss is more likely to occur in this situation than when a comfortable protector is used that provides only a modest amount of attenuation.

Bigger is not always better. Because one protector has an NRR 1 or 2 dB higher than another, does not mean that it will work out that way in actual use, as Figure 10-20 amply demonstrates. In fact, the laboratory NRR seems to bear relatively little relationship to the attenuation experienced on the job. The OHC, the professional supervisor, and the employee being fitted must all use their best judgment and experience to weigh the different factors entering into the decision of selecting the best hearing protector for each individual's situation.

---

[52] See NIOSH Criteria Document, p. 63.

[53] OHCs should not be misled into thinking that the practice of having subjects fit their own protectors can be generalized to the workplace. The laboratory is one situation and the factory floor is quite another. OHCs should always provide workers with hands-on assistance in the initial fitting and insertion of hearing protectors.

Procedures for Checking Attenuation

To date there is no *standard* method for checking the attenuation of hearing protectors in the field, but there are procedures that OHCs can use that will give an indication of how much help a protector is providing. These procedures can also be useful educational tools.

One procedure is to give a group of workers an audiometric test before the beginning of the work shift and then again at the end of the shift. If the hearing threshold levels in certain workers show a deterioration in the second test (in other words, TTS), then the hearing protectors are not providing sufficient attenuation or they are not being worn. Counseling, refitting, and retraining should improve the situation, and the tests can be repeated at a later date.

Another procedure that assesses attenuation more directly applies only to earplugs. The OHC approaches a worker during the work shift and hands the worker a sign that says "Please don't touch your earplugs" and "Follow me." The OHC takes the worker to the audiometric test room and proceeds to test his or her hearing using a conventional audiometer and with the plugs in place. After that the OHC instructs the worker to remove the plugs and conducts another audiometric test. The difference between the two audiograms represents the amount of attenuation that the worker is receiving at each test frequency. Although this procedure may not be as exact as the laboratory tests, it gives both the OHC and the worker a useful indication of how the worker is doing with the earplugs.[54]

In recent years, fit-check devices have been developed, some of which are commercially available. There are fit-check devices that are designed to be used in relatively quiet areas in the workplace, which could mean that a trip to the audiometric test booth might not be necessary. Most of these devices are meant to be used with earplugs, but there is a system available now to evaluate the attenuation of earmuffs as well (Michael, 1999; Michael and Byrne, 2000).

---

[54] There is some evidence that this method may not work as well with premolded plugs as with the user-molded or custom-molded varieties. Premolded plugs with a relatively long stem are especially liable to interfere with the test by making contact with the earphone's receiver.

References

Anku, L. (1987). "Use of Walkman radio." OSHA Standards Interpretations and Compliance Letters, 4-14-87.

ANSI (1997). American National Standard Methods for Measuring the Real-Ear Attenuation of Hearing Protectors. ANSI S12.6-1997. Acoustical Society of America, Melville, NY.

Berg, G., and Hiselius, P. (2000). "Uniform-attenuation hearing protectors provide superior protection for hearing-impaired wearers." *Spectrum*, 17(1), 16–18.

Berger, E.H. (1987). "EARLog #18—Can hearing aids provide hearing protection?" *Am. Ind. Hyg. Assoc. J.*, 48(1), A20–A21.

Berger, E.H. (2000). "Hearing protection devices." Chapter 10 in E.H. Berger, L.H. Royster, J.D. Royster, D.P. Driscoll, and M. Layne, (Eds.), *The Noise Manual, Fifth Edition*. American Industrial Hygiene Assoc., Fairfax, VA.

Dolan, T.G., and Maurer, J.F. (October 2000). "Hearing aids in occupational settings: Safety and management issues." *Occupational Safety and Health*.

Hörmann, H., Lazarus-Mainka, G., Schubeius, M., and Lazarus, H. (1984). "The effect of noise and the wearing of ear protectors on verbal communication." *Noise Control Engineering J.*, 23, 69–77.

Laroche, C., Ross, M.-J., Lefebvre, L., and Larocque, R. (1995). Determination des caracteristques acoustiques optimales des alarmes de recul. Etudes et Recherches, R-117. (IRSST) Institut de recherche en sante et en securite du travail du Quebec. Quebec, Canada.

Lazarus, H. (1983). "Literature review 1978–1984." In G. Rossi, (Ed.), *Proceedings of the Fourth International Congress on Noise as a Public Health Problem*. Centro Ricerche e Studi Amplifon, Milan, Italy.

Michael, K. (1999). "Measurement of insert-type hearing protector attenuation on the end-user: A practical alternative to relying on the NRR." *Spectrum, 16*(4), 13–17.

Michael, K.L., and Byrne, D.C. (2000). "Industrial noise and conservation of hearing." Chapter 19 in R.L. Harris, (Ed.), *Patty's Industrial Hygiene, Fifth Edition, Vol. 2*, John Wiley & Sons, New York.

Miles, J.B. (1983). "One type of muff and plug available for employee hearing protector selection." OSHA Standards Interpretations and Compliance Letters, 10-17-83.

Miles, J.B. (1994). "Questions and answers relative to the noise standard." OSHA Standards Interpretations and Compliance Letters, 5-8-94.

Nichols, M.W., and Teaster, E.C. (October 5, 2000). "Noise enforcement policy." Program Policy Letter No. P00-IV-4/P00-V-3. Mine Safety and Health Administration.

NIOSH (1975). "List of personal hearing protectors and attenuation data." U.S. Dept HEW (NIOSH) 76–120. Dept. Health and Human Services, Public Health Service, National Institute for Occupational Safety and Health.

NIOSH (1998). "Criteria for a recommended standard: Occupational noise exposure: Revised criteria, 1998." DHHS (NIOSH) 98–126. Dept. Health and Human Services, Public Health Service.

OSHA (1983). OSHA Instruction CPL 2-2.35, Nov. 9, 1983. "Guidelines for noise enforcement." Dept. Labor, Occupational Safety and Health Administration.

Suter, A.H. (1992). "Communication and job performance in noise: A review." *ASHA Monographs No. 28*. American Speech-Language-Hearing Assoc., Rockville, MD.

Tufts, J. (2002). "Measures of speech production in noise with and without HPDs." Paper presented at the 27th Annual Hearing Conservation Conference, National Hearing Conservation Association, Denver, CO.

Quiz

1. Most premolded earplugs come in a variety of sizes. (True or False)

2. Large-volume earmuffs provide somewhat more attenuation in the _____ _____ frequencies than the small-volume type.

3. What is the best type of noise environment for using semi-insert protectors?

4. When OSHA considers the combination of an earmuff with an earplug, what is the increase in attenuation assumed to be over the protector with the higher attenuation?

5. An active hearing protector uses _____ _____ to allow the passage of low and moderate levels of sound into the earcanal while attenuating high sound levels.

6. Why is the wearing of personal radios (and tape and disk players) on the job not recommended for employees in a hearing conservation program?

7. One of the advantages of user-molded earplugs is that they are easier to use in intermittent noise conditions. (True or False)

8. Inserting user-molded earplugs should always be done with _____ hands.

9. Although earmuffs do not come in a variety of sizes, they must still be fitted to individual wearers. (True or False)

10. What is the name of the effect when a person's own voice sounds low-pitched and rather hollow when wearing a hearing protector? In which conditions is this effect most pronounced?

11. What are the two main circumstances in which people have difficulty communicating when they are wearing hearing protectors?

12. Earmuffs may cause difficulties in localizing sounds, particularly in the _____ plane.

13. Hearing protectors with _____ attenuation can make communication easier than protectors that attenuate heavily in the high frequencies.

14. A small amount of cerumen should not interfere with the use of an earplug. (True or False)

15. Inexperienced fitters tend to select earplugs that are too _____. (tight or loose)

16. When should foam earplugs be disposed of?

17. The OSHA regulation requires that hearing protectors attenuate at least to a _____ dBA TWA for most employees. What level would you choose?

18. If C-weighting is not available and the A-weighting network is used, _____ dB must be subtracted from the protector's NRR. This subtraction is to account for the absence of a proper assessment of the low-frequency noise which is obtained using C-weighting. (True or False)

19. Studies of the field attenuation of hearing protectors indicate that workers receive only about _____ to _____ of the attenuation obtained in the laboratory.

20. When considering whether to cite a company for the absence of feasible engineering controls, OSHA inspectors will derate a hearing protector's NRR by _____ percent.

Abbreviations Used in Chapter X

ANSI	American National Standards Institute
dB	Decibels
dBA	Decibels measured on the A scale of the sound level meter (or dosimeter)

EPA	Environmental Protection Agency
Hz	Hertz
MSHA	Mine Safety and Health Administration
NHCA	National Hearing Conservation Association
NIOSH	National Institute for Occupational Safety and Health
NRR	Noise Reduction Rating
OHC	Occupational Hearing Conservationist
OSHA	Occupational Safety and Health Administration
STS	Standard threshold shift
TTS	Temporary threshold shift
TWA	Time-weighted average exposure level

Recommended Reading

Berger, E.H. The "EARLog" series, available from Aearo Co., 5457 W. 79th St., Indianapolis, IN or on the internet at **www.e-a-r.com**.

Berger, E.H. (2000). "Hearing protection devices." Chapter 10 in E.H. Berger, L.H. Royster, J.D. Royster, D.P. Driscoll, and M. Layne, (Eds.), *The Noise Manual., Fifth Edition*. American Industrial Hygiene Assoc., Fairfax, VA.

Franks, J.R., Stephenson, M.R., and Merry, C.J. (1996). "Personal hearing protection devices." In *Preventing Occupational Hearing Loss—A Practical Guide*. DHHS (NIOSH) 96–110. Department of Health and Human Services, Public Health Service, National Institute for Occupational Safety and Health, Cincinnati, OH.

Garrett, B.R.B., (2001). "The challenge of hearing protection for the hearing-impaired." *Baseline, NHCA Spectrum, 18*(1).

NIOSH (1998). "Hearing protectors," Chapter 6 in *Criteria for a Recommended Standard: Occupational Noise Exposure: Revised Criteria, 1998*. DHHS (NIOSH) 98–126. Dept. Health and Human Services, Public Health Service.

OSHA (November 9, 1983). Instruction CPL 2-2.35, "Guidelines for noise enforcement." OSHA Office of Health Compliance Assistance, Washington, DC.

Websites

www.msha.gov
Mine Safety and Health Administration

www.hearingconservation.org
National Hearing Conservation Association (NHCA)

www.cdc.gov/niosh
National Institute for Occupational Safety and Health (NIOSH)

www.osha.gov
Occupational Safety and Health Administration (OSHA)

www.osha-slc.gov/OshDoc/toc.interps.html
OSHA Interpretations
(type in: noise standards)

www.osha-slc.gov/dts/osta/otm/otm_iii/otm_iii_5.html
OSHA Technical Manual, Section III Chapter 5—Noise Measurement

Chapter XI

Training and Motivation

By this time the reader knows, as do most hearing conservation professionals, that hearing protectors can't simply be handed out with the expectation that they will be worn effectively. In fact, you can't be assured of their effectiveness even if protectors are initially sized, fitted, and inserted correctly. Employees must be trained and motivated in an ongoing program, otherwise the entire program may be an empty exercise. Without a good understanding of the purposes and procedures of the whole program, employees may be tempted to take the easy way out—by removing equipment panels or coverings meant to control noise, by modifying their hearing protectors to make them more comfortable, or by not wearing hearing protectors at all. Training and motivation present a challenge to the OHC and may represent the deciding factor in the success of the hearing conservation program.

Who Should Train?

The person who performs the training should be well-versed in every part of an effective hearing conservation program, including some details about hearing, the ear and how it operates, and especially about hearing protection devices. It would also be helpful for this individual to be familiar with the workers, the work process and environment, and the company's policies. The likely candidate for the job will be the OHC.

The company may hire a hearing conservation professional to do parts of the training, in which case this person should be instructed about the com-

pany's policies so that she or he does not recommend something that would contradict them. In any case, OHCs should always participate because they will have the most knowledge of the company and the work environment. Also, it is usually the OHC who must provide the oversight and follow-up.

The person who performs the training should be sincere and genuinely interested in the hearing conservation program and in the employees' welfare. This person should also be capable of gaining employees' attention and respect. To be effective the hearing conservation program must be taken seriously.

Including Managers and Supervisors

All employees whose TWAs exceed 85 dBA need to receive training at least once a year, according to the OSHA regulation. But there are others who also should receive training, namely supervisors and managers. If the word "training" sounds too undignified, perhaps "educational seminars" or "briefing sessions" would do. At any rate, it is a good idea for the OHC or other trainer to meet with supervisors and managers at least once a year to explain the program and to update them on its progress.

If management officials are going to give these programs their full support, they need to know about the hazards of noise, the costs and benefits of hearing conservation programs, and the pertinent regulatory requirements. In addition, they need to know about the questions and concerns of the workers, as well as the importance of always wearing

119

hearing protectors in noisy areas. Management should be given periodic progress reports on hearing conservation in the different areas of the company.

Foremen and supervisors may be very helpful allies of the OHC since these individuals will sometimes provide day-to-day supervision of the wearing of hearing protectors. They need to be given the same kinds of information as management officials and workers. They especially need to understand that improperly fitted or inserted hearing protectors may provide little or no attenuation, even though the protectors may look acceptable at first glance.

Techniques

To the extent possible, training sessions for workers should not interfere with production schedules. This may mean that training should be performed in a number of small segments rather than all at once. As a rule sessions should not be long, lasting only about 15 to 25 minutes, 30 minutes maximum.

Hearing conservation training may be done in conjunction with regularly scheduled safety meetings if the group is not too large. Small groups are probably the best medium, composed of people who have similar noise exposures. Training sessions should be in a seminar rather than lecture format, to give employees the opportunity to ask questions and to share their experiences.

Although audiovisual presentations and written materials may be helpful supplements to the training, they can never take the place of live, face-to-face interaction. This way, not only do workers have the opportunity to ask questions and discuss their problems, but they will also understand that the program is a human one rather than something automatic and sterile.

The material should be kept simple and meaningful and, to the extent possible, it should apply to the specific group of workers being trained—their jobs and individual noise environments. Demonstrations can help to make the program more relevant, such as the informal inspection of hearing protector insertion, tests with hearing protector fit-check devices, and the audiometric tests before and after the work shift (to identify TTS) described in Chapter X. Demonstrations also include showing workers their actual hearing threshold levels and comparing these levels to their previous audiograms, especially baseline audiograms, or to a population of non-noise-exposed people.

Employees should be given feedback often, praising them when they are wearing hearing protection successfully and cautioning them when they are not. The OHC needs to spend "quality" time with employees, helping them to adjust to hearing pro-tectors, reminding them how it sounds and feels to insert protectors effectively, and teaching employees to recognize the signs of wear.

Training Tips

Former CAOHC Council member George Krafcisin, representing the National Safety Council, developed some useful tips on effective training (see the Fall 2000 issue of *UPDATE*). He reminds OHCs of several important points, which are paraphrased below:

- Adults have a lot going on in their lives and jobs. Hearing conservation training may not be a high priority, so OHCs should give them a good reason to invest their time. Telling them that OSHA-required training will take place would not be as motivating as announcing an information session that will help them protect their hearing.
- People want to learn things that will be of direct value. How the decibel is derived will not be as motivating as how to select and insert earplugs that will be comfortable.
- Many workers will have an extensive base of knowledge and experience that can be very useful if shared with others.
- Older workers often can't hear or see as well as younger ones, so you may have to speak up or use a microphone and have handouts in large type.
- Some people learn best from hearing the spoken word, others from reading, and others from pictures. Important points should use all three modes.
- Not everybody speaks and reads English. Try to use instruction in the audience's native language. This may necessitate getting some help.
- Trainers should prepare thoroughly, organize the material into simple steps, and repeat important points frequently.
- You can best maintain control of the session by starting and ending on time, sticking to the subject, and insisting on discipline. Nobody benefits from a chaotic classroom.
- People remember 70% of what they hear in the first twenty minutes of a training session but only 15% of what they hear in the last twenty minutes. Go over the most important material first.
- Break up the energy flow by changing presentation style frequently: talk for a while, then have a discussion, then a video, then a practice session, etc.
- It's a good idea to get feedback on the training session. Give a short quiz and have the participants fill out an evaluation form to measure how much they have learned and how to improve future training sessions.

Content of the Employee Training Program

OSHA's Requirements

Section (k) of the OSHA noise regulation requires employers to institute a training program for all employees whose TWAs equal or exceed 85 dBA. The program must be repeated at least annually and it must be updated periodically to be consistent with changes in work processes and hearing protection devices.

The training must include information about the effects of noise on hearing and the purpose of audiometric testing, along with an explanation of the test procedures. Employees must also be given instruction on the purposes of hearing protectors, the advantages, disadvantages, and attenuation of various types, and their selection, fitting, use, and care.

Materials used in the training program must be made available to workers and to OSHA inspectors upon request.

MSHA's Requirements

The training provisions in Part 62.180 of the MSHA regulation are similar to OSHA's except that there is a requirement that the mine operator provide training within 30 days of a miner's enrollment into a hearing conservation program, and at least yearly after that. In addition to the OSHA provisions, MSHA also requires that the training include both the mine operator's and the miner's tasks in maintaining noise controls. The mine operator must certify the date and type of training given each miner.

Effects of Noise

Preventing noise-induced hearing loss is the major rationale for the hearing conservation program, and although hearing loss from noise may be a rather abstract concept, workers need to be well aware of its potential in their specific workplaces. It is usually helpful to hear from some of the older workers who have developed permanent hearing losses: how their hearing loss developed gradually; how difficult it is to communicate with family members and to try to socialize in a group of people; and how they wish they had taken better care of their hearing. This kind of testimonial can make hearing impairment less abstract and workers are more likely to take it seriously and personally.

Although it is not required by regulations, it is a good idea to mention some of the other adverse effects of noise, such as fatigue and jangled nerves, so that the trainer can point out that the attenuation provided by hearing protectors should alleviate these potential effects, sometimes substantially. Some employees report that they feel less irritable at home and they even sleep better at night once they start wearing hearing protectors on the job. Additional benefits may surface during the discussion.

The trainer should discuss hearing losses from other causes, particularly from non-occupational noise sources, and how to prevent them by avoiding these noise sources or by wearing adequately selected, fitted, and inserted hearing protectors.

Audiometric Testing

The audiometric test provides an excellent opportunity for a brief training session, where the OHC can counsel the worker about the status of his/her hearing, whether there has been any deterioration, and if so, what steps may be taken to prevent any further impairment. It is also an ideal time to check the hearing protectors, make sure they are comfortable, in good condition, and *used*.

Occasionally employees will refuse to take the audiometric test. This usually happens due to a lack of understanding because they are afraid that their hearing losses might be used to discriminate against them. The OHC should use the training session as an opportunity to reassure employees that they will not be dismissed or demoted because of the their hearing status. Of course, the trainer needs to have the support of the company in making this statement.[55] When a group of employees refuses to take the hearing test it is usually an indication of serious labor–management problems, which may need to be worked out above the level of the OHC.

Sometimes employees may misunderstand the purpose of the audiometric testing program and somehow believe that the test itself actually prevents hearing loss. OHCs need to be careful not to imply that audiometric testing *saves* their hearing, but instead that it attempts to identify small hearing losses so that steps may be taken to intervene before these losses become handicapping. Better yet, it attempts to identify temporary hearing losses before they become permanent. Of course, audiometric testing can only serve this function if it is done carefully, regularly, and according to the standards outlined in Chapters VII and VIII.

---

[55] If the employer were to fire or demote employees on the basis of their audiograms, this could be considered discrimination by the courts. The *Americans with Disabilities Act*, discussed in Chapter VI, makes it more difficult for employers to dismiss or demote workers on the basis of their hearing threshold levels. Instead, employers need to define the communication skills necessary for a particular job before hiring a person for that job, or if communication is of paramount importance, an existing employee who has developed a hearing loss on the job must be accommodated in some way. These are complex issues and often necessitate legal advice.

As mentioned above, demonstrations involving workers' own audiograms can be very helpful. While it is better not to discuss individual workers' audiograms in front of the group, hypothetical examples may be used, or a composite audiogram may be developed, representing the average hearing threshold levels of the members of the particular group being trained. The hypothetical example or composite audiogram may then be compared to a group of individuals with normal hearing for that approximate age group. OHCs should be aware that there are differing opinions as to what constitutes "normal" hearing, so these comparisons should be taken "with a grain of salt." The best individual counseling is to compare a worker's current audiogram to his or her past audiograms, applaud the success when no change has occurred, and convey the potential seriousness of the problem if there has been a decrease in hearing. This is especially important when a TTS has been identified, the warning sign that steps (or further steps) need to be taken before the loss becomes permanent.

Hearing Protectors

Training about hearing protectors should constitute the major portion of the training effort. The OSHA and MSHA regulations are explicit about including information on the purposes of hearing protectors and the advantages, disadvantages, and attenuation of various types, as well as their selection, fitting, use, and care. This means that the OHC needs to be well informed. It also means that the OHC should have a generous variety of appropriate protectors from which the employees may choose. The initial selection and subsequent training should involve hands-on fitting by the trainer and trainees.

The session should cover the signs of age and wear in the hearing protectors used by the employees being trained and should include examples of worn-out protectors. If the OHC is able to do the kind of on-site earplug checking described in the previous chapter, she or he should use the training session to explain the procedures and the fact that the test will be performed at random intervals with no warning. A fit-check procedure can also be incorporated into the regular training program.

A useful resource, "Tips for Fitting Hearing Protectors," (Berger, 2000) is included as Appendix L of this manual.

Noise Monitoring and Engineering Controls

The OSHA/MSHA regulations do not specifically require employers to include noise monitoring results as part of the training program, but OSHA's section (e) does require employers to notify each employee exposed at or above an 8-hour TWA of 85 dBA of the results of the monitoring. Section (f) requires employers to provide workers or their representatives with the opportunity to observe noise measurements. MSHA's requirements in section 62.110 are similar. For these reasons, OHCs should make sure that the subject of noise exposure monitoring is included in a periodic training program. In addition, it is helpful for workers to know the approximate level of their noise exposures and the particular hazards to which they are exposed.

It is also good practice to explain the basic principles of noise control with special emphasis on any noise control program that the company may have in place. As suggested in Chapter IX, some workers may have good ideas about practical and inexpensive noise control solutions for their particular equipment. The training session would be the logical time to discuss noise control measures that have already been implemented, solicit comments about how these controls are working, and request that workers refrain from removing devices like mufflers or enclosures. The OHC can communicate any problems with these devices to the industrial hygienist, noise control engineer, or other appropriate source.

Warning Signs

Although not strictly an element of the training program, a discussion of warning signs is often included in this topic area because these signs can reinforce the need to use hearing protection. Both OSHA and MSHA are silent on the subject of warning signs.[56] Perhaps one reason is because the regulations are more concerned with *exposures* than with noise *levels*, which may or may not affect workers directly. There is, however, a good use for warning signs in areas where people work intermittently and where it is clear that noise levels are hazardous and would contribute significantly to workers' exposures. Examples would be engine rooms, boiler rooms, or places where people are using pneumatic tools. (Of course these are not the only areas where hearing protectors would be required.) It is good practice to post warning signs at the entrance to all high-noise areas as a reminder to put on hearing protectors.

The NIOSH Criteria Document recommends that warning signs contain the following information:

WARNING
NOISE AREA
HEARING HAZARD
Use of Hearing Protectors Required

---

[56] Washington OSHA requires warning signs in areas where workers are exposed to noise levels at 115 dBA or above, and NIOSH recommends warning signs for areas where noise exposures are routinely at or above a TWA of 85 dBA.

Workers who do not speak English should be instructed verbally in their own language, or a graphic symbol of hearing protectors could be incorporated into the sign. Warning signs in multiple languages may be needed.

Materials

Audiovisual and written materials may be a useful adjunct to the training program but, as stated above, they cannot take the place of face-to-face interaction. If they are used, they should comprise a relatively small part of the training session. These materials may be helpful for individual viewing while waiting for audiometric tests or during some other free time.

Appendix A of this manual lists websites, many of which provide training materials and information. There are some interesting audio demonstrations that simulate hearing impairments of various degrees, which could be helpful in explaining why good hearing is so valuable. The website **www.e-a-r.com** contains an extensive list of videos, including descriptions, of over 50 commercially available films and videos: Certain other manufacturers of hearing protection list their own videos and training materials on their websites (information available from product distributors).

OHCs should keep in mind that new materials are continually appearing on the market and they should keep abreast of the safety, industrial hygiene, and hearing conservation publications to see these materials advertised and reviewed. The CAOHC *UPDATE* and the National Hearing Conservation Association (NHCA) publication, *Spectrum*, are excellent sources of information about current training materials. Also, quite a few manufacturers of hearing protectors and noise measurement equipment produce educational brochures and booklets intended for noise-exposed workers. The OHC should always review these materials before presenting them to employees to make sure that their quality is adequate and that they are appropriate to the situation. To keep training programs from becoming stale, OHCs should update their materials at least once a year.

As mentioned in Chapter VI, both OSHA and MSHA require employers to make certain kinds of materials readily available to workers. Section (l) of the OSHA regulation requires employers to post a copy of the regulation in the workplace (interpreted to mean available without workers having to ask for it), and also to make all of their training materials available to OSHA and NIOSH if these agencies should request them. Section 62.130 of the MSHA regulation requires mine operators to post on the mine bulletin board any procedures used in administrative controls, and to provide a copy of these procedures to the affected miner.

In addition to the regulatory requirements, the OHC may want to post information or write-ups about the company's hearing conservation program on the bulletin board. Such information may include the availability of a new kind of hearing protector, the scheduling of audiometric tests, or articles of general interest. It could also include the results of a particular department's audiometric testing in the form of a composite audiogram, hearing protector fit-checks, or TTS testing with names removed.

Motivation

No amount of education and training will be worthwhile if workers are not motivated to use their knowledge. Looking at the situation pragmatically, the OHC should make sure that workers are rewarded for wearing hearing protection and using it effectively, and *not* rewarded for using it ineffectively. This means that the OHC must be very attentive to the employees' needs and practices.

Rewards

Rewards should at least include praise for wearing and inserting the protectors properly. If the worker has been wearing an uncomfortable protector, changing to a better fitting, more comfortable protector will, by itself, be rewarding. Another reward that is a direct outcome of wearing hearing protectors effectively will be the reduction of fatigue and annoyance from loud noise. If the worker has been experiencing TTS and tinnitus, these adverse consequences should also be reduced or eliminated. Sometimes these benefits will not be readily apparent and the OHC will need to call them to the attention of employees.

Some companies have institutionalized rewards by giving out cash awards or lottery tickets to employees who have excellent records for wearing safety equipment. Other companies have given rewards to departments with good safety records, including good hearing conservation practices. Recent research, however, has shown that these kinds of "rewards" may produce disappointing results over the long haul and sometimes even backfire. A NIOSH report (Franks et al., 1996) discusses this research and points out that reward and punishment systems can lead to destructive competition between workers and animosity between worker groups and the managers who supervise them. These practices can actually damage worker self-esteem and decrease productivity. If an incentive system is desired by management *and* workers, it is most likely to succeed if it is designed and carried out by the affected workers themselves.

"Negative Rewards"

The OHC should try to make sure that employees are *not* rewarded for failure to wear hearing protectors or for wearing them incorrectly. An example of this kind of reward is the approval of fellow workers for being "man enough" not to use safety equipment. The OHC should try to counter any peer pressure or macho attitudes against wearing these devices. Detrimental rewards can also be realized by modifying plugs or muffs (and decreasing their attenuation) to make them more comfortable. These kinds of negative rewards are not easy to counteract. They require time, attention, and sometimes imagination on the part of the vigilant OHC. This is where the positive rewards, described above, come in. This is also where the OHC needs to be sensitive to unspoken fears, such as safety hazards due to communication difficulties, the perceived possibility of ear infections, and fears about not conforming to the prevailing macho attitude. And of course, the OHC needs to counter hearing protector modification by supplying as many other types and brands of protectors as necessary until the worker experiences both comfort and the appropriate attenuation.

Disciplinary actions should be used only as a last resort when all other measures have been exhausted. These measures may be written into company policy, but the OHC should be careful never to blame OSHA for them. The OSHA noise regulation has no provisions for transferring workers or any disciplinary action. *Before instituting these measures the employer needs to make sure that the worker does not have a legitimate complaint, such as a painful ear, an improperly fitted or inserted protector, or a problem with being unable to hear necessary speech communication or warning signals.*

According to the NIOSH report referenced above, there are well-documented negative side-effects from relying on punishment for failure to follow safety rules (Franks et al., 1996). Punishment only works if the behavior is closely monitored. Moreover, it does not encourage desired behavior. For example, if workers are punished for not wearing earplugs, they may cut them in half so that only the exterior portion shows and the plugs provide virtually no attenuation. Finally, the person who has to deal out the punishment may be the OHC, which could damage the relationship between OHC and workers, severely limiting the OHC's effectiveness.

The Older Worker

Older workers, who already have some hearing impairment, may be particularly difficult to motivate. They are likely to feel that they have already lost their hearing so the wearing of hearing protection is a useless exercise. The OHC should tell them that it is possible to lose more hearing if they are not protected and should stress the importance of keeping whatever hearing they still have. Hearing loss from aging will nearly always increase the existing impairment, and the idea is to prevent workers from being handicapped in their later years.

These workers may have significant difficulties hearing speech and warning signals while wearing hearing protectors, and the company should seriously consider fitting them with hearing protectors with uniform attenuation across the frequency spectrum or level-dependent protectors, as appropriate. If communication is an integral part of the job, active attenuators or communication headsets would be indicated.

Family Involvement

Companies should consider involving employees' family members in the hearing conservation program. They could set aside a time and place for audiometric tests for workers' spouses and school-age children. Audiometric testing of children could reveal hearing problems that may not have been discovered before. It would also provide an opportunity for husbands and wives to discuss the status of their hearing and the particulars of the hearing conservation program. This would enable the spouses to provide input on how the employee's hearing loss may affect the whole family, and to receive counseling from the OHC and/or a professional in hearing conservation. This kind of family involvement has been shown to increase the motivation for an effective hearing conservation program, as well as provide a useful service to employees and their families.

The Safety Climate

Recent research points to the fact that increasing the knowledge of workers and providing them with appropriate protective equipment is not enough. In the 1996 version of the NIOSH "Practical Guide," the authors state that a positive **safety climate** is a necessary ingredient to any personal protection program (Franks et al., 1996). This occurs when the hearing conservation program is fully embraced by workers as well as management, and workers play the pivotal role in the program, facilitating and reinforcing its provisions. The degree to which workers will do this depends on: (1) how firmly they believe they will benefit from the protection measures; (2) the amount of control they feel they have over their own health and well being; and (3) their beliefs about the barriers to protecting themselves. Barriers to using hearing protectors include many of the problems discussed earlier, such as difficulty with communication, negative peer pressure, and discomfort.

Although research on the safety climate is somewhat new, the ingredients that make up a good safety climate are not, and the OHC would do well to take these concepts seriously. (See especially pp. 55–59 of the *NIOSH Practical Guide*.)

Another useful resource is an article by CAOHC member Elliott Berger (2001), which gives useful tips for motivating workers to protect their hearing. The article is available at **www.e-a-r.com** (click on Industrial Safety, Hearing Protection, under Technical Literature click on "The Ardent Hearing Conservationist").

References

Berger, E.H. (2000). EARLog #19, "Tips for fitting hearing protectors." Aearo Co., 5457 W. 79th St., Indianapolis, IN.

Berger, E.H. (2001). "The ardent hearing conservationist," (abstract). *Spectrum, Suppl. 1, 18*, 17–18. Full paper available at **www.aearo.com**.

Franks, J.R., Stephenson, M.R., and Merry, C.J. (Eds.) (1996). "Education and motivation," and "Emerging trends and technologies." In *Preventing Occupational Hearing Loss—A Practical Guide*. DHHS (NIOSH) 96–110. Department of Health and Human Services, Public Health Service, National Institute for Occupational Safety and Health, Cincinnati, OH.

Krafcisin, G. (2000). "Some tips on effective training." CAOHC *UPDATE, 11*(3), 3.

Quiz

1. Besides noise-exposed workers, what other groups need to receive training on the hearing conservation program (or at least "educational seminars" or "briefing sessions")?

2. What is the desirable length of a worker training program?

3. Which is best for hearing conservation training—the lecture format or the seminar format?

4. Since workers may not want their hearing thresholds to be identified in front of a group, what other techniques can the OHC use to describe the hearing losses of the group being trained?

5. When would be a good time for workers to view a hearing conservation video?

6. What is a good way of making company hearing conservation information available to employees?

7. During the training session, what is the best time to introduce the most important material?

8. Give two reasons why institutionalized reward and punishment programs are often unsuccessful. When is an incentive program more likely to succeed?

Abbreviations Used in Chapter XI

dBA	Decibels measured on the A scale of the sound level meter (or dosimeter)
MSHA	Mine Safety and Health Administration
NIOSH	National Institute for Occupational Safety and Health
OHC	Occupational Hearing Conservationist
OSHA	Occupational Safety and Health Administration
TTS	Temporary threshold shift
TWA	Time-weighted average exposure

Recommended Reading

Berger, E.H. (2001). "The ardent hearing conservationist," (abstract). *Spectrum Suppl. 1, 18*, 17–18. Full paper available at **www.aearo.com**.

Franks, J.R., Stephenson, M.R., and Merry, C.J. (1996). "Education and motivation,"and "Emerging trends and technologies." In *Preventing Occupational Hearing Loss—A Practical Guide*. DHHS (NIOSH) 96–110. Department of Health and Human Services, Public Health Service, National Institute for Occupational Safety and Health, Cincinnati, OH.

Krafcisin, G. (Fall 2000). "Some tips on effective training." CAOHC *UPDATE, 11*(3) 3.

NIOSH (1998). Chapters 1 and 5 in *Criteria for a Recommended Standard: Occupational Noise Exposure: Revised Criteria, 1998*. DHHS (NIOSH) 98–126. Dept. Health and Human Services, Public Health Service.

Royster, L.H., and Royster, J.D. (2000). "Education and motivation." Chapter 8 in E.H. Berger, L.H. Royster, J.D. Royster, D.P. Driscoll, and M. Layne, (Eds.), *The Noise Manual, Fifth Edition*. American Industrial Hygiene Assoc., Fairfax, VA.

Websites

www.aearo.com or **www.e-a-r.com**
E·A·R/Aearo Company

www.hearingconservation.org
National Hearing Conservation Association

www.nsc.org
National Safety Council

Chapter XII

Recordkeeping and Program Evaluation

Why Bother to Keep Records?

Everyone who reads this manual will have a lot of other things to do and, probably, numerous responsibilities in addition to hearing conservation. The other parts of the program usually involve face-to-face contact with employees and are much more interesting than keeping records. So why bother? There are many reasons, important ones, and experienced OHCs could probably testify to all of them. Accurate and complete records are the only form of evidence that the hearing conservation program is working correctly and consistently.

First, the keeping of certain records is required by law. If a government inspector visits a company, she or he will want to know about employees' noise exposure levels. The inspector will also need to look at records to see if workers are losing their hearing; to find out which ones have experienced an STS and whether the audiometric testing was done properly—by trained technicians, with calibrated equipment, and in a room with sufficiently low background noise levels. Only with clear and complete records will the regulatory requirements be satisfied.

Accurate audiometric records are critical for comparing periodic test results to the baseline audiogram. Without them, this comparison is meaningless, and once again the program will be in violation of government regulations. Comparison of records is the only way to tell if an STS has occurred or if hearing is gradually deteriorating. Records are also necessary to assess the effectiveness of the overall hearing conservation program, which will be discussed in greater detail later in this chapter.

Other reasons for keeping good records are to assess priorities for engineering controls, for use in training and motivation (described in Chapter XI), and for providing the audiogram reviewer with the required information. According to OSHA and MSHA, the reviewer needs, at a minimum, a copy of the noise regulation, records of the employee's baseline and most recent hearing threshold levels, measurements of the background sound levels in the audiometric test environment, and records of audiometer calibrations. The OHC should also keep in mind that individual employees or their representatives are entitled to copies of their records on request.

Another important use of records is to create a "paper trail" in case any of the information is needed for worker compensation claims, a dispute involving OSHA or another employer, or a court case. Although all of an employee's records may be necessary, the pre-employment or first audiogram and the exit audiogram may be of particular importance.

Characteristics of Good Records

The most important features of good records should be accuracy, thoroughness, organization, and legibility. (If no one can read them they won't be very useful.) If on paper, they should be typed or neatly written in pen, with no erasures. If computerized, they should be easily retrievable. The OHC should keep in mind that these records may be scrutinized by company officials, government inspectors, workers, and other individuals in the medical or safety departments.

In addition, records need to be consistent with the company's policies and procedures. For example, some companies request workers to sign their audiometric test records and case histories to enhance the authenticity of these records.

Regulatory Requirements

Record Retention

OSHA: Section (m)(3) of the OSHA regulation requires minimum periods for retaining records: Records of noise exposure measurements must be retained for at least two years, and audiometric test records must be retained for the duration of the employee's employment. These relatively short durations are not in the best interest of either management or employees. The NIOSH Criteria Document recommends that employers keep records of noise surveys for 30 years, audiometric test records for the duration of employment plus 30 years, audiometric calibration records for 5 years, and records of hearing protector utilization for 30 years.

There is an OSHA regulation that specifically deals with recordkeeping titled, "Access to Employee Exposure and Medical Records," (29 CFR 1910.1020.) This regulation mandates a 30-year retention time. However, an OSHA interpretation states that specific regulations, including the noise regulation, take precedence over the general requirements of 1910.1020. And the "bare-bones" requirements of the noise regulation are the ones that OSHA will enforce. *Despite this, OHCs should be on notice that OSHA's retention periods are not nearly long enough and the best practice would be to keep records for at least several years after the employee's separation or retirement.*

MSHA's retention requirements are slightly different. Section 62.110 requires mine operators to keep copies of miner notification of noise exposures for the duration of exposure at or above the action level and for at least 6 months thereafter. Section 62.171 states that a miner's audiometric test records must be retained for the duration of the miner's exposure plus 6 months, and Section 62.175 requires mine operators to keep a record of a miner's training certificate as long as the miner is enrolled in the hearing conservation program plus 6 months.

Access to Records

OSHA states in Section (m)(4) that all records required by the regulation must be provided upon request to employees, former employees, their designated representatives, and to OSHA.

MSHA's requirements in Section 62.190 are similar, except that mine operators are given 15 days in which to grant the request, and this section specifies that the first copy must be provided at no cost to the miner and any additional copies be provided at reasonable cost.

Transfer of Records

OSHA: Section (m)(5) requires that employers who cease to do business must transfer all records required by this regulation to a successor employer, who must retain them for the same periods as prescribed by the regulation.

MSHA: Section 62.190 adds a requirement that the successor mine operator use the baseline (or revised baseline) audiogram obtained by the original mine operator to determine the existence of an STS or a reportable hearing loss.

Confidentiality

OSHA makes no mention of this issue.

MSHA, in Section 62.172, directs mine operators to instruct the reviewing physician, audiologist, or technician not to reveal to the mine operator any findings or diagnoses unrelated to the miner's occupational hearing loss or the wearing of hearing protectors without the written consent of the miner.

Types of Records

Computers are increasingly being used to trigger follow-up steps automatically, as well as being an efficient means to store and provide easy access to records, date them, and generate hard copy. Computerized recordkeeping will also facilitate long retention periods for all types of hearing conservation records. Computer software provides a means of integrating all aspects of the program—noise monitoring results, audiograms, records of hearing protector type and use, and attendance at training sessions. This way every aspect of the program may be linked to every other aspect so that the OHC can be alerted to take whatever steps are needed to prevent further hearing loss.

Noise Exposure Measurements

OSHA requires the employer to notify all employees whose TWAs exceed 85 dBA of the results of the noise exposure monitoring. This notification does not need to be in writing but, for the sake of clarity, it is usually a good idea to do so.

Records of noise exposure measurements need to be kept. These records should identify the employees that should be included in the hearing conservation program, the employees who must wear hearing protection (over 90 dBA), and the ones for which hearing protection must be provided, but where the use is optional (between 85 and 90 dBA). Part of this record may be a noise map of the plant, showing noise levels and identifying the areas where the use of hearing protection is mandatory.

OSHA requires the employer to maintain the employee's most recent noise exposure measurements with the record of an employee's audiometric test. This requirement has been interpreted to mean that the noise exposure measurement need not necessarily be written directly on the audiogram, but must be kept along with the audiogram so that it is readily available to audiogram reviewers, OSHA inspectors, individual employees, and others who may need to view the audiometric results in conjunction with the noise exposure measurements. Computerized recordkeeping can greatly facilitate this activity.

Although MSHA does not specifically require mine operators to keep copies of noise exposure measurements, this action is implied by the requirement to keep copies of the annual notification letters they must give to miners, stating not only the exposure determination but the corrective action the mine operator is taking.

Audiometric Records

Records should be kept of each audiometer's make, model, and serial number. This information also needs to be entered onto an employee's audiometric record (or made readily available) so that the OHC and the professional reviewer know exactly which audiometer was used for each test of every employee. This information is important because peculiar-looking threshold shifts may occur in whole groups of workers, which may be explained by a faulty audiometer or one whose calibration has been recently changed.

Audiometer calibration records also need to be kept. Records of the daily calibration should include a list of the items checked, such as earphones, cords, attenuator, etc., as well as a serial record of the hearing threshold levels of a non-noise-exposed listener who is regularly tested. Although the OHC will probably not perform the acoustic and exhaustive calibrations, these records should also be kept with the audiometer or should be readily available for inspection.

If the audiometric testing program is to be of any value, accurate records of hearing threshold levels must be kept, and the records of past audiograms should be available at the time of any audiometric test. The most convenient way to store these records is with the help of a computer, but you can also keep them by hand in the form of an audiogram chart or in tabular form. The tabular form is more convenient for making comparisons to baselines and calculating

STS, while the chart form may be easier to demonstrate to employees. However, recording thresholds on a graph-like audiogram (X's and O's) is not practical in making year-to-year comparisons. Also, microprocessor audiometers that print results on a small, built-in printer would best be manually recorded onto the tabular audiogram for easy comparison and analysis, since keeping the small printouts can become cumbersome.

OSHA requires employers to keep audiometric test records that include the employee's name and job classification, the date of the audiogram, the examiner's name, and the date of the last acoustic or exhaustive calibration of the audiometer. This information could be supplemented with some kind of employee identifying number, as well as the test date, time, and hours since the employee's last noise exposure. And, as mentioned above, information on noise exposure levels, hearing protection, and training attendance should also be available at the time of the annual audiometric test. If there are any gaps in these areas, the OHC can make sure that the necessary activity is carried out.

Audiometric records are medical records and should be treated with the same degree of integrity and confidentiality as other types of health records. OHCs should make sure that they are available only to those implementing the program, employees or their representatives, and government inspectors. Familiarity with OSHA's medical records regulation (29 CFR 1910.1020) would be helpful.

The OHC should also keep a record of any referral to an otolaryngologist or audiologist, especially when a particular employee may need ongoing medical treatment. In addition to a record of any STS, it is good practice for the OHC to keep records of audiogram interpretations, notifications, and counseling sessions, including notes on what transpired.

Evidence of Technician Competence

Although OSHA does not require that an audiometric technician show evidence of certification, the regulation does state that the person must either be certified by CAOHC or have "satisfactorily demonstrated competence in administering audiometric examinations...." The OSHA inspector will want to see evidence of this competence and that usually means a CAOHC certificate or at least written documentation of training and competence from the reviewing audiologist or physician.[57]

---

[57] If the testing is performed by a licensed or certified audiologist, otolaryngologist, or other physician, CAOHC certification is not required. It would be a good idea, however, to keep some sort of certificate on hand with the professional's credentials.

History

The OHC will want to keep a record of the employee's otological history, including ear infections, diseases, and any other ear problems, as well as familial hearing loss, recreational noise exposure, and, of course, the occupational noise exposure history. This information should be kept with the audiometric information and should be retained as long as the audiograms.

It would also be useful to add any available information about the employee's exposure to chemicals or other substances that are potentially ototoxic, such as organic solvents, heavy metals, and asphyxiants, as explained in Chapter II.

Visual Inspection

It is also a good idea to keep a record showing that the OHC has performed a visual inspection of the concha and earcanal. She or he should note whether or not an otoscope was used, the presence of any redness or swelling of the external ear, excessive cerumen, or other abnormalities. The OHC should remember not to diagnose, but refer to an audiologist or otolaryngologist any observations other than a normal appearance.

Audiometric Notification Letters to Employees

The employer is required by OSHA to notify employees in writing, within 21 days, of the determination of an STS (MSHA gives mine operators 30 days). Some companies give employees a letter every time their hearing is tested, regardless of the outcome. Other companies prefer to notify the employee only when there has been a change of hearing threshold level. This notification may occur even when the change has not been as great as an OSHA/MSHA STS, such as a NIOSH STS, or simply a steady deterioration. Notification letters may include one or more of the following, specifying right, left, and/or both ears:

- Your hearing threshold levels are within normal limits
- Your hearing threshold levels show a mild (moderate, or severe) degree of hearing loss
- Your hearing threshold levels appear to be decreasing
- Your hearing threshold levels show no change from the previous test
- Your hearing threshold levels show an OSHA (or MSHA) standard threshold shift (STS) when compared to the baseline audiogram
- You need to see an audiologist (otolaryngologist, or physician) for further evaluation

Hearing Protector Information

Although it is not mentioned in government regulations, the OHC will find it useful to keep records on employees' hearing protector information. Such records should include the type and brand selected, as well as the initial sizing, fitting, and any notes about the worker's acceptance of the device and the ability to insert it correctly. After that, the OHC may add notes resulting from periodic supervision, results of any hearing protector fit-checks, and any problems relating to rejection, communication difficulties, or destructive modification of the device. These kinds of notes should always be preceded by the date of each observation.

Training

Although training records are not required by OSHA, MSHA does require a record of training certification. In any case, it is also a good idea to keep a record of the dates of training sessions, the names of attendees, an outline of the topics discussed, and any audiovisual or written materials used. Even if the OHC gives an informal training session to an individual employee at the time of the audiometric test or while checking the hearing protectors, it is wise to enter a note to that effect in the employee's record.

Program Evaluation Information

Periodic reports of the hearing conservation program's progress should also be kept, including checklists completed and any statistical information on audiometric results of the noise-exposed employees. Such information could include the number of workers incurring an OSHA/MSHA or NIOSH STS (or a more sensitive measure of hearing deterioration), a computerized trend analysis, or any other statistical information about hearing threshold levels, and possibly the number of workers with compensable hearing losses.

Recording/Reporting Hearing Loss to Regulatory Agencies

OSHA

The 1981 version of OSHA's hearing conservation amendment required employers to record the existence of a permanent STS on the OSHA log (then called the Form 200) when the audiologist, otolaryngologist, or qualified physician reviewing the audiogram determined that the shift was work-related. In 1983, when the regulation was revised, this provision was deleted. The regulation's preamble explained that it was an unnecessary provision in the noise regulation because another OSHA regulation, 29 CFR 1904.2, already required the recording of work-related injuries and illnesses on the OSHA Form 200.

For many years, however, employers were unclear about what kinds of hearing losses they were supposed to record on the OSHA Form 200, if any. OSHA enforced the provision only sporadically. For a while OSHA maintained that employers should record all work-related, permanent STSs. Then in 1991, the agency issued a memo to its regional offices stating that they should require employers to record work-related shifts in hearing (from baseline) of an average of 25 dB or more at 2000, 3000, and 4000 Hz in either ear on the OSHA log, with age adjustments allowed. *The OHC should note that this policy did nothing to change the existing (10-dB average) definition of STS or the required follow-up actions under the noise regulation.*

As described in Chapter VI, OSHA has recently revised its requirements for recording hearing loss on the Form 300 (OSHA, 2002). The new rule requires employers to record a work-related STS, a 10-dB average shift from baseline (or the revised baseline) in either ear at 2000, 3000, and 4000 Hz if the shift plus the employee's baseline hearing thresholds at those same frequencies totals 25 dB or greater above audiometric zero. Age corrections may be used, but only when determining whether or not an STS has occurred and not when determining if the employee's current average hearing level is 25 dB or greater in relation to audiometric zero.

OSHA gives employers the opportunity to retest within 30 days before recording a work-related STS. If the retest confirms the STS, the hearing loss must be recorded within 7 days of the retest. If the retest does not confirm the STS, then the case need not be recorded. Also, if later testing reveals that the recorded STS is not permanent, the entry may be erased or lined-out.

OSHA defines a work-related hearing loss as one that is caused or contributed to by an event or exposure in the work environment, or a pre-existing hearing loss that is significantly aggravated by the work environment. If a physician or other licensed health care professional determines that the hearing loss is not work-related or has not been significantly aggravated by occupational noise, the employer is not required to record the loss on the OSHA Form 300.

The new rule will become effective on January 1, 2003. There is, however, one element that is not yet final as of this printing, and that is the exact location on which the employer must record the hearing loss. OSHA is considering adding a separate column for hearing loss on the Form 300. Until OSHA makes its final decision, employers must record the hearing loss in Column M5, "All other illnesses."

Despite the fact that several state-plan states have been requiring employers to record permanent, work-related STSs all along, without any 25 dB requirement, (Megerson, 2001), the new rule mandates all state programs to have exactly the same hearing loss recording requirements as federal OSHA.

MSHA

MSHA has codified its reporting requirements by stating that mine operators must report a change from baseline of 25 dB or more averaged over 2000, 3000, and 4000 Hz in either ear. This change must be reported on the MSHA Form 7000-14 unless a physician or audiologist determines that the loss is not work-related or aggravated by occupational noise exposure. Once again, this does not change MSHA's 10-dB average definition of STS.

Hearing Conservation Program Evaluation

Unfortunately, compliance with every part of OSHA's hearing conservation regulation does not necessarily keep workers from losing their hearing. It is not enough to go through the motions. Employers must also take a hard look at the effectiveness of the hearing conservation program. First one needs to examine an individual's series of audiograms, since each audiogram serves as a "marker" of the effectiveness of a program (NIOSH, 1998). But there are also two principal ways to look at the program as a whole: one is to perform an informal, practical survey or inventory of the program and the other is to evaluate it using statistical procedures.

On this very important matter there is no regulatory guidance. OSHA recognized the need for program evaluation in the 1981 version of the hearing conservation regulation and asked for comments from the public. When the regulation was revised in 1983 the agency was still unable to make any requirements or even any recommendations. Therefore, employers must use the advice of hearing conservation professionals and any guidelines from consensus and professional organizations.

OHCs need to be willing to devote the time and energy to evaluate their programs and get help from their audiometric program professional supervisors or consultants when necessary. Management needs to provide OHCs with the time and resources to perform program evaluation, and must be willing to acknowledge and solve any problems when the results show that the program is not working well enough (Franks et al., 1996). OHCs may need to call on their own capacities for persistence and diplomatic skill to obtain the time, resources, and commitment to get the job done.

Practical Survey

The first step is to make sure that the program complies with the OSHA or MSHA regulation, as appropriate. For this the OHC may consult the OSHA Compliance Checklist in Appendix D or the MSHA Program Checklist in Appendix G. But, as stated many times before, compliance with regulations is not enough, so a practical survey of the program is available as the "Program Evaluation Checklist" printed in Appendix H.

There are many practical questions to address in this program inventory. Examples would be: Are workers accepting their hearing protectors and are they wearing them effectively? Are supervisors and foremen involved? Is progress being made on the noise control program? Are employees being referred for medical treatment or audiological evaluation when necessary? Are they actually obtaining the treatment and evaluation? Have they been followed-up to see if the treatment was successful?

Probably the most important and yet the most difficult of the questions that will come up in hearing conservation program evaluation is whether workers' hearing is being saved. One popular way of looking at it is whether they are incurring STSs and, if so, what percentage of the exposed workers have an STS each year. But it has become clear that the OSHA/MSHA STS is not a very satisfactory way of judging a hearing loss prevention program because it allows substantial amounts of hearing loss to occur, especially when presbycusis adjustments are included. With a more conservative definition, such as the NIOSH definition (15 dB at any frequency if confirmed by a retest), STS[58] becomes a more useful measure.

Certain factors can cause STS rates to appear unrealistically low, for example, high rates of employee turnover, pre-existing hearing loss, and prior STSs (Royster and Royster, 1999). If we look at STS rates, or any shift rates for that matter, the question arises as to how many STSs are acceptable. Hearing conservation professionals have suggested criteria for acceptability ranging from 3 to 6 percent annually of the noise-exposed population. The NIOSH Criteria Document recommends an annual incidence of STS no greater than 3 percent.

Actually, no STS should be acceptable if it is caused by occupational noise. But hearing loss from aging, non-occupational noise exposure, and medical problems are likely to contribute some amount of STS, and it is often very difficult to distinguish among them. At this time there is no professional consensus on the acceptable rate of STS except that the rate should be small.

Statistical Procedures

Companies with more than about 30 employees should consider using audiometric database analysis to evaluate the effectiveness of their hearing conservation programs. Now that many of the larger companies (and even some of the smaller ones) use computer-based audiometers, these kinds of procedures are becoming increasingly feasible. The method involves examining audiograms taken over a period of at least five or six years. First, one looks for a possible "learning effect," a slight improvement in hearing threshold levels that commonly occurs over the first four or five years of testing. The presence of a learning effect should indicate that workers are not losing their hearing and the program is an effective one.

Other criteria include test–retest comparisons, in which the proportion of improving thresholds is compared to the proportion that is deteriorating. Another comparison is the sequential test–retest comparison, where each audiogram is compared to the results of the preceding year. By examining the combined results of these comparisons, the OHC or professional supervisor should be able to judge the overall effectiveness of the hearing conservation program.

These audiometric database analyses are considerably more sensitive than the OSHA/MSHA STS criterion, and they may provide information on the quality of the audiometric testing program, as well as the conservation of hearing.

An ANSI report, "Evaluating the Effectiveness of Hearing Conservation Programs" (ANSI S12.13-2002), details these procedures as well as the history and rationale for their development. The report is reprinted as Appendix P of this manual.

Other statistical methods are available for examining audiometric data. OHCs can consult with their audiometric program supervisors to learn more about these methods.

Wrap-up

By this time your head may be spinning with facts, suggestions, procedures, admonitions, and ideas. Some of you may be charged up and ready to go, while others may feel overloaded. Most of you will have busy schedules, in which hearing conservation is only one of a number of health-related duties.

Hopefully, you will keep this manual nearby, consult it often and, when in doubt, ask your audiological or medical supervisors for assistance. But before long, you should find that your confidence has grown, along with your experience. Indeed, as an OHC, your knowledge of workers' practices, problems, and successes places you in a unique and invaluable position to carry out an effective hearing conservation program.

---

[58] NIOSH refers to its definition of shift as "significant" rather than "standard."

References

Franks, J.R., Stephenson, M.R., and Merry, C.J. (1996). "Program evaluation." In *Preventing Occupational Hearing Loss—A Practical Guide*. DHHS (NIOSH) 96–110. Department of Health and Human Services, Public Health Service, National Institute for Occupational Safety and Health, Cincinnati, OH.

Megerson, S.C. (2001). "Update on hearing loss recordability: OSHA call for comments." CAOHC *UPDATE*, *13*(2), 2.

NIOSH (1998). "Criteria for a recommended standard: Occupational noise exposure: Revised criteria, 1998." DHHS (NIOSH) 98–126. Dept. Health and Human Services, Public Health Service.

OSHA (2002). "Occupational injury and illness recording and reporting requirements: Final rule." Dept. Labor, Occupational Safety and Health Administration, *67 Fed. Reg.*, 44037–44048.

Royster, J.D., and Royster, L.H. (September 1999). "How can we evaluate the effectiveness of occupational hearing conservation programs?" *The Hearing Review*.

Quiz

1. What is the minimum information that OSHA and MSHA require the professional reviewer to be provided with?

2. How long does OSHA require employers to keep audiograms? How long does MSHA require they should be kept? How long should they be kept?

3. It is good practice to keep a record of the visual examination of the employee's earcanals, noting whether or not an otoscope was used. (True or False)

4. OSHA requires the employer to notify employees in writing of the results of the noise monitoring. (True or False) Does MSHA?

5. What are the most important characteristics of good records?

6. Does OSHA's policy for recording hearing loss on the Form 300 change the existing threshold shift requirements for identifying an STS? Does MSHA's reporting requirement change its definition of STS?

7. Practical guidance for evaluating hearing conservation programs are found in which documents and appendices?

8. High rates of employee turnover can cause STS rates to be unrealistically low. (True or False)

9. Statistical procedures for evaluating hearing conservation program effectiveness may be used in companies with at least _____ employees.

10. Who is in a unique and invaluable position to carry out an effective hearing conservation program?

Abbreviations Used in Chapter XII

ANSI	American National Standards Institute
dB	Decibels
dBA	Decibels measured on the A scale of the sound level meter (or dosimeter)
Hz	Hertz
MSHA	Mine Safety and Health Administration
NIOSH	National Institute for Occupational Safety and Health
OHC	Occupational Hearing Conservationist
OSHA	Occupational Safety and Health Administration
STS	Standard threshold shift
TWA	Time-weighted average exposure level

Recommended Reading

Franks, J.R., Stephenson, M.R., and Merry, C.J. (1996). "Recordkeeping" and "Program evaluation." In *Preventing Occupational Hearing Loss—A Practical Guide*. DHHS (NIOSH) 96–110. Department of Health and Human Services, Public Health Service, National Institute for Occupational Safety and Health, Cincinnati, OH.

Megerson, S.C. (Summer 2001). "Update on hearing loss recordabilitiy: OSHA call for comments." CAOHC *UPDATE*, *13*(2) 2.

OSHA (June 4, 1991). Memorandum for Regional Administrators from Patricia Clark, Director, Directorate of Compliance Programs, "Recording of hearing loss and cumulative trauma disorders (CTDS) on the OSHA 200 Log."

Royster, J.D., and Royster, L.H. (2000). "Evaluating hearing conservation program effectiveness." Chapter 12 in E.H. Berger, L.H. Royster, J.D. Royster, D.P. Driscoll, and M. Layne, (Eds.), *The Noise Manual, Fifth Edition*. American Industrial Hygiene Assoc., Fairfax, VA.

Appendix A
Websites

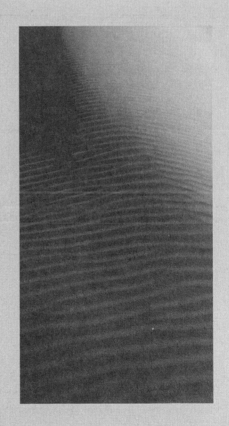

Websites

http://asa.aip.org	Acoustical Society of America (for information on ANSI standards etc.) (ASA)
www.entnet.org	American Academy of Otolaryngology—Head and Neck Surgery (AAO-HNS)
www.aaohn.org	American Association of Occupational Health Nurses (AAOHN)
www.acoem.org	American College of Occupational and Environmental Medicine (ACOEM)
www.aiha.org	American Industrial Hygiene Association (AIHA)
www.asse.org	American Society of Safety Engineers (ASSE)
www.asha.org	American Speech-Language-Hearing Association (ASHA)
www.ata.org	American Tinnitus Association (ATA)
www.AudiologyOnLine.com	Audiology Online
www.caohc.org	**Council for Accreditation in Occupational Hearing Conservation (CAOHC)**
www.e-a-r.com	E-A-R Aearo Co.
www.farmnoise.on.net	Farm Noise and Hearing Project (Australia)
www.hearnet.com	Hearing Education Awareness for Rockers (HEAR)
www.ince.org	Institute of Noise Control Engineering (INCE)
www.lhh.org	League for the Hard of Hearing (LHH)
www.lhsfna.org	Laborers' Health and Safety Fund of North America (LHFNA)
www.militaryaudiology.org	Military Audiology Association (MAA)
www.msha.gov	Mine Safety and Health Administration (MSHA)
www.msha.gov/1999noise/Surface/noisesurface.htm	MSHA Surface Equipment Noise Control
http://www-nehc.med.navy.mil/special/audspldr.htm	Navy Audiology Society Home Page
www.nased.com	National Association of Special Equipment Distributors (NASED)
www.hearingconservation.org	National Hearing Conservation Association (NHCA)
www.cdc.gov/niosh	National Institute for Occupational Safety and Health (NIOSH)
www.nidcd.nih.gov	National Institute on Deafness and Other Communication Disorders (NIDCD)
http://chid.nih.gov	NIDCD Information Clearing House: Combined Health Information Database
www.nsc.org	National Safety Council (NSC)
www.nonoise.org	Noise Pollution Clearinghouse
www.osha.gov	Occupational Safety and Health Administration (OSHA)
www.osha-slc.gov/Firm_osha_data/100007.html	OSHA Field Inspection Reference Manual, Section 7, Chapter III: Inspection (see section C.3.b)
www.osha.gov/SLTC/noisehearingconservation/index.html	(scroll to Standards Interpretations and Compliance Letters and click on SEARCH) OSHA Interpretations
www.osha-slc.gov/dts/osta/otm/otm_iii/otm_iii_5.html	OSHA Technical Manual, Section III Chapter 5—Noise Measurement
www.safe-at-work.com	Safe at Work
www.safetyline.wa.gov.au/sub30.htm	WorkSafe Western Australia Noise Page

**For descriptions of the CAOHC website links,
see following summary from the Fall 1999 issue of the *UPDATE*:**

Hearing Conservation: Internet Information & Training Resources

by Merrie L. Healy, RN MPH
CAOHC Representative of the National Safety Council

Anyone who has responsibility for an occupational hearing conservation program is aware of the need to obtain up-to-date information and training materials. In an effort to support that, this article will provide a summary of resources. Bearing in mind that not all persons have Internet access, addresses and phone numbers will be provided whenever possible. *(The inclusion of the following organizations and resources are not meant to be an endorsement by CAOHC.)*

CAOHC Website Links:
(www.caohc.org/related-websites.html)

The CAOHC website (www.caohc.org) provides information that includes a definition of CAOHC; lists the Component Professional Organizations (CPO); and provides directions on certification for occupational hearing conservationists and course directors. Resource information provides a sampling of past UPDATE newsletters and ordering of the Hearing Conservation Manual. *A new section, supplementary course director educational materials, has been added. Links to related websites provide additional resource access. This article begins with a summary of those website links:*

Acoustical Society of America (ASA)
2 Huntington Quadrangle
Melville, NY 11747-4502
516/576-2360
FAX: 516/576-2377
http://asa.aip.org

The website offers a "Listen to Sounds" program; and an available compact disc of auditory demonstrations.

Hearing Education Awareness for Rockers (HEAR)
P.O. Box 460847
San Francisco, CA 94146
415/773-9590
FAX: 415/552-4296
www.hearnet.com

Educational and information materials include "Can't Hear You Knocking" (VHS video); and sign songs. Devices and gizmos include audio materials such as a CD self-hearing test and "Tinnitus Away!" (cassette). Posters and hearing protection ordering information are also available.

League for Hard of Hearing (LHH)
71 W. 23rd Street
New York, NY 10010-4162
917/305-7700
FAX: 917/305-7888
TTY: 917/305-7999
www.llh.org

This is the organization that sponsors a national "Noise Awareness Day" (see UPDATE, Spring 1999 article). A packet of information regarding the impact of noise on hearing in a fun, easy format is available to promote this event.

National Hearing Conservation Association (NHCA)
9101 Kenyon Avenue, Suite #3000
Denver, CO 80237
303/224-9022
FAX: 303/770-1812
www.hearingconservation.org

This organization offers educational materials such as posters and slides.

National Institute for Occupational Safety & Health (NIOSH)
Hubert H. Humphrey Building
200 Independence Ave., S.W.
Room 715H
Washington, DC 20201
1-800-356-4674
www.cdc.gov/niosh/homepage.html

National Institute on Deafness & Other Communication Disorders (NIDCD)
National Institute of Health
31 Center Drive, MSC 2320
Bethesda, MD 20892-2320
www.nih.gov/nidcd

The following documents are available from **NIDCD** and **NIOSH**:

NIOSH Criteria Document

NIDCD Fact Sheet on Noise-Induced Hearing Loss

NIOSH: Preventing Hearing Loss –A Practical Guide (Note: this document describes the elements of an effective Hearing Loss Prevention Program and has an appendix that lists vendors with educational materials, specifying video titles.)

NIDCD bookmark "How Loud is Loud" (English/Spanish)

NIDCD bookmark "Ten Ways to Recognize Hearing Loss" (English/Spanish)

NIDCD Directory of Information Resources for Human Communication Disorders

Combined Health Information Database (CHID)
http://chid.nih.gov

A search using "hearing conservation" elicited 153 citations.

Internet Information

**Noise Pollution
Clearinghouse (NPC)**
P.O. Box 1137
Montpelier, VT 05601-1137
1-888-8332
www.nonoise.org

This site has a library of resources.

**Occupational Safety & Health
Administration (OSHA)**
U.S. Department of Labor
200 Constitution Avenue, N.W.
Room N-3647
Washington, DC 20210
202/219-8151
FAX: 202/219-5986
www.osha.gov

OSHA provides regulatory information related to compliance with the hearing conservation standard (29 CFR 1910.95). A search using "hearing conservation" resulted in 184 citations. Program and services include consultation and education programs. OSHA also links to other government and safety and health internet sites.

FYI: Other Hearing Conservation Resources

Audiology Forum: Video Otoscopy
www.li.net/~sullivan/ears.htm

This site offers a multitude of educational, informational articles and visual materials which can be used as teaching aids.

Navy Audiology Society Home Page
www-nmcp.med.navy.mil/audio/
nashome.html

This site offers PowerPoint presentations for hearing conservation programs.

Military Audiology Association
www.military/audiology.org

The Auditory Readiness Information Center offers a slide presentation educational package.

Safe at Work
517/349-5205
www.safe-at-work.com

This site provides information about sound exposure monitoring and control, and the hearing loss prevention process. Be sure to check the "REFERENCE" section. A slide presentation "Hearing Loss Prevention as a Business Process" includes speaker notes.

E•A•R/Aearo Company
Berger, EH (1979-1999) E-A-RLog Series of Technical Monographs on Hearing and Hearing Protection, Nos. 1-21. Contact Customer Service at 1-800-225-9038, or visit: www.e-a-r.com

Film and videotape information: Contact Elliott Berger (317/692-3031).

Noise & Hearing Conservation-References for Good Practice: Standards, Regulations, and Recommended References Pertaining to Noise, Vibration, and Noise-Induced Hearing Loss (AIHA and NHCA),

This document was prepared by the American Industrial Hygiene Association (AIHA) and the National Hearing Conservation Association (NHCA). It cites over 200 references organized in the following sections: Overview; Hearing Conservation Program Administration Guidelines; Quick References; Professional Organizations, Publications, and Home Pages; TLVs; Guidelines, Position Statements, and Criteria Documents; National and International Standards; Databases and Programs; Handbooks, Textbooks and Review Articles; U.S. Government Regulations and Reports; and Other Regulations and Reports.

The first three sections are available on the NHCA website (previously mentioned in this article). The entire document is free to NHCA members and can be purchased by non-members for $50.

Information Please!!

Those of you "in the trenches" involved with training and education have probably found some very useful resources and tools. CAOHC requests that you share information about such materials for publication in a future UPDATE. We often learn best from each other! Information can be sent to:

UPDATE Editor
Council for Accreditation in Occupational Health Conservation
611 E. Wells Street
Milwaukee, WI 53202
Phone: 414/276-5338
FAX: 414/276-2146
E-Mail: info@caohc.org

Appendix B
Information and Materials
Available from CAOHC

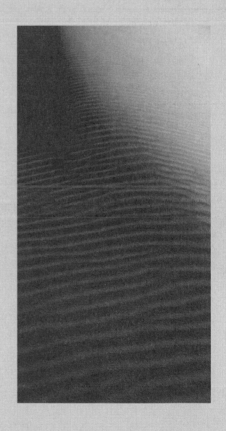

Information and Materials Available from CAOHC

- **CAOHC Website www.caohc.org**
  Home page describes CAOHC services, information, and materials.
  On-line forms (including OHC certification and recertification applications; manual order form; video order form; address correction).
  List of component professional organizations.
  List of related websites.
  List of prior issues of *UPDATE.*

- **Pamphlets about CAOHC**
  "The Stamp of Approval for Occupational Hearing Conservation"
  "CAOHC Q&A"

- **Newsletters**

  UPDATE
  Newsletter published by CAOHC. Very informative for OHCs, CDs, and anyone interested in occupational hearing conservation. Some key articles available on our website at **www.caohc.org**

  CABLE
  Newsletter for Course Directors available on-line quarterly.

- **Manual**
  The *Hearing Conservation Manual, 4th Edition,* by Alice Suter, PhD was completely rewritten in 2002. See order form enclosed.

- **Video**
  "Anatomy, Physiology, and Diseases of the Ear" Course Curriculum Package.
  A 20-minute video and instructional packet. See description and ordering information following.

Most of the above items are available without charge.

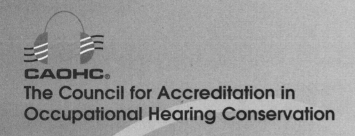

CAOHC®
The Council for Accreditation in
Occupational Hearing Conservation

~Presents~
Anatomy, Physiology
& Diseases of the Ear
Course Curriculum Package

- Provides audiometric technicians, industrial workers, CAOHC students and others with solid background information about the anatomy and physiology of the human ear.

- Instructs on the parts of the ear, how sound is processed, types of hearing loss and how they can be prevented.

- Increases knowledge about the effects of noise – encouraging workers to be more receptive to hearing conservation programs.

- Allows CAOHC Course Directors to substitute the otolaryngologist instructor in a 20-hour certification course.

- This curriculum includes a 22 minute video written and produced by CAOHC and supplemental materials that include interactive teaching techniques that will get your students involved in the learning process.

Curriculum package: $300.00 + $7.50 UPS shipping
Discounted to CAOHC Course Directors: $200.00 + $7.50 UPS shipping

This video is narrated by Robert Dobie, MD while professor and Chairman of the Department of Otolaryngology of the University of Texas Health Science Center. Dr. Dobie served on the CAOHC Council for ten years as the representative of the American Academy of Otolaryngology-Head and Neck Surgery. He is the author of the book <u>Medical-Legal Evaluation of Hearing Loss.</u>

CAOHC®

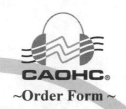

~Order Form ~

THE ANATOMY, PHYSIOLOGY AND DISEASES OF THE HUMAN EAR
VIDEO CURRICULUM PACKAGE

This video is narrated by Robert Dobie, MD while Professor and Chairman of the Department of Otolaryngology of the University of Texas Health Science Center. Dr.Dobie served on the CAOHC Council for ten years as the representative of the American Academy of Otolaryngology-Head and Neck Surgery. He is the author of the book <u>Medical-Legal Evaluation of Hearing Loss</u>. The Anatomy Video Curriculum includes a 22 minute video tape written and produced by CAOHC and supplemental materials that will help you involve your students, health staff, industrial workers, and others in the learning process .

This Anatomy Curriculum will:

- **Provide audiometric technicians, industrial workers & CAOHC students with solid background information about the anatomy and physiology of the human ear.**
- **Instruct on the parts of the ear, how sound is processed, types of hearing loss and how they can be prevented.**
- **Increase knowledge about the effects of noise - encouraging workers to be more receptive to hearing conservation programs.**
- **Allows CAOHC Course Directors to substitute the physician instructor in a 20-hour certification course. (If you are a CAOHC Course Director and using this video curriculum in a CAOHC approved OHC course, please consult the CD Handbook 2000 to meet course requirements.)**

Curriculum package: $ 300.00 + *UPS shipping*
Discounted to CAOHC Course Directors: $ 200.00 + *UPS shipping*

Quantity	Curriculum Price	+ UPS Shipping	Total
	$	$	$

Name _____

Company Name _____

Address (No PO Boxes please) _____

City/State/Zip _____

Method of Payment   ☐ MC   ☐ VA   ☐ Check/Money Order/Cash

Name on Card _____ Exp Date _____

CAOHC 611 E. Wells Street Milwaukee, WI 53202 Phone: 414/276-5338 Fax 414/276-2146 E-Mail: info@caohc.org

Appendix C
OSHA Noise Regulation

29 CFR 1910.95

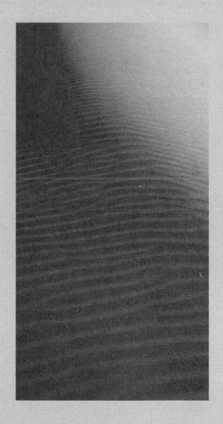

U.S. Department of Labor Regulations (Standards – 29 CFR)

Occupational noise exposure. — 1910.95

Regulations (Standards – 29 CFR)

– Table of Contents

- **Part Number:** 1910
- **Part Title:** Occupational Safety and Health Standards
- **Subpart:** G
- **Subpart Title:** Occupational Health and Environment Control
- **Standard Number:** 1910.95
- **Title:** Occupational noise exposure.
- **Appendix:** A, B, C, D, E, F, G, H, I

1910.95(a)

Protection against the effects of noise exposure shall be provided when the sound levels exceed those shown in Table G–16 when measured on the A scale of a standard sound level meter at slow response. When noise levels are determined by octave band analysis, the equivalent A-weighted sound level may be determined as follows:

FIGURE G–9 — Equivalent A-Weighted Sound Level

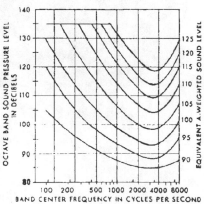

Equivalent sound level contours. Octave band sound pressure levels may be converted to the equivalent A-weighted sound level by plotting them on this graph and noting the A-weighted sound level corresponding to the point of highest penetration into the sound level contours. This equivalent A-weighted sound level, which may differ from the actual A-weighted sound level of the noise, is used to determine exposure limits from Table G–16.

1910.95(b)
1910.95(b)(1)

When employees are subjected to sound exceeding those listed in Table G–16, feasible administrative or engineering controls shall be utilized. If such controls fail to reduce sound levels within the levels of Table G–16, personal protective equipment shall be provided and used to reduce sound levels within the levels of the table.

1910.95(b)(2)

If the variations in noise level involve maxima at intervals of 1 second or less, it is to be considered continuous.

TABLE G–16 — PERMISSIBLE NOISE EXPOSURES [1]

Duration per day, hours	Sound level dBA slow response
8	90
6	92
4	95
3	97
2	100
1 1/2	102
1	105
1/2	110
1/4 or less	115

[1]When the daily noise exposure is composed of two or more periods of noise exposure of different levels, their combined effect should be considered, rather than the individual effect of each. If the sum of the following fractions: $C_1/T_1 + C_2/T_2 \ C_n/T_n$ exceeds unity, then, the mixed exposure should be considered to exceed the limit value. C_n indicates the total time of exposure at a specified noise level, and T_n indicates the total time of exposure permitted at that level. Exposure to impulsive or impact noise should not exceed 140 dB peak sound pressure level.

1910.95(c)

"Hearing conservation program."

1910.95(c)(1)

The employer shall administer a continuing, effective hearing conservation program, as described in paragraphs (c) through (o) of this section, whenever employee noise exposures equal or exceed an 8-hour time-weighted average sound level (TWA) of 85 decibels measured on the A scale (slow response) or, equivalently, a dose of fifty percent. For purposes of the hearing conservation program, employee noise exposures shall be computed in accordance with appendix A and Table G–16a, and without regard to any attenuation provided by the use of personal protective equipment.

1910.95(c)(2)

For purposes of paragraphs (c) through (n) of this section, an 8-hour time-weighted average of 85 decibels or a dose of fifty percent shall also be referred to as the action level.

1910.95(d)

"Monitoring."

1910.95(d)(1)

When information indicates that any employee's exposure may equal or exceed an 8-hour time-weighted average of 85 decibels, the employer shall develop and implement a monitoring program.

1910.95(d)(1)(i)

The sampling strategy shall be designed to identify employees for inclusion in the hearing conservation program and to enable the proper selection of hearing protectors.

1910.95(d)(1)(ii)

Where circumstances such as high worker mobility, significant variations in sound level, or a significant component of impulse noise make area monitoring generally inappropriate, the employer shall use representative personal sampling to comply with the monitoring requirements of this paragraph unless the employer can show that area sampling produces equivalent results.

1910.95(d)(2)
1910.95(d)(2)(i)
All continuous, intermittent and impulsive sound levels from 80 decibels to 130 decibels shall be integrated into the noise measurements.

1910.95(d)(2)(ii)
Instruments used to measure employee noise exposure shall be calibrated to ensure measurement accuracy.

1910.95(d)(3)
Monitoring shall be repeated whenever a change in production, process, equipment or controls increases noise exposures to the extent that:

1910.95(d)(3)(i)
Additional employees may be exposed at or above the action level; or

1910.95(d)(3)(ii)
The attenuation provided by hearing protectors being used by employees may be rendered inadequate to meet the requirements of paragraph (j) of this section.

1910.95(e)
"Employee notification." The employer shall notify each employee exposed at or above an 8-hour time-weighted average of 85 decibels of the results of the monitoring.

1910.95(f)
"Observation of monitoring." The employer shall provide affected employees or their representatives with an opportunity to observe any noise measurements conducted pursuant to this section.

1910.95(g)
"Audiometric testing program."

1910.95(g)(1)
The employer shall establish and maintain an audiometric testing program as provided in this paragraph by making audiometric testing available to all employees whose exposures equal or exceed an 8-hour time-weighted average of 85 decibels.

1910.95(g)(2)
The program shall be provided at no cost to employees.

1910.95(g)(3)
Audiometric tests shall be performed by a licensed or certified audiologist, otolaryngologist, or other physician, or by a technician who is certified by the Council for Accreditation in Occupational Hearing Conservation, or who has satisfactorily demonstrated competence in administering audiometric examinations, obtaining valid audiograms, and properly using, maintaining and checking calibration and proper functioning of the audiometers being used. A technician who operates microprocessor audiometers does not need to be certified. A technician who performs audiometric tests must be responsible to an audiologist, otolaryngologist or physician.

1910.95(g)(4)
All audiograms obtained pursuant to this section shall meet the requirements of Appendix C: "Audiometric Measuring Instruments."

1910.95(g)(5)
"Baseline audiogram."

1910.95(g)(5)(i)
Within 6 months of an employee's first exposure at or above the action level, the employer shall establish a valid baseline audiogram against which subsequent audiograms can be compared.

1910.95(g)(5)(ii)
"Mobile test van exception." Where mobile test vans are used to meet the audiometric testing obligation, the employer shall obtain a valid baseline audiogram within 1 year of an employee's first exposure at or above the action level. Where baseline audiograms are obtained more than 6 months after the employee's first exposure at or above the action level, employees shall wear hearing protectors for any period exceeding six months after first exposure until the baseline audiogram is obtained.

1910.95(g)(5)(iii)
Testing to establish a baseline audiogram shall be preceded by at least 14 hours without exposure to workplace noise. Hearing protectors may be used as a substitute for the requirement that baseline audiograms be preceded by 14 hours without exposure to workplace noise.

1910.95(g)(5)(iv)
The employer shall notify employees of the need to avoid high levels of non-occupational noise exposure during the 14-hour period immediately preceding the audiometric examination.

1910.95(g)(6)
"Annual audiogram." At least annually after obtaining the baseline audiogram, the employer shall obtain a new audiogram for each employee exposed at or above an 8-hour time-weighted average of 85 decibels.

1910.95(g)(7)
"Evaluation of audiogram."

1910.95(g)(7)(i)
Each employee's annual audiogram shall be compared to that employee's baseline audiogram to determine if the audiogram is valid and if a standard threshold shift as defined in paragraph (g)(10) of this section has occurred. This comparison may be done by a technician.

1910.95(g)(7)(ii)
If the annual audiogram shows that an employee has suffered a standard threshold shift, the employer may obtain a retest within 30 days and consider the results of the retest as the annual audiogram.

1910.95(g)(7)(iii)
The audiologist, otolaryngologist, or physician shall review problem audiograms and shall determine whether there is a need for further evaluation. The employer shall provide to the person performing this evaluation the following information:

1910.95(g)(7)(iii)(A)
A copy of the requirements for hearing conservation as set forth in paragraphs (c) through (n) of this section;

1910.95(g)(7)(iii)(B)
The baseline audiogram and most recent audiogram of the employee to be evaluated;

1910.95(g)(7)(iii)(C)
Measurements of background sound pressure levels in the audiometric test room as required in Appendix D: Audiometric Test Rooms.

1910.95(g)(7)(iii)(D)
Records of audiometer calibrations required by paragraph (h)(5) of this section.

1910.95(g)(8)
"Follow-up procedures."

1910.95(g)(8)(i)
If a comparison of the annual audiogram to the baseline audiogram indicates a standard threshold shift as defined in paragraph (g)(10) of this section has occurred, the employee shall be informed of this fact in writing, within 21 days of the determination.

1910.95(g)(8)(ii)
Unless a physician determines that the standard threshold shift is not work related or aggravated by occupational noise exposure, the employer shall ensure that the following steps are taken when a standard threshold shift occurs:

1910.95(g)(8)(ii)(A)
Employees not using hearing protectors shall be fitted with hearing protectors, trained in their use and care, and required to use them.

1910.95(g)(8)(ii)(B)

Employees already using hearing protectors shall be refitted and retrained in the use of hearing protectors and provided with hearing protectors offering greater attenuation if necessary.

1910.95(g)(8)(ii)(C)

The employee shall be referred for a clinical audiological evaluation or an otological examination, as appropriate, if additional testing is necessary or if the employer suspects that a medical pathology of the ear is caused or aggravated by the wearing of hearing protectors.

1910.95(g)(8)(ii)(D)

The employee is informed of the need for an otological examination if a medical pathology of the ear that is unrelated to the use of hearing protectors is suspected.

1910.95(g)(8)(iii)

If subsequent audiometric testing of an employee whose exposure to noise is less than an 8-hour TWA of 90 decibels indicates that a standard threshold shift is not persistent, the employer:

1910.95(g)(8)(iii)(A)

Shall inform the employee of the new audiometric interpretation; and

1910.95(g)(8)(iii)(B)

May discontinue the required use of hearing protectors for that employee.

1910.95(g)(9)

"Revised baseline." An annual audiogram may be substituted for the baseline audiogram when, in the judgment of the audiologist, otolaryngologist or physician who is evaluating the audiogram:

1910.95(g)(9)(i)

The standard threshold shift revealed by the audiogram is persistent; or

1910.95(g)(9)(ii)

The hearing threshold shown in the annual audiogram indicates significant improvement over the baseline audiogram.

1910.95(g)(10)

"Standard threshold shift."

1910.95(g)(10)(i)

As used in this section, a standard threshold shift is a change in hearing threshold relative to the baseline audiogram of an average of 10 dB or more at 2000, 3000, and 4000 Hz in either ear.

1910.95(g)(10)(ii)

In determining whether a standard threshold shift has occurred, allowance may be made for the contribution of aging (presbycusis) to the change in hearing level by correcting the annual audiogram according to the procedure described in Appendix F: "Calculation and Application of Age Correction to Audiograms."

1910.95(h)

"Audiometric test requirements."

1910.95(h)(1)

Audiometric tests shall be pure tone, air conduction, hearing threshold examinations, with test frequencies including as a minimum 500, 1000, 2000, 3000, 4000, and 6000 Hz. Tests at each frequency shall be taken separately for each ear.

1910.95(h)(2)

Audiometric tests shall be conducted with audiometers (including microprocessor audiometers) that meet the specifications of, and are maintained and used in accordance with, American National Standard Specification for Audiometers, S3.6-1969, which is incorporated by reference as specified in Sec. 1910.6.

1910.95(h)(3)

Pulsed-tone and self-recording audiometers, if used, shall meet the requirements specified in Appendix C: "Audiometric Measuring Instruments."

1910.95(h)(4)

Audiometric examinations shall be administered in a room meeting the requirements listed in Appendix D: "Audiometric Test Rooms."

1910.95(h)(5)

"Audiometer calibration."

1910.95(h)(5)(i)

The functional operation of the audiometer shall be checked before each day's use by testing a person with known, stable hearing thresholds, and by listening to the audiometer's output to make sure that the output is free from distorted or unwanted sounds. Deviations of 10 decibels or greater require an acoustic calibration.

1910.95(h)(5)(ii)

Audiometer calibration shall be checked acoustically at least annually in accordance with Appendix E: "Acoustic Calibration of Audiometers." Test frequencies below 500 Hz and above 6000 Hz may be omitted from this check. Deviations of 15 decibels or greater require an exhaustive calibration.

1910.95(h)(5)(iii)

An exhaustive calibration shall be performed at least every two years in accordance with sections 4.1.2; 4.1.3.; 4.1.4.3; 4.2; 4.4.1; 4.4.2; 4.4.3; and 4.5 of the American National Standard Specification for Audiometers, S3.6-1969. Test frequencies below 500 Hz and above 6000 Hz may be omitted from this calibration.

1910.95(i)

"Hearing protectors."

1910.95(i)(1)

Employers shall make hearing protectors available to all employees exposed to an 8-hour time-weighted average of 85 decibels or greater at no cost to the employees. Hearing protectors shall be replaced as necessary.

1910.95(i)(2)

Employers shall ensure that hearing protectors are worn:

1910.95(i)(2)(i)

By an employee who is required by paragraph (b)(1) of this section to wear personal protective equipment; and

1910.95(i)(2)(ii)

By any employee who is exposed to an 8-hour time-weighted average of 85 decibels or greater, and who:

1910.95(i)(2)(ii)(A)

Has not yet had a baseline audiogram established pursuant to paragraph (g)(5)(ii); or

1910.95(i)(2)(ii)(B)

Has experienced a standard threshold shift.

1910.95(i)(3)

Employees shall be given the opportunity to select their hearing protectors from a variety of suitable hearing protectors provided by the employer.

1910.95(i)(4)

The employer shall provide training in the use and care of all hearing protectors provided to employees.

1910.95(i)(5)

The employer shall ensure proper initial fitting and supervise the correct use of all hearing protectors.

1910.95(j)

"Hearing protector attenuation."

1910.95(j)(1)

The employer shall evaluate hearing protector attenuation for the specific noise environments in which the protector will be used. The employer shall use one of the evaluation methods described in Appendix B: "Methods for Estimating the Adequacy of Hearing Protection Attenuation."

1910.95(j)(2)

Hearing protectors must attenuate employee exposure at least to an 8-hour time-weighted average of 90 decibels as required by paragraph (b) of this section.

1910.95(j)(3)

For employees who have experienced a standard threshold shift, hearing protectors must attenuate employee exposure to an 8-hour time-weighted average of 85 decibels or below.

1910.95(j)(4)

The adequacy of hearing protector attenuation shall be re-evaluated whenever employee noise exposures increase to the extent that the hearing protectors provided may no longer provide adequate attenuation. The employer shall provide more effective hearing protectors where necessary.

1910.95(k)

"Training program."

1910.95(k)(1)

The employer shall institute a training program for all employees who are exposed to noise at or above an 8-hour time-weighted average of 85 decibels, and shall ensure employee participation in such program.

1910.95(k)(2)

The training program shall be repeated annually for each employee included in the hearing conservation program. Information provided in the training program shall be updated to be consistent with changes in protective equipment and work processes.

1910.95(k)(3)

The employer shall ensure that each employee is informed of the following:

1910.95(k)(3)(i)

The effects of noise on hearing;

1910.95(k)(3)(ii)

The purpose of hearing protectors, the advantages, disadvantages, and attenuation of various types, and instructions on selection, fitting, use, and care; and

1910.95(k)(3)(iii)

The purpose of audiometric testing, and an explanation of the test procedures.

1910.95(l)

"Access to information and training materials."

1910.95(l)(1)

The employer shall make available to affected employees or their representatives copies of this standard and shall also post a copy in the workplace.

1910.95(l)(2)

The employer shall provide to affected employees any informational materials pertaining to the standard that are supplied to the employer by the Assistant Secretary.

1910.95(l)(3)

The employer shall provide, upon request, all materials related to the employer's training and education program pertaining to this standard to the Assistant Secretary and the Director.

1910.95(m)

"Recordkeeping."

1910.95(m)(1)

"Exposure measurements." The employer shall maintain an accurate record of all employee exposure measurements required by paragraph (d) of this section.

1910.95(m)(2)

"Audiometric tests."

1910.95(m)(2)(i)

The employer shall retain all employee audiometric test records obtained pursuant to paragraph (g) of this section:

1910.95(m)(2)(ii)

This record shall include:

1910.95(m)(2)(ii)(A)

Name and job classification of the employee;

1910.95(m)(2)(ii)(B)

Date of the audiogram;

1910.95(m)(2)(ii)(C)

The examiner's name;

1910.95(m)(2)(ii)(D)

Date of the last acoustic or exhaustive calibration of the audiometer; and

1910.95(m)(2)(ii)(E)

Employee's most recent noise exposure assessment.

1910.95(m)(2)(ii)(F)

The employer shall maintain accurate records of the measurements of the background sound pressure levels in audiometric test rooms.

1910.95(m)(3)

"Record retention." The employer shall retain records required in this paragraph (m) for at least the following periods.

1910.95(m)(3)(i)

Noise exposure measurement records shall be retained for two years.

1910.95(m)(3)(ii)

Audiometric test records shall be retained for the duration of the affected employee's employment.

1910.95(m)(4)

"Access to records." All records required by this section shall be provided upon request to employees, former employees, representatives designated by the individual employee, and the Assistant Secretary. The provisions of 29 CFR 1910.20 (a)-(e) and (g)-(i) apply to access to records under this section.

1910.95(m)(5)

"Transfer of records." If the employer ceases to do business, the employer shall transfer to the successor employer all records required to be maintained by this section, and the successor employer shall retain them for the remainder of the period prescribed in paragraph (m)(3) of this section.

1910.95(n)

"Appendices."

1910.95(n)(1)

Appendices A, B, C, D, and E to this section are incorporated as part of this section and the contents of these appendices are mandatory.

1910.95(n)(2)

Appendices F and G to this section are informational and are not intended to create any additional obligations not otherwise imposed or to detract from any existing obligations.

1910.95(o)

"Exemptions." Paragraphs (c) through (n) of this section shall not apply to employers engaged in oil and gas well drilling and servicing operations.

1910.95(p)

"Startup date." Baseline audiograms required by paragraph (g) of this section shall be completed by March 1, 1984.

Noise exposure computation — 1910.95 App A

This Appendix is Mandatory
I. Computation of Employee Noise Exposure

(1) Noise dose is computed using Table G–16a as follows:

(i) When the sound level, L, is constant over the entire work shift, the noise dose, D, in percent, is given by: $D = 100 \ C/T$ where C is the total length of the work day, in hours, and T is the reference duration corresponding to the measured sound level, L, as given in Table G-16a or by the formula shown as a footnote to that table.

(ii) When the workshift noise exposure is composed of two or more periods of noise at different levels, the total noise dose over the work day is given by:

$$D = 100 (C_1/T_1 + C_2/T_2 + \ldots + C_n/T_n)$$

where C_n indicates the total time of exposure at a specific noise level, and T_n indicates the reference duration for that level as given by Table G–16a.

(2) The eight-hour time-weighted average sound level (TWA), in decibels, may be computed from the dose, in percent, by means of the formula: $TWA = 16.61 \log_{10} (D/100) + 90$. For an eight-hour workshift with the noise level constant over the entire shift, the TWA is equal to the measured sound level.

(3) A table relating dose and TWA is given in Section II.

TABLE G–16A

A-weighted sound level, L (decibel)	Reference duration, T (hour)
80	32
81	27.9
82	24.3
83	21.1
84	18.4
85	16
86	13.9
87	12.1
88	10.6
89	9.2
90	8
91	7.0
92	6.1
93	5.3
94	4.6
95	4
96	3.5
97	3.0
98	2.6
99	2.3
100	2
101	1.7
102	1.5
103	1.3
104	1.1
105	1
106	0.87
107	0.76
108	0.66
109	0.57
110	0.5
111	0.44
112	0.38
113	0.33
114	0.29
115	0.25
116	0.22
117	0.19
118	0.16
119	0.14
120	0.125
121	0.11
122	0.095
123	0.082
124	0.072
125	0.063
126	0.054
127	0.047
128	0.041
129	0.036
130	0.031

In the preceding table the reference duration, T, is computed by

$$T = \frac{8}{2^{(L - 90)/5}}$$

where L is the measured A-weighted sound level.

II. Conversion Between "Dose" and "8-Hour Time-Weighted Average"

Sound Level

Compliance with paragraphs (c)−(r) of this regulation is determined by the amount of exposure to noise in the workplace. The amount of such exposure is usually measured with an audio-dosimeter which gives a readout in terms of "dose." In order to better understand the requirements of the amendment, dosimeter readings can be converted to an "8-hour time-weighted average sound level" (TWA).

In order to convert the reading of a dosimeter into TWA, see Table A–1, below. This table applies to dosimeters that are set by the manufacturer to calculate dose or percent exposure according to the relationships in Table G-16A. So, for example, a dose of 91 percent over an eight-hour day results in a TWA of 89.3 dB, and, a dose of 50 percent corresponds to a TWA of 85 dB.

If the dose as read on the dosimeter is less than or greater than the values found in Table A–1, the TWA may be calculated by using the formula: $TWA = 16.61 \log_{10} (D/100) + 90$, where TWA = 8-hour time-weighted average sound level and D = accumulated dose in percent exposure.

TABLE A–1 — CONVERSION FROM "PERCENT NOISE EXPOSURE" OR "DOSE" TO "8-HOUR TIME-WEIGHTED AVERAGE SOUND LEVEL" (TWA)

Dose or percent noise exposure	TWA
10	73.4
15	76.3
20	78.4
25	80.0
30	81.3
35	82.4
40	83.4
45	84.2
50	85.0
55	85.7
60	86.3
65	86.9
70	87.4
75	87.9
80	88.4
81	88.5
82	88.6
83	88.7
84	88.7
85	88.8
86	88.9
87	89.0
88	89.1
89	89.2
90	89.2
91	89.3

TABLE A–1 — CONVERSION FROM "PERCENT NOISE EXPOSURE" OR "DOSE" TO "8-HOUR TIME-WEIGHTED AVERAGE SOUND LEVEL" (TWA) —CONTINUED

Dose or percent noise exposure	TWA
92	89.4
93	89.5
94	89.6
95	89.6
96	89.7
97	89.8
98	89.9
99	89.9
100	90.0
101	90.1
102	90.1
103	90.2
104	90.3
105	90.4
106	90.4
107	90.5
108	90.6
109	90.6
110	90.7
111	90.8
112	90.8
113	90.9
114	90.9
115	91.1
116	91.1
117	91.1
118	91.2
119	91.3
120	91.3
125	91.6
130	91.9
135	92.2
140	92.4
145	92.7
150	92.9
155	93.2
160	93.4
165	93.6
170	93.8
175	94.0
180	94.2
185	94.4
190	94.6
195	94.8
200	95.0
210	95.4
220	95.7
230	96.0
240	96.3
250	96.6
260	96.9
270	97.2
280	97.4
290	97.7
300	97.9
310	98.2
320	98.4
330	98.6
340	98.8
350	99.0
360	99.2
370	99.4
380	99.6
390	99.8
400	100.0
410	100.2
420	100.4
430	100.5
440	100.7
450	100.8

Dose or percent noise exposure	TWA
460	101.0
470	101.2
480	101.3
490	101.5
500	101.6
510	101.8
520	101.9
530	102.0
540	102.2
550	102.3
560	102.4
570	102.6
580	102.7
590	102.8
600	102.9
610	103.0
620	103.2
630	103.3
640	103.4
650	103.5
660	103.6
670	103.7
680	103.8
690	103.9
700	104.0
710	104.1
720	104.2
730	104.3
740	104.4
750	104.5
760	104.6
770	104.7
780	104.8
790	104.9
800	105.0
810	105.1
820	105.2
830	105.3
840	105.4
850	105.4
860	105.5
870	105.6
880	105.7
890	105.8
900	105.8
910	105.9
920	106.0
930	106.1
940	106.2
950	106.2
960	106.3
970	106.4
980	106.5
990	106.5
999	106.6

Methods for estimating the adequacy of hearing protector attenuation — 1910.95 App B

This Appendix is Mandatory

For employees who have experienced a significant threshold shift, hearing protector attenuation must be sufficient to reduce employee exposure to a TWA of 85 dB. Employers must select one of the following methods by which to estimate the adequacy of hearing protector attenuation.

The most convenient method is the Noise Reduction Rating (NRR) developed by the Environmental Protection Agency (EPA). According to EPA regulation, the NRR must be shown on the hearing protector package. The NRR is then related to an individual worker's noise environment in order to assess the adequacy of the attenuation of a given hearing protector. This appendix describes four methods of using the NRR to determine whether a particular hearing protector provides adequate protection within a given exposure environment. Selection among the four procedures is dependent upon the employer's noise measuring instruments.

Instead of using the NRR, employers may evaluate the adequacy of hearing protector attenuation by using one of the three methods developed by the National Institute for Occupational Safety and Health (NIOSH), which are described in the "List of Personal Hearing Protectors and Attenuation Data," HEW Publication No. 76–120, 1975, pages 21–37. These methods are known as NIOSH methods No. 1, No. 2 and No. 3. The NRR described below is a simplification of NIOSH method No. 2. The most complex method is NIOSH method No. 1, which is probably the most accurate method since it uses the largest amount of spectral information from the individual employee's noise environment. As in the case of the NRR method described below, if one of the NIOSH methods is used, the selected method must be applied to an individual's noise environment to assess the adequacy of the attenuation. Employers should be careful to take a sufficient number of measurements in order to achieve a representative sample for each time segment.

NOTE: The employer must remember that calculated attenuation values reflect realistic values only to the extent that the protectors are properly fitted and worn.

When using the NRR to assess hearing protector adequacy, one of the following methods must be used:

(i) When using a dosimeter that is capable of C-weighted measurements:

(A) Obtain the employee's C-weighted dose for the entire workshift, and convert to TWA (see appendix A, II).

(B) Subtract the NRR from the C-weighted TWA to obtain the estimated A-weighted TWA under the ear protector.

(ii) When using a dosimeter that is not capable of C-weighted measurements, the following method may be used:

(A) Convert the A-weighted dose to TWA (see appendix A).

(B) Subtract 7 dB from the NRR.

(C) Subtract the remainder from the A-weighted TWA to obtain the estimated A-weighted TWA under the ear protector.

(iii) When using a sound level meter set to the A-weighting network:

(A) Obtain the employee's A-weighted TWA.

(B) Subtract 7 dB from the NRR, and subtract the remainder from the A-weighted TWA to obtain the estimated A-weighted TWA under the ear protector.

(iv) When using a sound level meter set on the C-weighting network:

(A) Obtain a representative sample of the C-weighted sound levels in the employee's environment.

(B) Subtract the NRR from the C-weighted average sound level to obtain the estimated A-weighted TWA under the ear protector.

(v) When using area monitoring procedures and a sound level meter set to the A-weighing network.

(A) Obtain a representative sound level for the area in question.

(B) Subtract 7 dB from the NRR and subtract the remainder from the A-weighted sound level for that area.

(vi) When using area monitoring procedures and a sound level meter set to the C-weighting network:

(A) Obtain a representative sound level for the area in question.

(B) Subtract the NRR from the C-weighted sound level for that area.

Audiometric measuring instruments – 1910.95 App C

This Appendix is Mandatory

1. In the event that pulsed-tone audiometers are used, they shall have a tone on-time of at least 200 milliseconds.

2. Self-recording audiometers shall comply with the following requirements:

(A) The chart upon which the audiogram is traced shall have lines at positions corresponding to all multiples of 10 dB hearing level within the intensity range spanned by the audiometer. The lines shall be equally spaced and shall be separated by at least 1/4 inch. Additional increments are optional. The audiogram pen tracings shall not exceed 2 dB in width.

(B) It shall be possible to set the stylus manually at the 10-dB increment lines for calibration purposes.

(C) The slewing rate for the audiometer attenuator shall not be more than 6 dB/sec except that an initial slewing rate greater than 6 dB/sec is permitted at the beginning of each new test frequency, but only until the second subject response.

(D) The audiometer shall remain at each required test frequency for 30 seconds (+ or − 3 seconds). The audiogram shall be clearly marked at each change of frequency and the actual frequency change of the audiometer shall not deviate from the frequency boundaries marked on the audiogram by more than + or − 3 seconds.

(E) It must be possible at each test frequency to place a horizontal line segment parallel to the time axis on the audiogram, such that the audiometric tracing crosses the line segment at least six times at that test frequency. At each test frequency the threshold shall be the average of the midpoints of the tracing excursions.

Audiometric test rooms — 1910.95 App D

This Appendix is Mandatory

Rooms used for audiometric testing shall not have background sound pressure levels exceeding those in Table D–1 when measured by equipment conforming at least to the Type 2 requirements of American National Standard Specification for Sound Level Meters, S1.4-1971 (R1976), and to the Class II requirements of American National Standard Specification for Octave, Half-Octave, and Third-Octave Band Filter Sets, S1.11-1971 (R1976).

TABLE D–1 — MAXIMUM ALLOWABLE OCTAVE-BAND SOUND PRESSURE LEVELS FOR AUDIOMETRIC TEST ROOMS

Octave-band center frequency (Hz)	500	1000	2000	4000	8000
Sound pressure level (dB)	40	40	47	57	62

Acoustic calibration of audiometers – 1910.95 App E

This Appendix is Mandatory

Audiometer calibration shall be checked acoustically, at least annually, according to the procedures described in this appendix. The equipment necessary to perform these measurements is a sound level meter, octave-band filter set, and a National Bureau of Standards 9A coupler. In making these measurements, the accuracy of the calibrating equipment shall be sufficient to determine that the audiometer is within the tolerances permitted by American Standard Specification for Audiometers, S3.6-1969.

(1) "Sound Pressure Output Check"

A. Place the earphone coupler over the microphone of the sound level meter and place the earphone on the coupler.

B. Set the audiometer's hearing threshold level (HTL) dial to 70 dB.

C. Measure the sound pressure level of the tones at each test frequency from 500 Hz through 6000 Hz for each earphone.

D. At each frequency the readout on the sound level meter should correspond to the levels in Table E–1 or Table E–2, as appropriate, for the type of earphone, in the column entitled "sound level meter reading."

(2) "Linearity Check"

A. With the earphone in place, set the frequency to 1000 Hz and the HTL dial on the audiometer to 70 dB.

B. Measure the sound levels in the coupler at each 10-dB decrement from 70 dB to 10 dB, noting the sound level meter reading at each setting.

C. For each 10-dB decrement on the audiometer the sound level meter should indicate a corresponding 10 dB decrease.

D. This measurement may be made electrically with a voltmeter connected to the earphone terminals.

(3) "Tolerances"

When any of the measured sound levels deviate from the levels in Table E–1 or Table E–2 by + or − 3 dB at any test frequency between 500 and 3000 Hz, 4 dB at 4000 Hz, or 5 dB at 6000 Hz, an exhaustive calibration is advised. An exhaustive calibration is required if the deviations are greater than 15 dB or greater at any test frequency.

TABLE E–1 — REFERENCE THRESHOLD LEVELS FOR TELEPHONICS — TDH–39 EARPHONES

Frequency, Hz	Reference threshold level for TDH-39 earphones, dB	Sound level meter reading, dB
500	11.5	81.5
1000	7	77
2000	9	79
3000	10	80
4000	9.5	79.5
6000	15.5	85.5

TABLE E–2 — REFERENCE THRESHOLD LEVELS FOR TELEPHONICS — TDH–49 EARPHONES

Frequency, Hz	Reference threshold level for TDH-49 earphones, dB	Sound level meter reading, dB
500	13.5	83.5
1000	7.5	77.5
2000	11	81.0
3000	9.5	79.5
4000	10.5	80.5
6000	13.5	83.5

Calculations and application of age corrections to audiograms – 1910.95 App F

This Appendix Is Non-Mandatory

In determining whether a standard threshold shift has occurred, allowance may be made for the contribution of aging to the change in hearing level by adjusting the most recent audiogram. If the employer chooses to adjust the audiogram, the employer shall follow the procedure described below. This procedure and the age correction tables were developed by the National Institute for Occupational Safety and Health in the criteria document entitled "Criteria for a Recommended Standard . . . Occupational Exposure to Noise," ((HSM)-11001).

For each audiometric test frequency;

(i) Determine from Tables F–1 or F–2 the age correction values for the employee by:

(A) Finding the age at which the most recent audiogram was taken and recording the corresponding values of age corrections at 1000 Hz through 6000 Hz;

(B) Finding the age at which the baseline audiogram was taken and recording the corresponding values of age corrections at 1000 Hz through 6000 Hz.

(ii) Subtract the values found in step (i)(B) from the value found in step (i)(A).

(iii) The differences calculated in step (ii) represent that portion of the change in hearing that may be due to aging.

EXAMPLE: Employee is a 32-year-old male. The audiometric history for his right ear is shown in decibels below.

Employee's age	Audiometric Test Frequency (Hz)				
	1000	2000	3000	4000	6000
26	10	5	5	10	5
*27	0	0	0	5	5
28	0	0	0	10	5
29	5	0	5	15	5
30	0	5	10	20	10
31	5	10	20	15	15
*32	5	10	10	25	20

The audiogram at age 27 is considered the baseline since it shows the best hearing threshold levels. Asterisks have been used to identify the baseline and most recent audiogram. A threshold shift of 20 dB exists at 4000 Hz between the audiograms taken at ages 27 and 32.

(The threshold shift is computed by subtracting the hearing threshold at age 27, which was 5, from the hearing threshold at age 32, which is 25.) A retest audiogram has confirmed this shift. The contribution of aging to this change in hearing may be estimated in the following manner:

Go to Table F–1 and find the age correction values (in dB) for 4000 Hz at age 27 and age 32.

	Frequency (Hz)				
	1000	2000	3000	4000	6000
Age 32	6	5	7	10	14
Age 27	5	4	6	7	11
Difference	1	1	1	3	3

The difference represents the amount of hearing loss that may be attributed to aging in the time period between the baseline audiogram and the most recent audiogram. In this example, the difference at 4000 Hz is 3 dB. This value is subtracted from the hearing level at 4000 Hz, which in the most recent audiogram is 25, yielding 22 after adjustment. Then the hearing threshold in the baseline audiogram at 4000 Hz (5) is subtracted from the adjusted annual audiogram hearing threshold at 4000 Hz (22). Thus the age-corrected threshold shift would be 17 dB (as opposed to a threshold shift of 20 dB without age correction).

TABLE F–1 — AGE CORRECTION VALUES IN DECIBELS FOR MALES

Years	Audiometric Test Frequency (Hz)				
	1000	2000	3000	4000	6000
20 or younger	5	3	4	5	8
21	5	3	4	5	8
22	5	3	4	5	8
23	5	3	4	6	9
24	5	3	5	6	9
25	5	3	5	7	10
26	5	4	5	7	10
27	5	4	6	7	11
28	6	4	6	8	11
29	6	4	6	8	12
30	6	4	6	9	12
31	6	4	7	9	13
32	6	5	7	10	14
33	6	5	7	10	14
34	6	5	8	11	15
35	7	5	8	11	15
36	7	5	9	12	16
37	7	6	9	12	17
38	7	6	9	13	17
39	7	6	10	14	18
40	7	6	10	14	19
41	7	6	10	14	20
42	8	7	11	16	20
43	8	7	12	16	21
44	8	7	12	17	22
45	8	7	13	18	23
46	8	8	13	19	24
47	8	8	14	19	24
48	9	8	14	20	25
49	9	9	15	21	26
50	9	9	16	22	27
51	9	9	16	23	28
52	9	10	17	24	29
53	9	10	18	25	30
54	10	10	18	26	31
55	10	11	19	27	32
56	10	11	20	28	34
57	10	11	21	29	35
58	10	12	22	31	36
59	11	12	22	32	37
60 or older	11	13	23	33	38

TABLE F–2 — AGE CORRECTION VALUES IN DECIBELS FOR FEMALES

Years	Audiometric Test Frequency (Hz)				
	1000	2000	3000	4000	6000
20 or younger	7	4	3	3	6
21	7	4	4	3	6
22	7	4	4	4	6
23	7	5	4	4	7
24	7	5	4	4	7
25	8	5	4	4	7
26	8	5	5	4	8
27	8	5	5	5	8
28	8	5	5	5	8
29	8	5	5	5	9
30	8	6	5	5	9
31	8	6	6	5	9
32	9	6	6	6	10
33	9	6	6	6	10
34	9	6	6	6	10
35	9	6	7	7	11
36	9	7	7	7	11
37	9	7	7	7	12
38	10	7	7	7	12
39	10	7	8	8	12
40	10	7	8	8	13
41	10	8	8	8	13
42	10	8	9	9	13
43	11	8	9	9	14
44	11	8	9	9	14
45	11	8	10	10	15
46	11	9	10	10	15
47	11	9	10	11	16
48	12	9	11	11	16
49	12	9	11	11	16
50	12	10	11	12	17
51	12	10	12	12	17
52	12	10	12	13	18
53	13	10	13	13	18
54	13	11	13	14	19
55	13	11	14	14	19
56	13	11	14	15	20
57	13	11	15	15	20
58	14	12	15	16	21
59	14	12	16	16	21
60 or older	14	12	16	17	22

Monitoring noise levels non-mandatory informational appendix — 1910.95 App G

This appendix provides information to help employers comply with the noise monitoring obligations that are part of the hearing conservation amendment.

WHAT IS THE PURPOSE OF NOISE MONITORING?

This revised amendment requires that employees be placed in a hearing conservation program if they are exposed to average noise levels of 85 dB or greater during an 8 hour workday. In order to determine if exposures are at or above this level, it may be necessary to measure or monitor the actual noise levels in the workplace and to estimate the noise exposure or "dose" received by employees during the workday.

WHEN IS IT NECESSARY TO IMPLEMENT A NOISE MONITORING PROGRAM?

It is not necessary for every employer to measure workplace noise. Noise monitoring or measuring must be conducted only when exposures are at or above 85 dB. Factors which suggest that noise exposures in the workplace may be at this level include employee complaints about the loudness of noise, indications that employees are losing their hearing, or noisy conditions which make normal conversation difficult. The employer should also consider any information available regarding noise emitted from specific machines. In addition, actual workplace noise measurements can suggest whether or not a monitoring program should be initiated.

HOW IS NOISE MEASURED?

Basically, there are two different instruments to measure noise exposures: the sound level meter and the dosimeter. A sound level meter is a device that measures the intensity of sound at a given moment. Since sound level meters provide a measure of sound intensity at only one point in time, it is generally necessary to take a number of measurements at different times during the day to estimate noise exposure over a workday. If noise levels fluctuate, the amount of time noise remains at each of the various measured levels must be determined.

To estimate employee noise exposures with a sound level meter it is also generally necessary to take several measurements at different locations within the workplace. After appropriate sound level meter readings are obtained, people sometimes draw "maps" of the sound levels within different areas of the workplace. By using a sound level "map" and information on employee locations throughout the day, estimates of individual exposure levels can be developed. This measurement method is generally referred to as "area" noise monitoring.

A dosimeter is like a sound level meter except that it stores sound level measurements and integrates these measurements over time, providing an average noise exposure reading for a given period of time, such as an 8-hour workday. With a dosimeter, a microphone is attached to the employee's clothing and the exposure measurement is simply read at the end of the desired time period. A reader may be used to read-out the dosimeter's measurements. Since the dosimeter is worn by the employee, it measures noise levels in those locations in which the employee travels. A sound level meter can also be positioned within the immediate vicinity of the exposed worker to obtain an individual exposure estimate. Such procedures are generally referred to as "personal" noise monitoring.

Area monitoring can be used to estimate noise exposure when the noise levels are relatively constant and employees are not mobile. In workplaces where employees move about in different areas or where the noise intensity tends to fluctuate over time, noise exposure is generally more accurately estimated by the personal monitoring approach.

In situations where personal monitoring is appropriate, proper positioning of the microphone is necessary to obtain accurate measurements. With a dosimeter, the microphone is generally located on the shoulder and remains in that position for the entire workday. With a sound level meter, the microphone is stationed near the employee's head, and the instrument is usually held by an individual who follows the employee as he or she moves about.

Manufacturer's instructions, contained in dosimeter and sound level meter operating manuals, should be followed for calibration and maintenance. To ensure accurate results, it is considered good professional practice to calibrate instruments before and after each use.

HOW OFTEN IS IT NECESSARY TO MONITOR NOISE LEVELS?

The amendment requires that when there are significant changes in machinery or production processes that may result in increased noise levels, remonitoring must be conducted to determine whether additional employees need to be included in the hearing conservation program. Many companies choose to remonitor periodically (once every year or two) to ensure that all exposed employees are included in their hearing conservation programs.

WHERE CAN EQUIPMENT AND TECHNICAL ADVICE BE OBTAINED?

Noise monitoring equipment may be either purchased or rented. Sound level meters cost about $500 to $1,000, while dosimeters range in price from about $750 to $1,500. Smaller companies may find it more economical to rent equipment rather than to purchase it. Names of equipment suppliers may be found in the telephone book (Yellow Pages) under headings such as: "Safety Equipment," "Industrial Hygiene," or "Engineers-Acoustical." In addition to providing information on obtaining noise monitoring equipment, many companies and individuals included under such listings can provide professional advice on how to conduct a valid noise monitoring program. Some audiological testing firms and industrial hygiene firms also provide noise monitoring services. Universities with audiology, industrial hygiene, or acoustical engineering departments may also provide information or may be able to help employers meet their obligations under this amendment.

Free, on-site assistance may be obtained from OSHA-supported state and private consultation organizations. These safety and health consultative entities generally give priority to the needs of small businesses.

Availability of referenced documents — 1910.95 App H

Paragraphs (c) through (o) of 29 CFR 1910.95 and the accompanying appendices contain provisions which incorporate publications by reference. Generally, the publications provide criteria for instruments to be used in monitoring and audiometric testing. These criteria are intended to be mandatory when so indicated in the applicable paragraphs of 1910.95 and appendices.

It should be noted that OSHA does not require that employers purchase a copy of the referenced publications. Employers, however, may desire to obtain a copy of the referenced publications for their own information.

The designation of the paragraph of the standard in which the referenced publications appear, the titles of the publications, and the availability of the publications are as follows:

Paragraph designation	Referenced publication	Available from —
Appendix B	"List of Personal Hearing Protectors and Attenuation Data," HEW Pub. No. 76-120, 1975. NTIS-PB267461.	National Technical Information Service, Port Royal Road, Springfield, VA 22161.
Appendix D	"Specification for Sound Level Meters," S1.4-1971 (R1976).	American National Standards Institute, Inc., 1430 Broadway, New York, NY 10018.
1910.95(k)(2), Appendix E	"Specifications for Audiometers," S3.6-1969.	American National Standards Institute, Inc., 1430 Broadway, New York, NY 10018.
Appendix D	"Specification for Octave, Half-Octave and Third-Octave Band Filter Sets," S1.11-1971 (R1976).	Back Numbers Department, Dept. STD, American Institute of Physics, 333 E. 45th St., New York, NY 10017; American National Standards Institute, Inc., 1430 Broadway, New York, NY 10018.

The referenced publications (or a microfiche of the publications) are available for review at many universities and public libraries throughout the country. These publications may also be examined at the OSHA Technical Data Center, Room N2439, United States Department of Labor, 200 Constitution Avenue, N.W., Washington, DC 20210, (202) 219-7500 or at any OSHA Regional Office (see telephone directories under United States Government — Labor Department).

Definitions — 1910.95 App I

These definitions apply to the following terms as used in paragraphs (c) through (n) of 29 CFR 1910.95.

Action level — An 8-hour time-weighted average of 85 decibels measured on the A-scale, slow response, or equivalently, a dose of fifty percent.

Audiogram — A chart, graph, or table resulting from an audiometric test showing an individual's hearing threshold levels as a function of frequency.

Audiologist — A professional, specializing in the study and rehabilitation of hearing, who is certified by the American Speech-Language-Hearing Association or licensed by a state board of examiners.

Baseline audiogram — The audiogram against which future audiograms are compared.

Criterion sound level — A sound level of 90 decibels.

Decibel (dB) — Unit of measurement of sound level.

Hertz (Hz) — Unit of measurement of frequency, numerically equal to cycles per second.

Medical pathology — A disorder or disease. For purposes of this regulation, a condition or disease affecting the ear, which should be treated by a physician specialist.

Noise dose — The ratio, expressed as a percentage, of (1) the time integral, over a stated time or event, of the 0.6 power of the measured SLOW exponential time-averaged, squared A-weighted sound pressure and (2) the product of the criterion duration (8 hours) and the 0.6 power of the squared sound pressure corresponding to the criterion sound level (90 dB).

Noise dosimeter — An instrument that integrates a function of sound pressure over a period of time in such a manner that it directly indicates a noise dose.

Otolaryngologist — A physician specializing in diagnosis and treatment of disorders of the ear, nose and throat.

Representative exposure — Measurements of an employee's noise dose or 8-hour time-weighted average sound level that the employers deem to be representative of the exposures of other employees in the workplace.

Sound level — Ten times the common logarithm of the ratio of the square of the measured A-weighted sound pressure to the square of the standard reference pressure of 20 micropascals. Unit: decibels (dB). For use with this regulation, SLOW time response, in accordance with ANSI S1.4-1971 (R1976), is required.

Sound level meter — An instrument for the measurement of sound level.

Time-weighted average sound level — That sound level, which if constant over an 8-hour exposure, would result in the same noise dose as is measured.

Appendix D
OSHA Compliance Checklist

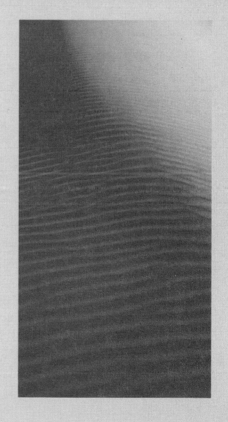

J.R. Franks, M.R. Stephenson, and C.J. Merry. (1996). "OSHA Noise Standard Compliance Checklist." Appendix A in *Preventing Occupational Hearing Loss — A Practical Guide.* U.S. Dept. Health and Human Services, NIOSH, Cincinnati, OH.

OSHA NOISE STANDARD COMPLIANCE CHECKLIST*

PURPOSE
This checklist summarizes the OSHA noise standard. It is intended to assist companies conducting hearing loss prevention program evaluations to assess compliance with OSHA requirements and to determine program effectiveness. **It is not intended to be used as a substitute for the OSHA Standard**. Items listed under "comments" represent current NIOSH recommendations that differ from the OSHA Standard.

REFERENCE
Refer to OSHA Standard 29 CFR 1910.95(a)-(p) with accompanying appendices A-I, Occupational Noise Exposure Standard for the standard's specific requirements: Code of Federal Regulations, Title 29, Chapter XVII, Part 1910, Subpart G. (See also 36 FR 10466 and 10518, May 29, 1971; Amended 46 FR 4078-4179, Jan. 16, 1981; Revised 48 FR 9776-9785, Mar. 8, 1983).

No.	29 CFR 1910.95 Requirement	Paragraph No.	NIOSH Recommendation
	PROTECTION AGAINST NOISE		
1	Must be provided when sound levels exceed 90-dBA time-weighted average measured with slow response and 5 dB exchange rate	(a)	Must be provided when sound levels exceed *85-dBA TWA with a 3-dB exchange rate.*
	CONTROLS		
2	Feasible engineering or administrative controls for employees exceeding TWA 90 dBA	(b)(1)	*Feasible engineering or administrative controls for employees exceeding 85 dBL$_{Aeq}$*
3	Impulse or impact noise should not exceed 140 dB peak sound pressure level	(b)(2)	
	PROGRAM		
4	Include employees whose noise exposures exceed 85 dB TWA with 5-dB exchange rate	(c)(1) (c)(2)	85 dBL$_{Aeq}$ (3-dB exchange rate)
	MONITORING		
5	Conduct noise monitoring when 85-dBA TWA equaled or exceeded with 5 dB exchange rate	(d)(1)	Conduct noise monitoring when 85-dBA TWA equaled or exceeded with *3-dB exchange rate*
6	Use representative personal monitoring for highly mobile workers, significantly varying sound levels, and impulse noise exposure	(d)(1)(ii)	
7	Include all continuous, intermittent, and impulsive sound levels from 80–130 dBA in measurements	(d)(2)(I)	
8	Calibrate equipment	(d)(2)(ii)	
9	Repeat monitoring when noise exposure increases significantly	(d)(3)	
	EMPLOYEE NOTIFICATION		
10	Notify employees of noise monitoring results when exposure is at or above 85 dBA TWA with 5-dB exchange rate	(e)	*3-dB exchange rate*

No.	29 CFR 1910.95 Requirement	Paragraph No.	NIOSH Recommendation
	OBSERVATION OF MONITORING		
11	Employees or their representatives may observe noise monitoring	(f)	
	AUDIOMETRIC TEST PROGRAM		
12	Audiometric testing *available* to employees exposed at or above 85 dBA TWA	(g)(1)	Testing required.
13	Tests performed by professional or by competent technician *(certification recommended)*	(g)(3)	Use of *micro-processor* audiometers does not *exempt* technician from certification
14	Audiograms meet 1910.95 Appendix C requirements	(g)(4)	
	BASELINE AUDIOGRAM		
15	Establish within 6 months or within *l year* if using mobile van	(g)(5)(I)(ii)	W/in 30 days of enrollment in hearing loss prevention program
16	14-hour period without workplace noise before baseline (hearing protection *can* be substituted)	(g)(5)(iv)	Hearing protection *cannot* be substituted
17	Notify employees to avoid high non-occupational noise levels before baseline	(g)(5)(iv)	
	ANNUAL AUDIOGRAM		
18	Provide for all employees exposed at or above 85 dBA TWA with 5-dB exchange rate	(g)(6)	Provide for all employees exposed at or above 85 dBA TWA with 3-dB exchange rate
	AUDIOGRAM EVALUATION		
19	Compare each annual test to baseline for validity and to see if standard threshold shift (STS) exists (10 dB average at 2000, 3000, and 4000 Hz)	(g)(7)(I)	Hearing Loss Prevention Program effectiveness indicated by no more than 5% of workers showing significant threshold shift (15 dB twice, same ear, same frequency)
20	If STS, retest within *30 days (optional)*	(g)(7)(ii)	*Immediate retest*; if retest the same, schedule for 30-day confirmation audiogram
21	Audiologist, otolaryngologist, or physician reviews problem audiograms and determines need for further evaluation	(g)(7)(iii)	
	FOLLOW-UP		
22	Notify employees with STS in writing within *21 days*	(g)(8)(i)	*Immediate notification*

No.	29 CFR 1910.95 Requirement	Paragraph No.	NIOSH Recommendation
23	Actions to be taken (unless physician determines that STS is not work-related): Provide employees with hearing protectors (if not already wearing), train in care and use, and require them to be worn • Refit and retrain employees already using protectors • Refer as necessary for clinical evaluations or additional testing • Inform employees with non-work-related ear problems of need for otologic exam	(g)(8)(ii)	All employees exposed to 85 dB TWA with 3-dB exchange rate use hearing protection

REVISION OF BASELINE

No.	29 CFR 1910.95 Requirement	Paragraph No.	NIOSH Recommendation
24	Annual audiogram may become baseline as per OSHA criteria	(g)(9)	

STANDARD THRESHOLD SHIFT

No.	29 CFR 1910.95 Requirement	Paragraph No.	NIOSH Recommendation
25	Definition – change relative to baseline of *10 dB or more in average* hearing level at 2000, 3000, and 4000 Hz, either ear. Allowance for aging *optional* – Appendix F	(g)(10)	A shift of *15 dB* or more at 500, 1000, 2000, 3000, 4000, or 6000 Hz in either ear; and the same shift at the same test frequency in the same ear on an immediate retest. No correction allowance for aging

AUDIOMETRIC TEST REQUIREMENTS

No.	29 CFR 1910.95 Requirement	Paragraph No.	NIOSH Recommendation
26	Each ear tested at frequencies of 500, 1000, 2000, 3000, 4000, and 6000 Hz	(h)(1)	Test also at *8000 Hz*
27	Audiometers meet ANSI S3.6-1969	(h)(2)	ANSI S3.6-1996
28	Pulsed-tone and self-recording audiometers meet Appendix C requirements	(h)(3)	ANSI S3.6-1996
29	Test rooms meet *Appendix D* requirements	(h)(4)	Test rooms meet specifications of ANSI S3.1-1991
30	Audiometer calibration includes: • Functional checks before each day's use • Acoustical check annually according to Appendix E • Exhaustive calibration every 2 years	(h)(5)	

HEARING PROTECTORS

No.	29 CFR 1910.95 Requirement	Paragraph No.	NIOSH Recommendation
31	*Available to all employees exposed at or* above 85 dBA TWA and replaced as necessary	(i)(1)	*Worn at 85 dBA and above regardless* of exposure time

32	Worn by employees when:
	• Exposed to 90 dBA TWA or above
	• Exposed to 85 dBA TWA or above when
	  – no baseline after 6 months, or
	  – STS occurs
		(i)(2)	

33	Employees select from a variety of suitable hearing protectors	(i)(3)	
34	Employees trained in care and use	(i)(4)	
35	Employer ensures proper initial fitting and supervises correct use	(i)(5)	

No.	29 CFR 1910.95 Requirement	Paragraph No.	NIOSH Recommendation

HEARING PROTECTOR ATTENUATION

36	Evaluate attenuation for specific noise environments according to *Appendix B*	(j)(1)	Derate the NRR by 25% for earmuffs, 50% for formable slow-recovery foam earplugs and 75% for all other earplugs
37	Attenuate to at least *90 dBA,* or 85 dBA if STS experienced	(j)(2) (j)(3)	Attenuate to *85 dBA*
38	Re-evaluate attenuation as necessary	(j)(4)	

TRAINING PROGRAM

39	Provide training to employees exposed to 85 dBA TWA or above	(k)(1)	
40	Repeat annually and update materials	(k)(2)	
41	Training includes: • Effects of noise on hearing • Purpose of hearing protectors, advantages, disadvantages, attenuation; instructions on selection, fit, use, and care • Purpose and procedures of audiometric testing	(k)(3)	

ACCESS

42	Copies of OSHA standard available to employees or their representatives and posted in workplace	(l)(1)	
43	Information provided by OSHA available to employees	(l)(2)	
44	All records provided on request to employees, former employees, representatives, and OSHA	(m)(4)	

RECORDKEEPING

45	Maintain accurate records of noise exposure measurements	(m)(1)	
46	Maintain audiometric records with the following information: • Employee name and job classification • Date of audiogram • Examiner's name • Date of last acoustic or exhaustive calibration • Employee's most recent noise exposure assessment • Background noise levels in audio test rooms	(m)(2)	
47	Retain all noise exposure records for at least 2 years	(m)(3) (i)	
48	Retain all audiometric test records at least for duration of employment	(m)(3) (ii)	Retain all audiometric test records at least for duration of employment *plus 30 years*
49	Transfer all records to successor employer	(m)(5)	

No.	29 CFR 1910.95 Requirement	Paragraph No.	NIOSH Recommendation
	MANDATORY OSHA APPENDICES		
50	*Noise Exposure Computation*	Appen. A	*85 dBA 3-dB exchange*
51	Methods for Estimating the Adequacy of Hearing Protector Attenuation	Appen. B	*Derated NRR*
52	Audiometric Measuring Instruments	Appen. C	
53	Audiometric Test Rooms	Appen. D	Type 1 SLMs in accordance with ANSI S3.1-1991, Type 2 SLMs designed since 1989 may be substituted in most cases. Test room background noise levels must be equal to or less than ears-covered levels of ANSI S3.1-1991
54	Acoustic Calibration of Audiometers	Appen. E	
	NON-MANDATORY OSHA APPENDICES		
55	Calculations and Application of Age Corrections to Audiograms	Appen. F	*No age correction for* calculating STS
56	Monitoring Noise Levels	Appen. G	
57	Availability of Referenced Documents	Appen. H	
58	Definitions	Appen. I	

* Much of this material has been adapted from Gasaway, D. C. Evaluating and fine-tuning the elements that comprise a program. Chapter 15 in D. C. Gasaway, *Hearing Conservation: A Practical Manual and Guide*, Prentice Hall, Inc.: Englewood Cliffs, N.J., 1985.

Last Updated July 15, 1999

Appendix E
List of OSHA Interpretation and Compliance Letters

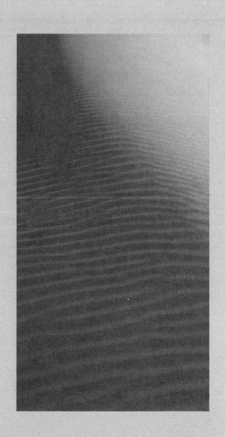

Found at **www.osha.gov/SLTC/noisehearing conservation/index.html**

(Scroll to Standards Interpretations and Compliance Letters and click on SEARCH. Individual letter may be obtained by clicking on the title of the desired letter.)

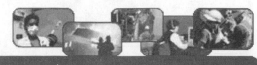
[Text Only]
Search Results

Standard Interpretations Search Results

"**noise**" matched **95** documents.

Relevance	Date	Title
Sorted	Sort by	Sort by
100%	24-Feb-1997	Placement of the noise dosimeter microphone for measuring the noise exposure of an employee using an airline respirator equipped with a shroud.
100%	23-Jan-1995	Occupational Noise Exposure Standard when an employee with a history of off-the-job noise exposure.
100%	09-May-1994	Hearing conservation standard questions.
100%	31-Aug-1993	Use of insert earphones for audiometric testing.
100%	06-Jan-1992	Welding and Noise in confined space
100%	05-Mar-1990	Observation of monitoring requirement at 1910.95(f) in the occupational noise exposure standard
100%	22-Feb-1985	Fast response noise dosimetry measurement not acceptable.
93%	08-May-1984	Questions and answers relative to the noise standard.
85%	01-Apr-1991	Occupational noise exposure limits
77%	01-Aug-1994	Clarification of the policy for classifying violations as repeated, as well as clarification of specific regulations.
69%	29-Jun-1992	Occupational noise, including hearing conservation, in construction work.
69%	16-Sep-1983	Applicability of the noise standard to portable ear muff type radios.
62%	14-Apr-1987	Use of Walkman Radio, Tape, or CD Players and Their Effect When Hearing Protection Is In Use
62%	01-May-1983	Noise regulations apply to all places of entertainment.
54%	24-Aug-1990	Product endorsement policy and telephone headsets.
54%	20-Nov-1987	Reduction of noise exposure for metal spray operations.
54%	10-Dec-1986	Calibration of noise dosimeters
54%	10-Apr-1986	General review of the OSHA noise standard.
54%	13-Mar-1984	"Laboratory-based noise reduction" defined.
54%	19-Jan-1982	Provisions to assure that workers are adequately protected from noise exposure.
46%	01-Feb-2001	Acceptability of Task-Based Noise Exposure Assessment Modeling (T-BEAM).
46%	28-Jul-1999	OSHA's rationale for the noise exposure PEL.
46%	12-Jul-1993	Reverse signal alarms for motor vehicles.
46%	14-Dec-1989	Noise inspection conducted at Robben's Roost, Louisville, Kentucky.
46%	09-Jun-1987	Requirement for instituting engineering and administrative controls for noise.
46%	10-Oct-1986	Field calibration of noise dosimeters.

46%	10-Jul-1986	Response to letter suggesting that the noise standard of 90 dB(A) is set at too high a level, and should be 85 dB(A) or less.
39%	26-Sep-2001	Differentiation between the 80 dBA threshold for hearing conservation and the 90 dBA PEL.
39%	17-Aug-2000	Noise exposure measurement records must be retained for 2 years.
39%	04-Aug-1992	Hearing conservation program.
39%	29-Mar-1988	Response to Freedom of Information Act request for standards and guidelines related to working around aircraft.
39%	15-Aug-1983	Citation guidelines in relation to monitoring programs.
39%	11-May-1983	Employee noise exposure assessment records are part of audiometric test record.
39%	03-Jun-1982	Hearing conservation standard in relation to poultry processing industry.
39%	15-Sep-1981	Compliance determination based on worst day noise exposure.
39%	11-Jul-1980	Regulations for back-up alarms.
31%	19-Mar-1999	Occupational noise exposure standard affords protection to landscape service industry employees.
31%	07-Dec-1987	Hearing conservation programs and "ear blasts" on communication headsets
31%	03-Dec-1987	Response to an inquiry about "ear blasts" on communications headsets.
31%	16-Jun-1986	The noise standard applies to environments with undue atmospheric pressure.
31%	10-Oct-1985	Noise standards applicable to Metra are under the jurisdiction of the Federal Railroad Administration.
31%	01-Feb-1984	Costs of employee training under the noise standard paid by employer.
31%	03-May-1983	Requirement to make a positive determination of work-relatedness of threshold shift revoked.
31%	26-Mar-1982	Question of whether the noise standard is adjusted for workshifts greater than 8 hours.
23%	23-Sep-1999	Protection of ground-level workers from lowering of aerial lift bucket.
23%	03-Nov-1998	Requirements for back-up alarms on construction vehicles.
23%	02-Jun-1998	Hearing conservation: referrals, financial responsibility, and documentation.
23%	26-Mar-1996	Requirements of the Occupational Noise Exposure Standard with regards to hearing protectors.
23%	23-Feb-1996	Baseline audiograms.
23%	03-Feb-1994	Employers' responsibilities towards temporary employees.
23%	20-Aug-1987	Horns and audible alarms.
23%	01-Apr-1987	Applicability of 1910.95 to cotton gins.
23%	15-Aug-1985	Some employers have banned portable stereo headsets.
23%	24-May-1983	Comparison to baseline audiograms and retest audiograms
23%	11-Jan-1982	Variable day to day exposures cannot be averaged for compliance with action level
23%	13-Aug-1976	Use of audible alarms in lieu of physical barriers.
15%	10-Nov-1999	OSHA policy regarding PEL adjustments for extended work shifts.
15%	30-Oct-1996	Enforcement of the Control of Hazardous Energy (LOTO).
15%	09-Jul-1993	Noise exposure standard and impairment adjustments.
15%	29-Oct-1991	Noise and potential hazard of backup alarms on equipment at construction sites.
15%	10-Jul-1989	Review of Policy on Section 4(b)(1) of the Act

15%	27-Jul-1987	Free audiometric testing for employees exposed over the action level.
15%	18-Jun-1985	Audiograms conducted in accordance with the hearing conservation amendment.
15%	06-Jun-1985	Interpretation of "effective hearing conservation program".
15%	03-Feb-1984	March 1, 1984 is the deadline for baseline audiograms
15%	03-Jan-1984	Use of the "hold" switch on audiometers when background noise levels exceed the criteria in Table D-1.
15%	29-Mar-1983	The hearing conservation amendment does not cover construction or agriculture.
15%	19-Mar-1975	Administrative controls and PPE used to reduce exposure below limits if engineering controls are not feasible.
8%	01-Apr-1999	Maintenance and preservation of employee exposure records.
8%	11-Sep-1995	Interpretation of OSHA requirements for personal protective equipment to be used during marine oil spill emergency response operations.
8%	24-May-1995	Compliance determination by OSHA concerning the use of radio-frequency-activated pagers for meeting the requirements of Employee alarm systems.
8%	14-Feb-1994	Recording of hearing loss on the OSHA Log 200.
8%	16-Sep-1993	Summary report on OSHA inspections conducted at superfund incinerator sites.
8%	18-May-1992	OSHA's regulations apply only to employer-employee relationship and not to employer activities that can affect the general public.
8%	11-Sep-1991	Recording hearing loss on the OSHA 200 Log
8%	04-Sep-1991	Standard Threshold Shift in hearing level
8%	29-Jul-1991	Committing a de minimis violation when using an insert earphone designated as ER-3A.
8%	04-Jun-1991	Recording Of Hearing Loss and Cumulative Trauma Disorders
8%	17-Nov-1989	Identification of a standard threshold shift (STS) for individuals with a very poor sense of hearing.
8%	09-Feb-1988	Posting of the Occupational Noise Exposure Standard.
8%	11-Dec-1987	Clarification of requirements for 40 hours of training.; Site specific training is required for employees who receive general training.
8%	15-Jun-1987	Recertifying tecnicians who do audiometric testing and pulmonary function testing.
8%	17-Feb-1987	OSHA has no standards for the design and implementation of video display workstations.
8%	18-Dec-1984	Use of an electronic back-up mirror used with a with a reverse audible alarm.
8%	14-Dec-1984	Regulations for the calibration of spirometers and audiometers;Regulations for the calibration of spirometers and audiometers.
8%	11-Sep-1984	Regulations for machine shop and press room safety.
8%	30-Aug-1984	Quest Bio Acoustic Simulator may be used for daily audiometer checks.
8%	17-Oct-1983	One type of muff and plug available for employee hearing protector selection.
8%	30-Sep-1983	Ear muffs and ear plugs are not both required if one offers protection
8%	27-Sep-1983	Notification requirements for standard threshold shifts.
8%	04-Aug-1983	Methods of training for microprocessor audiometer technicians.
8%	28-Jul-1982	Use or powered air purifying respirators for abrasive blasting.
8%	13-Jul-1982	Applicability of the noise standard to pulpwood logging.
8%	30-Jun-1981	Horns on construction equipment.
8%	23-Jul-1979	"Audible above" is a signal alarm distinguishable from the surrounding noise level.

Appendix F
MSHA Noise Regulation

30 CFR Part 62

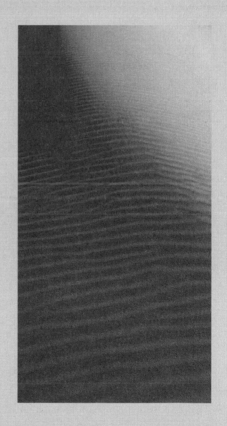

Subpart F—[Removed]

6. Subpart F (§§ 70.500 through 70.511) is removed.

PART 71—[AMENDED]

7. The authority citation for part 71 continues to read as follows:

Authority: 30 U.S.C. 811, 951, 957, 961.

Subpart I—[Removed]

8. Subpart I (§§ 71.800 through 71.805) is removed.

Subchapters M and N—[Redesignated]

9. Subchapter M is redesignated as Subchapter I, Subchapter N is redesignated as Subchapter K, and Subchapter N is reserved.

10. A new Subchapter M is added, "Uniform Mine Health Regulations."

11. A new part 62 is added to new Subchapter M to read as follows:

PART 62—OCCUPATIONAL NOISE EXPOSURE

Sec.
62.100   Purpose and scope; effective date
62.101   Definitions
62.110   Noise exposure assessment
62.120   Action level
62.130   Permissible exposure level
62.140   Dual hearing protection level
62.150   Hearing conservation program
62.160   Hearing protectors
62.170   Audiometric testing
62.171   Audiometric test procedures
62.172   Evaluation of audiograms
62.173   Follow-up evaluation when an audiogram is invalid
62.174   Follow-up corrective measures when a standard threshold shift is detected
62.175   Notification of results; reporting requirements
62.180   Training
62.190   Records
Appendix to part 62
Authority: 30 U.S.C. 811.

§ 62.100 Purpose and scope; effective date.

The purpose of these standards is to prevent the occurrence and reduce the progression of occupational noise-induced hearing loss among miners. This part sets forth mandatory health standards for each surface and underground metal, nonmetal, and coal mine subject to the Federal Mine Safety and Health Act of 1977. The provisions of this part become effective September 13, 2000.

§ 62.101 Definitions.

The following definitions apply in this part:

Access. The right to examine and copy records.

Action level. An 8-hour time-weighted average sound level (TWA$_8$) of 85 dBA, or equivalently a dose of 50%, integrating all sound levels from 80 dBA to at least 130 dBA.

Audiologist. A professional, specializing in the study and rehabilitation of hearing, who is certified by the American Speech-Language-Hearing Association (ASHA) or licensed by a state board of examiners.

Baseline audiogram. The audiogram recorded in accordance with § 62.170(a) of this part against which subsequent audiograms are compared to determine the extent of hearing loss.

Criterion level. The sound level which if constantly applied for 8 hours results in a dose of 100% of that permitted by the standard.

Decibel (dB). A unit of measure of sound pressure levels, defined in one of two ways, depending upon the use:

(1) For measuring sound pressure levels, the decibel is 20 times the common logarithm of the ratio of the measured sound pressure to the standard reference sound pressure of 20 micropascals μPa), which is the threshold of normal hearing sensitivity at 1000 Hertz (Hz).

(2) For measuring hearing threshold levels, the decibel is the difference between audiometric zero (reference pressure equal to 0 hearing threshold level) and the threshold of hearing of the individual being tested at each test frequency.

Dual Hearing Protection Level. A TWA$_8$ of 105 dBA, or equivalently, a dose of 800% of that permitted by the standard, integrating all sound levels from 90 dBA to at least 140 dBA.

Exchange rate. The amount of increase in sound level, in decibels, which would require halving of the allowable exposure time to maintain the same noise dose. For the purposes of this part, the exchange rate is 5 decibels (5 dB).

Hearing protector. Any device or material, capable of being worn on the head or in the ear canal, sold wholly or in part on the basis of its ability to reduce the level of sound entering the ear, and which has a scientifically accepted indicator of noise reduction value.

Hertz (Hz). Unit of measurement of frequency numerically equal to cycles per second.

Medical pathology. A condition or disease affecting the ear.

Miner's designee. Any individual or organization to whom a miner gives written authorization to exercise a right of access to records.

Qualified technician. A technician who has been certified by the Council for Accreditation in Occupational Hearing Conservation (CAOHC), or by another recognized organization offering equivalent certification.

Permissible exposure level. A TWA$_8$ of 90 dBA or equivalently a dose of 100% of that permitted by the standard, integrating all sound levels from 90 dBA to at least 140 dBA.

Reportable hearing loss. A change in hearing sensitivity for the worse, relative to the miner's baseline audiogram, or the miner's revised baseline audiogram where one has been established in accordance with § 62.170(c)(2), of an average of 25 dB or more at 2000, 3000, and 4000 Hz either ear.

Revised baseline audiogram. An annual audiogram designated to be used in lieu of a miner's original baseline audiogram in measuring changes in hearing sensitivity as a result of the circumstances set forth in §§ 62.170(c)(1) or 62.170(c)(2) of this part.

Sound level. The sound pressure level in decibels measured using the A-weighting network and a slow response, expressed in the unit dBA.

Standard threshold shift. A change in hearing sensitivity for the worse relative to the miner's baseline audiogram, or relative to the most recent revised baseline audiogram where one has been established, of an average of 10 dB or more at 2000, 3000, and 4000 Hz in either ear.

Time-weighted average-8 hour (TWA$_8$). The sound level which, if constant over 8 hours, would result in the same noise dose as is measured.

§ 62.110 Noise exposure assessment.

(a) The mine operator must establish a system of monitoring that evaluates each miner's noise exposure sufficiently to determine continuing compliance with this part.

(b) The mine operator must determine a miner's noise dose (D, in percent) by using a noise dosimeter or by computing the formula:

$$D = 100(C_1/T_1 + C_2/T_2 + \ldots + C_n/T_n),$$

where C_n is the total time the miner is exposed at a specified sound level, and T_n is the reference duration of exposure at that sound level shown in Table 62–1.

(1) The mine operator must use Table 62–2 when converting from dose readings to equivalent TWA$_8$ readings.

(2) A miner's noise dose determination must:

(i) Be made without adjustment for the use of any hearing protector;

(ii) Integrate all sound levels over the appropriate range;

(iii) Reflect the miner's full work shift;

(iv) Use a 90-dB criterion level and a 5-dB exchange rate; and

(v) Use the A-weighting and slow response instrument settings.

(c) *Observation of monitoring.* The mine operator must provide affected miners and their representatives with an opportunity to observe noise exposure monitoring required by this section and must give prior notice of the date and time of intended exposure monitoring to affected miners and their representatives.

(d) *Miner notification.* The mine operator must notify a miner of his or her exposure when the miner's exposure is determined to equal or exceed the action level, exceed the permissible exposure level, or exceed the dual hearing protection level, provided the mine operator has not notified the miner of an exposure at such level within the prior 12 months. The mine operator must base the notification on an exposure evaluation conducted either by the mine operator or by an authorized representative of the Secretary of Labor. The mine operator must notify the miner in writing within 15 calendar days of:

(1) The exposure determination; and

(2) the corrective action being taken.

(e) The mine operator must maintain a copy of any such miner notification, or a list on which the relevant information about that miner's notice is recorded, for the duration of the affected miner's exposure at or above the action level and for at least 6 months thereafter.

§ 62.120 Action level.

If during any work shift a miner's noise exposure equals or exceeds the action level the mine operator must enroll the miner in a hearing conservation program that complies with § 62.150 of this part.

§ 62.130 Permissible exposure level.

(a) The mine operator must assure that no miner is exposed during any work shift to noise that exceeds the permissible exposure level. If during any work shift a miner's noise exposure exceeds the permissible exposure level, the mine operator must use all feasible engineering and administrative controls to reduce the miner's noise exposure to the permissible exposure level, and enroll the miner in a hearing conservation program that complies with § 62.150 of this part. When a mine operator uses administrative controls to reduce a miner's exposure, the mine

operator must post the procedures for such controls on the mine bulletin board and provide a copy to the affected miner.

(b) If a miner's noise exposure continues to exceed the permissible exposure level despite the use of all feasible engineering and administrative controls, the mine operator must continue to use the engineering and administrative controls to reduce the miner's noise exposure to as low a level as is feasible.

(c) The mine operator must assure that no miner is exposed at any time to sound levels exceeding 115 dBA, as determined without adjustment for the use of any hearing protector.

§ 62.140 Dual hearing protection level.

If during any work shift a miner's noise exposure exceeds the dual hearing protection level, the mine operator must, in addition to the actions required for noise exposures that exceed the permissible exposure level, provide and ensure the concurrent use of both an ear plug and an ear muff type hearing protector. The following table sets out mine operator actions under MSHA's noise standard.

Provision	Condition	Action required by the mine operator
§ 62.120	Miner's noise exposure is less than the action level.	None.
§ 62.120	Miner's exposure equals or exceeds the action level, but does not exceed the permissible exposure level (PEL).	Operator enrolls the miner in hearing conservation program (HCP) which includes (1) a system of monitoring, (2) voluntary, with two exceptions, use of operator-provided hearing protectors, (3) voluntary audiometric testing, (4) training, and (5) recordkeeping.
§ 62.130	Miner's exposure exceeds the PEL.	Operator uses/continues to use all feasible engineering and administrative controls to reduce exposure to PEL; enrolls the miner in a HCP including ensured use of operator-provided hearing protectors; posts administrative controls and provides copy to affected miner; must never permit a miner to be exposed to sound levels exceeding 115 dBA.
§ 62.140	Miner's exposure exceeds the dual hearing protection level.	Operator enrolls the miner in a HCP, continues to meet all the requirements of § 62.130, ensures concurrent use of earplug and earmuff.

§ 62.150 Hearing conservation program.

A hearing conservation program established under this part must include:

(a) A system of monitoring under § 62.110 of this part;

(b) The provision and use of hearing protectors under § 62.160 of this part;

(c) Audiometric testing under §§ 62.170 through 62.175 of this part;

(d) Training under § 62.180 of this part; and

(e) Recordkeeping under § 62.190 of this part.

§ 62.160 Hearing protectors.

(a) A mine operator must provide a hearing protector to a miner whose

noise exposure equals or exceeds the action level under § 62.120 of this part.

In addition, the mine operator must:

(1) Train the miner in accordance with § 62.180 of this part;

(2) Allow the miner to choose a hearing protector from at least two muff types and two plug types, and in the event dual hearing protectors are required, to choose one of each type;

(3) Ensure that the hearing protector is in good condition and is fitted and maintained in accordance with the manufacturer's instructions;

(4) Provide the hearing protector and necessary replacements at no cost to the miner; and

(5) Allow the miner to choose a different hearing protector(s), if

wearing the selected hearing protector(s) is subsequently precluded due to medical pathology of the ear.

(b) The mine operator must ensure, after satisfying the requirements of paragraph (a) of this section, that a miner wears a hearing protector whenever the miner's noise exposure exceeds the permissible exposure level before the implementation of engineering and administrative controls, or if the miner's noise exposure continues to exceed the permissible exposure level despite the use of all feasible engineering and administrative controls.

(c) The mine operator must ensure, after satisfying the requirements of paragraph (a) of this section, that a miner wears a hearing protector when the miner's noise exposure is at or above the action level, if:

(1) The miner has incurred a standard threshold shift; or

(2) More than 6 months will pass before the miner can take a baseline audiogram.

§ 62.170 Audiometric testing.

The mine operator must provide audiometric tests to satisfy the requirements of this part at no cost to the miner. A physician or an audiologist, or a qualified technician under the direction or supervision of a physician or an audiologist must conduct the tests.

(a) *Baseline audiogram.* The mine operator must offer miners the opportunity for audiometric testing of the miner's hearing sensitivity for the purpose of establishing a valid baseline audiogram to compare with subsequent annual audiograms. The mine operator may use an existing audiogram of the miner's hearing sensitivity as the baseline audiogram if it meets the audiometric testing requirements of § 62.171 of this part.

(1) The mine operator must offer and provide within 6 months of enrolling the miner in a hearing conservation program, audiometric testing which results in a valid baseline audiogram, or offer and provide the testing within 12 months where the operator uses mobile test vans to do the testing.

(2) The mine operator must notify the miner to avoid high levels of noise for at least 14 hours immediately preceding the baseline audiogram. The mine operator must not expose the miner to workplace noise for the 14-hour quiet period before conducting the audiometric testing to determine a baseline audiogram. The operator may substitute the use of hearing protectors for this quiet period.

(3) The mine operator must not establish a new baseline audiogram or a new revised baseline audiogram, where one has been established, due to changes in enrollment status in the hearing conservation program. The mine operator may establish a new baseline or revised baseline audiogram for a miner who is away from the mine for more than 6 consecutive months.

(b) *Annual audiogram.* After the baseline audiogram is established, the mine operator must continue to offer subsequent audiometric tests at intervals not exceeding 12 months for as long as the miner remains in the hearing conservation program.

(c) *Revised baseline audiogram.* An annual audiogram must be deemed to be a revised baseline audiogram when, in the judgment of the physician or audiologist:

(1) A standard threshold shift revealed by the audiogram is permanent; or (2) The hearing threshold shown in the annual audiogram indicates significant improvement over the baseline audiogram.

§ 62.171 Audiometric test procedures.

(a) All audiometric testing under this part must be conducted in accordance with scientifically validated procedures. Audiometric tests must be pure tone, air conduction, hearing threshold examinations, with test frequencies including 500, 1000, 2000, 3000, 4000, and 6000 Hz. Each ear must be tested separately.

(b) The mine operator must compile an audiometric test record for each miner tested. The record must include:

(1) Name and job classification of the miner tested;

(2) A copy of all of the miner's audiograms conducted under this part;

(3) Evidence that the audiograms were conducted in accordance with paragraph (a) of this section;

(4) Any exposure determination for the miner conducted in accordance with § 62.110 of this part; and

(5) The results of follow-up examination(s), if any.

(c) The operator must maintain audiometric test records for the duration of the affected miner's employment, plus at least 6 months, and make the records available for inspection by an authorized representative of the Secretary of Labor.

§ 62.172 Evaluation of audiograms.

(a) The mine operator must:

(1) Inform persons evaluating audiograms of the requirements of this part and provide those persons with a copy of the miner's audiometric test records;

(2) Have a physician or an audiologist, or a qualified technician who is under the direction or supervision of a physician or audiologist:

(i) Determine if the audiogram is valid; and

(ii) Determine if a standard threshold shift or a reportable hearing loss, as defined in this part, has occurred.

(3) Instruct the physician, audiologist, or qualified technician not to reveal to the mine operator, without the written consent of the miner, any specific findings or diagnoses unrelated to the miner's hearing loss due to occupational noise or the wearing of hearing protectors; and

(4) Obtain the results and the interpretation of the results of audiograms conducted under this part within 30 calendar days of conducting the audiogram.

(b)(1) The mine operator must provide an audiometric retest within 30 calendar days of receiving a determination that

an audiogram is invalid, provided any medical pathology has improved to the point that a valid audiogram may be obtained.

(2) If an annual audiogram demonstrates that the miner has incurred a standard threshold shift or reportable hearing loss, the mine operator may provide one retest within 30 calendar days of receiving the results of the audiogram and may use the results of the retest as the annual audiogram.

(c) In determining whether a standard threshold shift or reportable hearing loss has occurred, allowance may be made for the contribution of aging (presbycusis) to the change in hearing level. The baseline, or the revised baseline as appropriate, and the annual audiograms used in making the determination should be adjusted according to the following procedure:

(1) Determine from Tables 62–3 or 62–4 the age correction values for the miner by:

(i) Finding the age at which the baseline audiogram or revised baseline audiogram, as appropriate, was taken, and recording the corresponding values of age corrections at 2000, 3000, and 4000 Hz;

(ii) Finding the age at which the most recent annual audiogram was obtained and recording the corresponding values of age corrections at 2000, 3000, and 4000 Hz; and

(iii) Subtracting the values determined in paragraph (c)(1)(i) of this section from the values determined in paragraph (c)(1)(ii) of this section. The differences calculated represent that portion of the change in hearing that may be due to aging.

(2) Subtract the values determined in paragraph (c)(1)(iii) of this section from the hearing threshold levels found in the annual audiogram to obtain the adjusted annual audiogram hearing threshold levels.

(3) Subtract the hearing threshold levels in the baseline audiogram or revised baseline audiogram from the adjusted annual audiogram hearing threshold levels determined in paragraph (c)(2) of this section to obtain the age-corrected threshold shifts.

§ 62.173 Follow-up evaluation when an audiogram is invalid.

(a) If a valid audiogram cannot be obtained due to a suspected medical pathology of the ear that the physician or audiologist believes was caused or aggravated by the miner's occupational exposure to noise or the wearing of hearing protectors, the mine operator must refer the miner for a clinical-audiological evaluation or an otological examination, as appropriate, at no cost to the miner.

(b) If a valid audiogram cannot be obtained due to a suspected medical pathology of the ear that the physician or audiologist concludes is unrelated to the miner's occupational exposure to noise or the wearing of hearing protectors, the mine operator must instruct the physician or audiologist to inform the miner of the need for an otological examination.

(c) The mine operator must instruct the physician, audiologist, or qualified technician not to reveal to the mine operator, without the written consent of the miner, any specific findings or diagnoses unrelated to the miner's occupational exposure to noise or the wearing of hearing protectors.

§ 62.174 Follow-up corrective measures when a standard threshold shift is detected.

The mine operator must, within 30 calendar days of receiving evidence or confirmation of a standard threshold shift, unless a physician or audiologist determines the standard threshold shift is neither work-related nor aggravated by occupational noise exposure:

(a) Retrain the miner, including the instruction required by § 62.180 of this part;

(b) Provide the miner with the opportunity to select a hearing protector, or a different hearing protector if the miner has previously selected a hearing protector, from among those offered by the mine operator in accordance with § 62.160 of this part; and

(c) Review the effectiveness of any engineering and administrative controls to identify and correct any deficiencies.

§ 62.175 Notification of results; reporting requirements.

(a) The mine operator must, within 10 working days of receiving the results of an audiogram, or receiving the results of a follow-up evaluation required under § 62.173 of this part, notify the miner in writing of:

(1) The results and interpretation of the audiometric test, including any finding of a standard threshold shift or reportable hearing loss; and

(2) The need and reasons for any further testing or evaluation, if applicable.

(b) When evaluation of the audiogram shows that a miner has incurred a reportable hearing loss as defined in this part, the mine operator must report such loss to MSHA as

a noise-induced hearing loss in accordance with part 50 of this title, unless a physician or audiologist has determined that the loss is neither work-related nor aggravated by occupational noise exposure.

§ 62.180 Training.

(a) The mine operator must, within 30 days of a miner's enrollment into a hearing conservation program, provide the miner with training. The mine operator must give training every 12 months thereafter if the miner's noise exposure continues to equal or exceed the action level. Training must include:

(1) The effects of noise on hearing;

(2) The purpose and value of wearing hearing protectors;

(3) The advantages and disadvantages of the hearing protectors to be offered;

(4) The various types of hearing protectors offered by the mine operator and the care, fitting, and use of each type;

(5) The general requirements of this part;

(6) The mine operator's and miner's respective tasks in maintaining mine noise controls; and

(7) The purpose and value of audiometric testing and a summary of the procedures.

(b) The mine operator must certify the date and type of training given each miner, and maintain the miner's most recent certification for as long as the miner is enrolled in the hearing conservation program and for at least 6 months thereafter.

§ 62.190 Records.

(a) The authorized representatives of the Secretaries of Labor and Health and Human Services must have access to all records required under this part. Upon written request, the mine operator must provide, within 15 calendar days of the request, access to records to:

(1) The miner, or with the miner's written consent, the miner's designee, for all records that the mine operator must maintain for that individual miner under this part;

(2) Any representative of miners designated under part 40 of this title, to training certifications compiled under § 62.180(b) of this part and to any notice of exposure determination under § 62.110(d) of this part, for the miners whom he or she represents; and

(3) Any former miner, for records which indicate his or her own exposure.

(b) When a person with access to records under paragraphs (a)(1), (a)(2),

or (a)(3) of this section requests a copy of a record, the mine operator must provide the first copy of such record at no cost to that person, and any additional copies requested by that person at reasonable cost.

(c) Transfer of records. (1) The mine operator must transfer all records required to be maintained by this part, or a copy thereof, to a successor mine operator who must maintain the records for the time period required by this part.

(2) The successor mine operator must use the baseline audiogram, or revised baseline audiogram, as appropriate, obtained by the original mine operator to determine the existence of a standard threshold shift or reportable hearing loss.

Appendix to Part 62

TABLE 62–1.—REFERENCE DURATION

dBA	T (hours)
80	32.0
85	16.0
86	13.9
87	12.1
88	10.6
89	9.2
90	8.0
91	7.0
92	6.1
93	5.3
94	4.6
95	4.0
96	3.5
97	3.0
98	2.6
99	2.3
100	2.0
101	1.7
102	1.5
103	1.3
104	1.1
105	1.0
106	0.87
107	0.76
108	0.66
109	0.57
110	0.50
111	0.44
112	0.38
113	0.33
114	0.29
115	0.25

At no time shall any excursion exceed 115 dBA. For any value, the reference duration (T) in hours is computed by:

$$T = \frac{8}{2^{(L-90)/5}}$$ where L is the measured

A-weighted, slow-response sound pressure level.

TABLE 62–2.—"DOSE"/TWA$_8$ EQUIVALENT

Dose (percent)	TWA$_8$
25	80
29	81
33	82
38	83
44	84
50	85
57	86
66	87
76	88
87	89
100	90
115	91
132	92
152	93
174	94
200	95
230	96
264	97
303	98
350	99
400	100
460	101
530	102
610	103
700	104
800	105
920	106
1056	107
1213	108
1393	109
1600	110
1838	111
2111	112
2425	113
2786	114
3200	115

Interpolate between the values found in this Table, or extend the Table, by using the formula: TWA$_8$ = 16.61 log$_{10}$(D/100) + 90

TABLE 62–3.—AGE CORRECTION VALUE IN DECIBELS FOR MALES (SELECTED FREQUENCIES)

Age (years)	kHz 2	3	4
20 or less	3	4	5
21	3	4	5
22	3	4	5
23	3	4	6
24	3	5	6
25	3	5	7
26	4	5	7
27	4	6	7
28	4	6	8
29	4	6	8
30	4	6	9
31	4	7	9
32	5	7	10
33	5	7	10
34	5	8	11
35	5	8	11
36	5	9	12
37	6	9	12
38	6	9	13
39	6	10	14
40	6	10	14
41	6	10	14
42	7	11	16
43	7	12	16
44	7	12	17
45	7	13	18
46	8	13	19
47	8	14	19
48	8	14	20
49	9	15	21
50	9	16	22
51	9	16	23
52	10	17	24
53	10	18	25
54	10	18	26
55	11	19	27
56	11	20	28
57	11	21	29
58	12	22	31
59	12	22	32
60 or more	13	23	33

TABLE 62–4.—AGE CORRECTION VALUE IN DECIBELS FOR FEMALES (SELECTED FREQUENCIES)

Age (years)	kHz 2	3	4
20 or less	4	3	3
21	4	4	3
22	4	4	4
23	5	4	4
24	5	4	4
25	5	4	4
26	5	5	4
27	5	5	5
28	5	5	5
29	5	5	5
30	6	5	5
31	6	6	5
32	6	6	6
33	6	6	6
34	6	6	6
35	6	7	7
36	7	7	7
37	7	7	7
38	7	7	7
39	7	8	8
40	7	8	8
41	8	8	8
42	8	9	9
43	8	9	9
44	8	9	9
45	8	10	10
46	9	10	10
47	9	10	11
48	9	11	11
49	9	11	11
50	10	11	12
51	10	11	12
52	10	12	13
53	10	13	13
54	11	13	14
55	11	14	14
56	11	14	15
57	11	15	15
58	12	15	16
59	12	16	16
60 or more	12	16	17

[FR Doc. 99–22964 Filed 9-7-99; 8:45 am]
BILLING CODE 4510–33–P

Appendix G
MSHA Regulation Checklist

from Associates in Acoustics, Inc., Evergreen, Co.

PROGRAM CHECKLIST FOR MSHA'S
OCCUPATIONAL NOISE EXPOSURE REGULATION

Company:_____   **Location:** _____

Reviewer: _____   **Date:** _____

This checklist is designed to help mine operators evaluate and ensure compliance with MSHA's noise exposure regulation, 30 CFR Part 62. Part 62 sets standards for surface and underground metal, nonmetal, and coal mines subject to the Federal Mine Safety and Health Act of 1977. An answer of "no" to any of the following questions indicates the need for further investigation and possible corrective action. Terms highlighted for the first time in ***bold and italics*** may be cross-referenced to the definitions section of the MSHA noise regulation. For details and further explanation, refer to the complete text and tables of 30 CFR Part 62, *Federal Register, Vol. 64, No. 176, September 13, 1999, 49630–49634.*

ITEM NO.	SECTION OF REG.	HEARING CONSERVATION PROGRAM COMPONENT	YES	NO	COMMENTS
		NOISE MONITORING			
1.	62.110 (a)	Is noise exposure assessment conducted when information indicates that any miner's exposure may equal or exceed the ***action level***, defined as an 8-hour ***time-weighted-average*** (TWA) of 85 dBA, or equivalently, a dose 50% of the ***Permissible Exposure Level*** (PEL)?			
2.	62.110 (a)(b)	Is the noise monitoring strategy designed to evaluate each miner's noise exposure sufficiently to determine continuing compliance with the rule, including: • Determining if a miner's noise exposure equals or exceeds the action level, exceeds the PEL, or exceeds the ***dual hearing protection level*** • Determining the effectiveness of the engineering and administrative controls • Identifying areas of the mine where ***hearing protectors*** are required, and • Ensuring that the audiometric test providers receive the necessary information to properly evaluate miners' audiograms?			
3.	62.101 62.110 (b)(2)(ii)	When determining whether a miner's TWA equals or exceeds the action level for inclusion in the HCP, are all ***sound levels*** from 80 to at least 130 dBA integrated into the TWA, or dose, determination?			
4.	62.101 62.110 (b)(2)(ii)	When determining whether a miner's TWA exceeds the PEL, are all sound levels from 90 to at least 140 dBA integrated into the TWA, or dose, determination?			

168

ITEM NO.	SECTION OF REG.	HEARING CONSERVATION PROGRAM COMPONENT	YES	NO	COMMENTS
5.	62.110 (b)(2)(i)	Are TWA determinations made without regard to the use of hearing protectors?			
6.	62.110 (b)(2)(iii)	Do TWA determinations reflect the miner's full work shift?			
7.	62.110 (b)(2)(iv)(v)	Are TWAs measured and/or determined using the following specifications: • a 90-dBA *criterion level* • a 5-dBA *exchange rate* • A-weighting and "slow" response settings of the instrumentation • an 80-dBA threshold level for HCP inclusion purposes, and • a 90-dBA threshold level for determining compliance with the PEL?			
8.	62.110 (c)	When noise monitoring is to be conducted, are miners and their representatives given prior notice of the date and time the survey is scheduled?			
9.	62.110 (c)	When noise monitoring is conducted, are miners and their representatives provided an opportunity to observe the monitoring process?			
10.	62.110 (d)	Are all miners* exposed to noise equal to or exceeding the action level, exceeding the PEL, or exceeding the dual hearing protection level notified of the monitoring results in writing, and any corrective actions being taken, within 15 calendar days of the exposure determination and corrective actions? * Note: it is not necessary to re-notify miners who have been informed of the same results within the prior 12 months.*			
		REDUCTION IN NOISE EXPOSURES			
11.	62.130(a)(b)	For all miner noise exposures that exceed the PEL, are feasible engineering or administrative controls used to reduce those exposures within acceptable limits, or to as low a level as feasible? *Note: MSHA considers the following factors when determining whether engineering and/or administrative controls are feasible: the nature and extent of the exposure, the demonstrated effectiveness of available technology, and whether the committed resources are wholly out of proportion to the expected results.*			
12.	62.130 (a)	When administrative controls are used, are the procedures posted on the mine bulletin board?			
13.	62.130 (a)	When administrative controls are used, is a copy of the procedures provided to affected miners?			

ITEM NO.	SECTION OF REG.	HEARING CONSERVATION PROGRAM COMPONENT	YES	NO	COMMENTS
14.	62.130 (c)	Are procedures or mechanisms in place to ensure no miner is exposed at any time to a sound level exceeding 115 dBA*? *Note: as determined without adjustment for the use of hearing protection.*			
		HEARING CONSERVATION PROGRAM (HCP)			
15.	62. 120 62.150	Whenever miner noise exposures equal or exceed the action level, is there a continuing and effective HCP in place that complies with the regulation, including: • a system of noise exposure monitoring • the provision and use of hearing protectors • audiometric testing • training, and • recordkeeping?			
		HEARING PROTECTORS			
16.	62.160 (a)	Are hearing protectors with scientifically accepted indicators of noise reduction, and necessary replacements, provided to all miners in the HCP at no cost? *Note: although hearing protectors must be provided and used if engineering and administrative controls fail to reduce the miner's exposure to the PEL, they are not accepted in lieu of such controls.*			
17.	62.160 (a)(2)	Is the miner allowed to choose the type of hearing protector from at least two muff and two plug type devices? *Note: although the type is selected by the miner, the size and fit of the device must be determined by the mine operator.*			
18.	62.140	Are miners with TWAs over 105 dBA, or equivalently a noise dose greater than 800% of the PEL, required to use dual hearing protection (concurrent use of an earplug and earmuff)? *Note: the TWA for this purpose must be determined integrating sound levels from 90 to at least 140 dB.*			
19.	62.160 (a)(2)	When dual hearing protectors are required, is the miner allowed to select one muff and one plug from at least two devices of each type?			
20.	62.160 (a)(3)	Is there a procedure in place to ensure that hearing protection is in good condition and replaced as needed?			
21.	62.160 (a)(3)	Is hearing protection fitted and maintained in accordance with the manufacturers' instructions?			
22.	62.160 (a)(5)	Is the miner allowed to choose a different hearing protector(s) if the initially selected hearing protector(s) is subsequently precluded due to **medical pathology** of the ear?			

ITEM NO.	SECTION OF REG.	HEARING CONSERVATION PROGRAM COMPONENT	YES	NO	COMMENTS
23.	62.160 (b)	Are all miners whose exposures exceed the PEL required to wear hearing protection devices? *Note: this requirement is in effect before engineering and/or administrative controls are implemented, or if the control measures do not reduce the TWAs below the PEL.*			
24.	62.160 (c)	Are hearing protection devices required to be worn by all miners in the HCP who: • will have more than 6 months pass before they can take a **baseline audiogram**, or • have incurred a **standard threshold shift** (STS) in hearing?			
		AUDIOMETRIC TESTING			
25.	62.170 (a)	If a prior hearing test was used to establish a baseline audiogram (first or "reference" audiometric test), were all test requirements of section 62.171 satisfied?			
26.	62.170 (a)	If a prior hearing test was not available or not used to establish the baseline audiogram, has each miner in the HCP been offered the opportunity to establish a valid baseline audiogram? *Note: MSHA has indicated that all baseline audiograms must be in place for miners in the HCP by March 13, 2001 (or September 13, 2001 if mobile van services are used)*			
27.	62.170 (a)(1) (3)	Are valid baseline audiograms for all miners in the HCP established within six months of first exposure at or above the action level, or within one year if mobile van services are utilized? *Note: a new baseline may be established for a miner who is away from the mine for more than six consecutive months.*			
28.	62.170 (a)(2)	Do miners receive prior notification of the need to avoid high levels of non-occupational noise exposure during the 14-hour period immediately preceding the *baseline* audiometric test?			
29.	62.170 (a)(2)	Is there a 14-hour period without exposure to workplace noise* prior to obtaining a baseline audiogram for each miner? ** Note: hearing protection may be used to satisfy this quiet period requirement.*			
30.	62.170 (b)	For all miners included in the HCP, are audiometric tests offered at least every 12 months after the baseline audiogram is established?			
31.	62.170 (c)	Is an annual audiogram deemed to be a *revised baseline audiogram* when in the judgement of the reviewing *audiologist* or physician, there is significant improvement over the baseline?			

ITEM NO.	SECTION OF REG.	HEARING CONSERVATION PROGRAM COMPONENT	YES	NO	COMMENTS
32.	62.170 (c)	Is an annual audiogram deemed to be a revised baseline audiogram when in the judgement of the reviewing physician or audiologist, a standard threshold shift (STS) has occurred and is considered permanent?			
33.	62.170	Are all audiometric tests provided at no cost to miners in the HCP?			
34.	62.170	Are all audiometric tests performed by an audiologist, physician, or a *qualified* (CAOHC-certified or equivalent) *technician*?			
35.	62.170	If audiometric tests are performed by a qualified (CAOHC-certified or equivalent) technician, is this individual under the direction and supervision of an audiologist or physician?			
36.	62.171 (a)	Do all audiometric tests consist of pure-tone, air-conduction, hearing threshold examinations at frequencies of 500, 1000, 2000, 3000, 4000, and 6000 *Hertz* (Hz) for each ear separately?			
37.	62.171 (a)	Are all audiometric tests conducted using scientifically validated procedures for conducting audiometric testing, calibrating audiometers, and qualifying audiometric test rooms?			
		EVALUATION OF AUDIOGRAMS and FOLLOW-UP			
38.	62.172 (a)(1)	Has the audiologist or physician evaluating the audiograms been informed of the requirements of 62.172 (Evaluation of Audiograms) and been provided a copy of the miner's audiometric test records?			
39.	62.172 (a)(2) (c)	Has a physician or audiologist, or a qualified (CAOHC-certified or equivalent) technician who is under the direction and supervision of a physician or audiologist: • determined if each audiogram is valid, and • determined if a standard threshold shift* (STS) or a *reportable hearing loss** has occurred? ** Note: allowance may be made for the contribution of aging (presbycusis), utilizing procedures specified in 62.172 (c).*			
40.	62.172 (a)(3) 62.173 (c)	Has the physician, audiologist, or qualified technician been instructed not to reveal to the mine operator, without the written consent of the miner, any specific findings or diagnoses unrelated to occupational noise exposure, hearing loss due to workplace noise, or the wearing of hearing protectors?			

ITEM NO.	SECTION OF REG.	HEARING CONSERVATION PROGRAM COMPONENT	YES	NO	COMMENTS
41.	62.172 (a)(4)	Have the results and interpretation of the results of audiograms been received by the mine operator within 30 calendar days of conducting the audiogram?			
42.	62.172 (b)(1)(2)	Are audiometric retests provided within 30 calendar days of receiving a determination that an audiogram is invalid, provided any medical pathology has improved to the point that a valid test may be obtained? *Note: the mine operator may provide one (optional) audiometric retest within 30 calendar days of receiving a determination that an STS or reportable hearing loss has occurred and may use this test as the annual audiogram.*			
43.	62.173 (a)	When a valid audiogram cannot be obtained due to a suspected work-related medical pathology of the ear, are affected miners *referred* for a clinical-audiological evaluation or an otological examination, at no cost to the employee?			
44.	62.173 (b)	When a valid audiogram cannot be obtained due to a suspected medical pathology of the ear that the physician or audiologist concludes is *unrelated* to the miner's occupational noise exposure or the wearing of hearing protection, is the audiologist or physician instructed to *inform* affected miners of the need for an otological examination?			
45.	62.174	Unless a physician or audiologist determines an STS is neither work related nor aggravated by exposure to workplace noise, are the following actions taken within 30 days of receiving evidence or confirmation of the STS: • retrain the affected miner as per requirements of 62.180, • provide the miner with the opportunity to select a hearing protector, or a different protector, from among those offered by the employer in accordance with 62.160, and • review the effectiveness of any engineering and administrative controls to identify and correct any deficiencies?			
46.	62.175 (a)	Is each miner notified in writing within 10 working days of the mine operator receiving the results of an audiogram or a follow-up audiogram (as required under 62.173) of: • the results and interpretation of the hearing test, including any finding of an STS or reportable hearing loss, and • the needs and reasons for further testing, if applicable?			

ITEM NO.	SECTION OF REG.	HEARING CONSERVATION PROGRAM COMPONENT	YES	NO	COMMENTS
47.	62.175 (b)	When evaluation of the audiograms show that a miner has incurred a reportable hearing loss, has this been reported to MSHA within 10 working days according to Part 50 (on Form 7000-1)? *Note: hearing losses need not be reported if a physician or audiologist determines that the loss is neither work-related nor aggravated by occupational noise exposure.*			
		TRAINING			
48.	62.180 (a)	Is training provided to each miner within 30 days of enrollment in the HCP?			
49.	62.180 (a)	Is training repeated for miners in the HCP at least every twelve months?			
50.	62.180 (a) 62.160 (a)(1)	Does initial and repeat training include information on all of the following items: • the effects of noise on hearing, • the purpose and value of wearing hearing protection devices, • the advantages and disadvantages of the hearing protectors offered, • the various types of hearing protectors offered and the care, fitting, and use of each type, • the general requirements of the regulation, • the mine operator's and miner's respective tasks in maintaining mine noise controls, and • the purpose and value of audiometric testing and an explanation of the test procedures?			
		RECORDS			
51.	62.110 (e)	When a miner is notified of his/her noise exposure, is a copy of this notification letter (or a comparable document) maintained for the duration of the miner's enrollment in the HCP plus 6 months?			
52.	62.171 (b)	Does each miner's audiometric test records contain the following: • name and job classification of the miner tested, • a copy of all of the miner's audiograms, • evidence that the audiograms were conducted in accordance with audiometric test requirements* [Section 171(a)], • any personal noise exposure determinations, and • the results of follow-up examinations, if any? *Note: evidence that a group of audiograms were conducted in accordance with requirements is sufficient, provided that the record makes clear which audiograms are involved.*			
53.	62.171 (c)	Are the audiometric test records kept for the duration of the affected miner's employment plus 6 months?			

174

ITEM NO.	SECTION OF REG.	HEARING CONSERVATION PROGRAM COMPONENT	YES	NO	COMMENTS
54.	62.180 (b)	Is the date and type of training given each miner documented, and the miner's most recent certification maintained for as long as the miner is enrolled in the HCP plus 6 months?			
55.	62.190 (a)	If applicable, have authorized representatives of the Secretaries of Labor and Health and Human Services been provided *access* to all records required under Part 62 upon request?			
56.	62.190 (a)(1)	If applicable, have all records maintained under Part 62 for an individual miner been provided to that miner, or with written consent to the *miner's designee*, within 15 calendar days of written request?			
57.	62.190 (a)(2)	If applicable, have HCP training certifications and notices of noise exposure determinations been provided to specific miner representatives as designated under Part 40, within 15 calendar days of written request?			
58.	62.190 (a)(3)	If applicable, have former miners been provided their records of previous noise exposures within 15 calendar days of written request?			
59.	62.190 (c)(1)	Is there a mechanism in place to transfer all records required to be maintained under the regulation to a successor mine operator?			
60.	62.190 (c)(2)	If applicable, if a successor mine operator has come into being, are all baseline, or revised baseline audiograms, obtained from the original mine operator and used for purposes of determining whether an STS or reportable hearing loss has occurred?			

Additional Comments: _____

_____

_____

Recommendations: _____

_____

_____

This document was prepared 05/02/00 by:

Associates in Acoustics, Inc.   **Ph. (303) 670-9270**
31385 Burn Lane   **Fax (303) 670-9937**
Evergreen, CO 80439   **www.esion.com**

Appendix H
Program Evaluation Checklist

J.R. Franks, M.R. Stephenson, and C.J. Merry. (1996). "Program Evaluation Checklist." Appendix B in *Preventing Occupational Hearing Loss — A Practical Guide.* U.S. Dept. Health and Human Services, NIOSH, Cincinnati, OH.

HEARING CONSERVATION PROGRAM
EVALUATION CHECKLIST

Training and Education

Failures or deficiencies in hearing conservation programs (hearing loss prevention programs) can often be traced to inadequacies in the training and education of noise-exposed employees and those who conduct elements of the program.

1. Has training been conducted at least once a year?
2. Was the training provided by a qualified instructor?
3. Was the success of each training program evaluated?
4. Is the content revised periodically?
5. Are managers and supervisors directly involved?
6. Are posters, regulations, handouts, and employee newsletters used as supplements?
7. Are personal counseling sessions conducted for employees having problems with hearing protection devices or showing hearing threshold shifts?

Supervisor Involvement

Data indicate that employees who refuse to wear hearing protectors or who fail to show up for hearing tests frequently work for supervisors who are not totally committed to the hearing loss prevention programs.

1. Have supervisors been provided with the knowledge required to supervise the use and care of hearing protectors by subordinates?
2. Do supervisors wear hearing protectors in appropriate areas?
3. Have supervisors been counseled when employees resist wearing protectors or fail to show up for hearing tests?
4. Are disciplinary actions enforced when employees repeatedly refuse to wear hearing protectors?

Noise Measurement

For noise measurements to be useful, they need to be related to noise exposure risks or the prioritization of noise control efforts, rather than merely filed away. In addition, the results need to be communicated to the appropriate personnel, especially when follow-up actions are required.

1. Were the essential/critical noise studies performed?
2. Was the purpose of each noise study clearly stated? Have noise-exposed employees been notified of their exposures and apprised of auditory risks?
3. Are the results routinely transmitted to supervisors and other key individuals?
4. Are results entered into health/medical records of noise exposed employees?
5. Are results entered into shop folders?
6. If noise maps exist, are they used by the proper staff?
7. Are noise measurement results considered when contemplating procurement of new equipment? Modifying the facility? Relocating employees?
8. Have there been changes in areas, equipment, or processes that have altered noise exposure? Have follow-up noise measurements been conducted?
9. Are appropriate steps taken to include (or exclude) employees in the hearing loss prevention programs whose exposures have changed significantly?

Engineering and Administrative Controls

Controlling noise by engineering and administrative methods is often the most effective means of reducing or eliminating the hazard. In some cases engineering controls will remove requirements for other components of the program, such as audiometric testing and the use of hearing protectors.

1. Have noise control needs been prioritized?
2. Has the cost-effectiveness of various options been addressed?
3. Are employees and supervisors apprised of plans for noise control measures? Are they consulted on various approaches?
4. Will in-house resources or outside consultants perform the work?
5. Have employees and supervisors been counseled on the operation and maintenance of noise control devices?
6. Are noise control projects monitored to ensure timely completion?
7. Has the full potential for administrative controls been evaluated? Are noisy processes conducted during shifts with fewer employees? Do employees have sound-treated lunch or break areas?

Monitoring Audiometry and Recordkeeping

The skills of audiometric technicians, the status of the audiometer, and the quality of audiometric test records are crucial to hearing loss prevention program success. Useful information may be ascertained from the audiometric records as well as from those who actually administer the tests.

1. Has the audiometric technician been adequately trained, certified, and recertified as necessary?
2. Do on-the-job observations of the technicians indicate that they perform a thorough and valid audiometric test, instruct and consult the employee effectively, and keep appropriate records?
3. Are records complete?
4. Are follow-up actions documented?
5. Are hearing threshold levels reasonably consistent from test to test? If not, are the reasons for inconsistencies investigated promptly?
6. Are the annual test results compared to baseline to identify the presence of an OSHA standard threshold shift?
7. Is the annual incidence of standard threshold shift greater than a few percent? If so, are problem areas pinpointed and remedial steps taken?
8. Are audiometric trends (deteriorations) being identified, both in individuals and in groups of employees? (NIOSH recommends no more than 5% of workers showing 15 dB Significant Threshold Shift, same ear, same frequency.)
9. Do records show that appropriate audiometer calibration procedures have been followed?
10. Is there documentation showing that the background sound levels in the audiometer room were low enough to permit valid testing?
11. Are the results of audiometric tests being communicated to supervisors and managers as well as to employees?
12. Has corrective action been taken if the rate of no-shows for audiometric test appointments is more than about 5%?
13. Are employees incurring STS notified in writing within at least 21 days? (NIOSH recommends immediate notification if retest shows 15 dB Significant Threshold Shift, same ear, same frequency.)

Referrals

Referrals to outside sources for consultation or treatment are sometimes in order, but they can be an expensive element of the hearing loss prevention program, and should not be undertaken unnecessarily.

1. Are referral procedures clearly specified?
2. Have letters of agreement between the company and consulting physicians or audiologists been executed?
3. Have mechanisms been established to ensure that employees needing evaluation or treatment actually receive the service (i.e., transportation, scheduling, reminders)?
4. Are records properly transmitted to the physician or audiologist, and back to the company?
5. If medical treatment is recommended, does the employee understand the condition requiring treatment, the recommendation, and methods of obtaining such treatment?
6. Are employees being referred unnecessarily?

Hearing Protection Devices

When noise control measures are infeasible, or until such time as they are installed, hearing protection devices are the only way to prevent hazardous levels of noise from damaging the inner ear. Making sure that these devices are worn effectively requires continuous attention on the part of supervisors and program implementors as well as noise-exposed employees.

1. Have hearing protectors been made available to all employees whose daily average noise exposures are 85 dBA or above? (NIOSH recommends requiring HPD use if noises equal or exceed 85 dBA regardless of exposure time.)
2. Are employees given the opportunity to select from a variety of appropriate protectors?
3. Are employees fitted carefully with special attention to comfort?
4. Are employees thoroughly trained, not only initially but at least once a year?
5. Are the protectors checked regularly for wear or defects, and replaced immediately if necessary?
6. If employees use disposable hearing protectors, are replacements readily available?
7. Do employees understand the appropriate hygiene requirements?
8. Have any employees developed ear infections or irritations associated with the use of hearing protectors? Are there any employees who are unable to wear these devices because of medical conditions? Have these conditions been treated promptly and successfully?
9. Have alternative types of hearing protectors been considered when problems with current devices are experienced?
10. Do employees who incur noise-induced hearing loss receive intensive counseling?
11. Are those who fit and supervise the wearing of hearing protectors competent to deal with the many problems that can occur?
12. Do workers complain that protectors interfere with their ability to do their jobs? Do they interfere with spoken instructions or warning signals? Are these complaints followed promptly with counseling, noise control, or other measures?
13. Are employees encouraged to take their hearing protectors home if they engage in noisy non-occupational activities?
14. Are new types of or potentially more effective protectors considered as they become available?
15. Is the effectiveness of the hearing protector program evaluated regularly?
16. Have at-the-ear protection levels been evaluated to ensure that either over or under protection has been adequately balanced according to the anticipated ambient noise levels?
17. Is each hearing protector user required to demonstrate that he or she understands how to use and care for the protector? The results documented?

Administrative

Keeping organized and current on administrative matters will help the program run smoothly.

1. Have there been any changes in federal or state regulations? Have hearing loss prevention program's policies been modified to reflect these changes?
2. Are copies of company policies and guidelines regarding the hearing loss prevention program available in the offices that support the various program elements? Are those who implement the program elements aware of these policies? Do they comply?
3. Are necessary materials and supplies being ordered with a minimum of delay?
4. Are procurement officers overriding the hearing loss prevention program implementor's requests for specific hearing protectors or other hearing loss prevention equipment? If so, have corrective steps been taken?
5. Is the performance of key personnel evaluated periodically? If such performance is found to be less than acceptable, are steps taken to correct the situation?
6. Safety: Has the failure to hear warning shouts or alarms been tied to any accidents or injuries? If so, have remedial steps been taken?

Appendix I
Hearing Loss Statutes in the U.S. and Canada

R.A. Dobie, and S.C. Megerson. (2000).
"Workers' Compensation." Chapter 18 in E.H.
Berger, L.H. Royster, J.D. Royster, D.P. Driscoll,
and M. Layne, (Eds.), *The Noise Manual, Fifth
Edition.* American Industrial Hyygiene Assoc.,
Fairfax, VA.

TABLE 18.1

Hearing loss statutes in the United States and Canada.

Jurisdiction	1. Is occupational hearing loss compensable?	2. Is minimum noise exposure required for filing?	3. Schedule in weeks (one ear).	4. Schedule in weeks (both ears).	5. Maximum compensation (one ear).	6. Maximum compensation (both ears).	7. Hearing impairment formula.	8. Waiting period.	9. Is deduction made for presbycusis?	10. Is award made for tinnitus?	11. Provision for hearing aid?	12. Credit for improvement with hearing aid?	13. Is hearing loss prior to employment considered in compensation claim?	14. Statute of limitations for hearing-loss claim.	15. Penalty for not wearing hearing protection devices?	16. Self-assessment of hearing impairment considered in rating/award?	Comments
Alabama	Yes	No	53	163	$11,660	$35,860	ME	No	No	Yes-I	Yes	No	Yes	2 yrs.	Yes-D	Poss	
Alaska	Yes	No	*	*	*	*	AAO-79	No	No	Yes-I	Yes	No*	No*	2 yrs.	No	No	**3-6:** awards based on temporary disability and permanent partial impairment according to AMA guidelines; **12:** unless hearing aid enables worker to return to work; **13:** as long as there has been substantial aggravation at work.
Arizona	Yes	No	86	260	$23,100	$69,300	ME	No	No	Yes-I	Yes	No	Yes	1 yr.	No	No	
Arkansas	Yes	No	42	158	$11,296	$42,502	AAO-79	No	Poss	No	Poss	No	Yes	Yes*	No	No	**14:** statute of limitations and other hearing loss issues currently before Board of Appeals.
California	Yes	No	50*	311*	$8,040*	$58,863*	AAO-79	No	No	Yes	Yes	Yes	Yes	1 yr.	Yes-P	Yes	**3-6:** awards modified by age and occupation at time of injury.
Colorado	Yes	No	35	139	$5,250	$20,850	AAO-79	No	Yes	Yes	Yes	No	Yes	Yes	Yes-P	No	
Connecticut	Yes	No	35	104	*	*	ME*	3 days	Poss	Poss	Poss	Poss	Poss	1 yr.	Yes-P	Poss	**5-6:** no maximum reported—award is number of weeks scheduled benefit at claimant's compensation rate; **7:** case law has supported AAO-79.
Delaware	Yes	No	75	175	$30,833	$71,944	ME	No	No	No	Yes	Yes	No	2 yrs.	No	No	
District of Columbia	Yes	No	39	150	$34,880	$134,170	AAO-79	6 mo.	Poss	Poss	Poss	Poss	Poss	1 yr.	Poss	Poss	
Florida	Yes	No	18	105	$8,892	$51,870	AAO-79	No	No	Yes-I	Yes	No	Yes	2 yrs.	Yes-P	No	
Georgia	Yes*	Yes*	NA	150	NA	NR	AAOO-59	6 mos.	NR	No	NR	NR	Yes	NR	Yes-D	NR	**1:** no awards granted for monaural hearing loss unless pre-existing deafness in other ear; **2:** 90 dBA for 90 days.
Hawaii	Yes	Yes	52	200	$26,416	$101,600	AAOO-59	No	No	Yes	Yes	No	No	2 yrs.	No	No	

State																	Comments
Idaho	Yes*	No	NR	175	NR	$42,639	ME	No	No	No	Yes-I	No	No	Yes	1 yr.	No	No	1: only hearing loss due to work-related trauma/injury is considered.
Illinois	Yes	Yes*	50-100	200	$43,989	$87,978	Other*	No	No	No	Yes-I	Yes	No	Yes	2-3 yrs.	No	No	2: 90 dBA TWA; 7: avg > 30 dB at 1000, 2000, and 3000 Hz, 1.82% per dB.
Indiana	Yes*	No	*	*	$12,500	$39,500	ME	No	Yes	NR	NR	No	NR	Yes	2 yrs.	Yes-D	Yes	1: only hearing loss due to work-related trauma/injury is compensable, but case law evolving--likely to consider NIHL in future; 3-4: awards paid for temp. disability (up to 500 wks) or permanent partial impairment based on % of max. awards.
Iowa	Yes	Yes	50	175	$43,600	$152,600	AAO-79	1 mon.	Yes	Yes	Yes	Yes	No	Yes	2 yrs.	Yes-D	No	
Kansas	Yes	No	30	110	$10,980	$40,260	AAO-79	No	Yes	Yes-I	Yes-I	Yes	Yes	Yes	200 days	Yes-D	No	
Kentucky	Yes	No	520	Life-time	*	*	ME	No	No	No	No	No	No	No	3-5 yrs.	No	No	5-6: award based on % impairment and average weekly wage.
Louisiana	Yes*	No	100	100	NR	$36,700	ME	No	No	Yes-I	Yes-I	No	No	Yes	1 yr.	Yes-D	No	1: only hearing loss due to work-related trauma/injury is considered.
Maine	Yes	Yes	50	200	$20,100	$80,400	AAOO-59	30 days	Yes*	Yes-I	Yes-I	Yes	Yes	Yes	Yes	Yes-D	No	9: 1/2 dB for each year over 40 yrs. of age.
Maryland	Yes	Yes*	125	250	NR	NR	AAOO-59	Yes	Poss	Poss	Poss	Yes	No	Yes	Yes	NR	Poss	2: exposure to harmful noise for 90 days or more.
Massachusetts	Yes	No	*	*	*	*	ME	No	Yes	Yes	Yes	Yes	NR	Yes	Yes	Yes	No	3-6: based on statewide average wage — maximum $700/week.
Michigan	No*																	1: no compensation for occupational hearing loss — employees are compensated only if an injury to the ear (that may or may not result in hearing loss) causes a loss of wages.
Minnesota	Yes	No	*	*	*	*	AAO-79	3 mos.	No	No	No	Yes	No	Yes	3 yrs.	No	No	
Mississippi	Yes	No	40	150	$11,191	$41,967	ME	No	No	Yes	Yes	Yes	No	No	Yes	No	Yes	
Missouri	Yes	No	49	180	$14,442	$53,051	AAOO-59	6 mo.	Yes*	Yes	Yes	Yes	No	Yes	No	Yes-P*	No	9: 1/2 dB per year over age 40 yrs.; 15: results in 15% penalty.
Montana	Yes	Yes*	40	200	NR	NR	AAOO-59	6 mo.	Yes*	No	No	No	No	Yes	No	No	No	2: 90 dB daily for 90 days or more; 9: 1/2 dB per year over age 40 years.
Nebraska	Yes	No	50	*	$22,200	*	ME	No	No	Poss	Poss	Yes	No	Yes	2 yrs.	No	No	4 and 6: average weekly wage x life expectancy.
Nevada	Yes	No	*	*	*	*	AAO-79	No	Poss	Yes	Yes	Yes	No	Yes	No	Yes-P	No	3-6: awards determined according to AMA guide and state statute.

table continued on next page.

Data compiled in 1998/1999 by Susan Megerson with assistance from Cyd Kladden.

KEY: Poss - possible; **NA** - non-applicable; **NR** - no response; ***** - see comments; **AAOO-59** - avg. > 25 dB at 500, 1000, and 2000 Hz; **AAO-79** - avg. > 25 dB at 500, 1000, 2000, and 3000 Hz; **I** - only if impairment also present; **D** - claim denied; **P** - penalty applied.
ME - medial evidence, hearing loss formula at discretion of consulting physician;

TABLE 18.1 — continued
Hearing loss statutes in the United States and Canada.

Jurisdiction	1. Is occupational hearing loss compensable?	2. Is minimum noise exposure required for filing?	3. Schedule in weeks (one ear).	4. Schedule in weeks (both ears).	5. Maximum compensation (one ear).	6. Maximum compensation (both ears).	7. Hearing impairment formula.	8. Waiting period.	9. Is deduction made for presbycusis?	10. Is award made for tinnitus?	11. Provision for hearing aid?	12. Credit for improvement with hearing aid?	13. Is hearing loss prior to employment considered in compensation claim?	14. Statute of limitations for hearing-loss claim.	15. Penalty for not wearing hearing protection devices?	16. Self-assessment of hearing impairment considered in rating/award?	Comments
New Hampshire	Yes	No	30	123	$25,200	$103,320	ME	No	No	No	Yes	No	Yes	2 yrs.	No	No	2: 90 dB TWA; 7: avg. > 30 dB at 1000, 2000, and 3000 Hz, 1.5% per dB.
New Jersey	Yes	Yes*	60	200	$8,280	$48,200	Other*	4 wks.	No.	Yes	Yes	Yes	Yes	2 yrs.	Yes-D	Yes	
New Mexico	Yes	No	40	150	$15,039	$56,397	ME	7 days	No	Yes	No	No	Yes	1 yr.	Poss-P	No	2: exposure to harmful noise for 90 days or more.
New York	Yes	Yes*	60	150	$24,000	$60,000	AAO-79	3 mos.	No	No	No	No	Yes	90 days	No	No	
North Carolina	Yes	Yes*	70	150	$37,240	$79,800	AAO-79*	6 mos.	No	No	Yes	No	Yes	2 yrs.	Yes-D	No	2: 90 dBA for at least 90 days; 7: if hearing loss due to injury, then "medical evidence" is utilized.
North Dakota	Yes	No	5	100	$695	$13,900	AAO-79	No	No	Yes-I	Yes	No	Yes	No	No	No	1: only permanent total hearing loss in one or both ears is compensable.
Ohio	Yes*	No	25	125	$13,525	$67,625	ME	No	Poss	No	Yes	No	No	2 yrs.	No	No	
Oklahoma	Yes	No	104	312	$22,194	$66,583	AAO-79	No	No	Yes*	Yes	No	Yes	2 yrs.	Yes-D	No	10: up to 5% for tinnitus in cases of unilateral hearing loss.
Oregon	Yes	No	*	*	$27,240	$87,168	Other*	No	Yes	Yes	Yes	No	Yes*	1 yr.	No	No	3-4: one time permanent partial disability award based on impairment; 7: avg > 25 dB at 500, 1000, 2000, 3000, 4000, and 6000 Hz, 1.5% per dB; 13: if baseline completed within 180 days of hire.
Pennsylvania	Yes	No*	60	260	*	*	AAO-79	No	No	No	No	No	Yes*	3 yrs.	No	No	2: case law has adopted OSHA standards as employer defense; 5 and 6: # weeks x 2/3 average wage; 13: only if pre-employment testing was performed at employer's expense.

186

Jurisdiction																	Comments
Rhode Island	Yes	Yes	17*	100*	$1,530*	$9,000*	AAO-79	6 mos.	Yes	Poss-I	Poss	No	No*	2 yrs.	No	No	**3:** 60 weeks if loss due to trauma; **4:** 200 weeks for trauma; **5:** $5400 for trauma; **6:** $18,000 for trauma; **13:** current employer is solely responsible for occupational loss.
South Carolina	Yes	No	80	165	$38,678	$79,773	AAO-79	No	No	No	No	No	Yes	No	No	No	
South Dakota	Yes	Yes*	50	150	$20,400	$61,200	AAO-79	No	Yes*	No	Yes	No	Yes	2 yrs.	Yes-D	No	**2:** 90 dBA TWA; **9:** 1/2 dB for each year over 45 yrs.
Tennessee	Yes	No	75	150	$38,625	$77,250	ME	No	Yes	Yes-I	Yes	Poss	Yes	1 yr.	Poss-D	Yes	
Texas	Yes	No	*	*	*	*	AAO-79	No	No	No	No	No	Yes	30 days	No	No	**3-6:** no maximum scheduled awards.
Utah	Yes	Yes*	NR	109	NR	$35,425	AAO-79	6 wks.	NR	NR	NR	NR	Yes	180 days	NR	NR	**2:** 90 dBA TWA or impact/impulsive noise 140 dB or greater.
Vermont	Yes	No	24	142	$17,448	$103,052	ME	No	No	Yes-I	Yes	No	No	Yes	Yes-D	No	
Virginia	Yes*	No	50	100	*	*	AAO-79	No	No	No	Poss	No	Yes	2-5 yrs.	No	No	**1:** only hearing loss due to work-related trauma or injury is considered; **5-6:** # weeks x average weekly wage.
Washington	Yes	No	N/A	N/A	$10,837	$65,023	AAO-79	No	No	Yes-I	Yes	No	Yes	2 yrs.	No	No	
West Virginia	Yes	No	*	*	*	*	AAO-79	2 mos.	Yes	No	Yes	No	Yes	3 yrs.	No	No	**3-6:** hearing loss compensation is based on a percentage of whole body impairment (max for both ears, 22.5% whole body).
Wisconsin	Yes	No	36	216	*	*	Other*	7 days	No	No*	Yes	No	Yes	No	No	No	**5-6:** depends on year of retirement; **7:** avg. ≥ 30 dB at 500, 1000, 2000, and 3000 Hz; **10:** not compensable since 1/1/92.
Wyoming	Yes	No	*	*	*	*	ME	No	NR	NR	No	No	Yes	Yes	Yes-D	NR	**3-6:** based upon rating of impairment.
U.S. DOL – FECA	Yes	Yes	52	52	NR	NR	AAO-79	No	No	No	Yes	No	No	3 yrs.	No	No	FECA - federal employees compensation act
U.S. DOL – Longshoremen	Yes	No	52	200	*	*	AAO-79	No	No	No	Yes	No	No	1 yr.	No	No	
Guam	Yes	No	52	200	$13,000	$50,000	ME	No	Yes	Yes-I	Yes	No	Yes	1 yr.	No	No	**5-6:** based upon compensation rate, increases annually.
Alberta	Yes*	NA	NA	NA	$3,184	$19,105	NR	No	No	Yes-I	Yes	No	Yes	5 yrs.	No	No	**2:** 85 dBA for 8 hrs.
British Columbia	Yes*	NA	NA	*	*	*	Other*	No	No	No	Yes	No	Yes	No	No	No	**2:** 85 dB L$_{EX,8h}$ for 2 yrs.; **5-6:** based on % of annual wage; **7:** avg > 28 dB at 500, 1000, and 2000 Hz; 2.5% per dB
Manitoba	Yes*	NA	NA	*	*	*	Other*	No	Yes*	No	Yes	No	Yes	No	Poss-D	No	**2:** 85 dB for 2 yrs.; **5-6:** lump sum paid based on %; **7:** avg ≥ 35 dB at 500, 1000, 2000, and 3000 Hz; **9:** 1/2 dB per year over 60 yrs. of age.

table continued on next page.

Data compiled in 1998/1999 by Susan Megerson with assistance from Cyd Kladden.

KEY: Poss - possible; **NA** - non-applicable; **NR** - no response; ***** - see comments; **AAOO-59** - avg. > 25 dB at 500, 1000, and 2000 Hz; **AAO-79** - avg. > 25 dB at 500, 1000, 2000, and 3000 Hz; **I** - only if impairment also present; **D** - claim denied; **P** - penalty applied.
ME - medial evidence, hearing loss formula at discretion of consulting physician.

TABLE 18.1 — continued
Hearing loss statutes in the United States and Canada.

Jurisdiction	1. Is occupational hearing loss compensable?	2. Is minimum noise exposure required for filing?	3. Schedule in weeks (one ear).	4. Schedule in weeks (both ears).	5. Maximum compensation (one ear).	6. Maximum compensation (both ears).	7. Hearing impairment formula.	8. Waiting period.	9. Is deduction made for presbycusis?	10. Is award made for tinnitus?	11. Provision for hearing aid?	12. Credit for improvement with hearing aid?	13. Is hearing loss prior to employment considered in compensation claim?	14. Statute of limitations for hearing-loss claim.	15. Penalty for not wearing hearing protection devices?	16. Self-assessment of hearing impairment considered in rating/award?	Comments
New Brunswick	Yes	No	NA	NA	*	*	ME	No	No	Yes-I	Yes	No	Yes	Yes*	No	No	5-6: depends on percent of disability; 14: prior to retirement.
NW Territories	Yes	Yes*	*	*	$147/month	$887/month	Other*	Yes*	No	No	Yes	No	Yes	1 yr.	No	No	2: 90 dB for 8 hrs/day for 2 yrs.; 3-4: no maximum time period; 7: avg ≥ 30 dB at 500, 1000, 2000, and 3000 Hz; 8: when removed from exposure.
Nova Scotia	Yes	Yes*	*	*	*	*	Other*	No	Yes*	Yes*	Yes	Yes	Yes	5 yrs.	No	No	2: 85 dB for 8 hrs/day for 5 yrs.; 3-6: awards based on pre-injury wages and % impairment with no maximums; 7: avg ≥ 35 at 500, 1000, 2000 and 3000 Hz; 9: 1/2 dB per year over age 60 yrs.; 10: 2-5% awarded if specific criteria are met.
Ontario	Yes	Yes*	NA	NA	*	*	AAO-79	No	Yes*	Yes	Yes	No	Yes	6 mo.	No	No	2: 90 dB for 5 yrs.; 5-6: lump sum awards based on % impairment, age at date of accident and maximum medical recovery; 9: 1/2 dB per year over age 60 yrs.
Prince Edward Island	Yes	Yes*	*	*	*	*	ME	No	Yes*	Yes*	Yes	No	Yes	No	No	No	2: 2 yrs. minimum; 3-6: lump sum awards based on % impairment; 9: 1/2 dB per year over age 60 yrs.; 10: 2% maximum.
Quebec	Yes	Yes*	*	*	*	*	ME	No	Yes	No	Yes	No	Yes	No	No	NR	2: 90 dB for 8 hrs/day for 2 yrs.; 3-6: lump sum award based on % impairment and age at time of injury.
Saskatchewan	Yes	No	*	*	$1,130	$13,560	Other *	No	No	Yes-I	Yes	No	Yes	No	No	No	3-4: lump sum pension and hearing aid costs; 7: avg ≥ 30 dB at 500, 1000, 2000, and 3000 Hz.
Yukon	Yes	Yes*	*	*	*	*	AAO-79	2-5 yrs.	Yes*	Yes-I	Yes	No	Yes	No	No	No	2: 85 dB for 8 hrs/day; 3-6: awards based on % impairment and ability to return to work; 9: maximum 2% for each year over age 45 yrs.

KEY: Poss - possible; NA - non-applicable; NR - no response; * - see comments; AAOO-59 - avg. > 25 dB at 500, 1000, and 2000 Hz; AAO-79 - avg. > 25 dB at 500, 1000, 2000, and 3000 Hz; ME - medical evidence, hearing loss formula at discretion of consulting physician; I - only if impairment also present; D - claim denied; P - penalty applied.

Appendix J
Hard to Test Workers

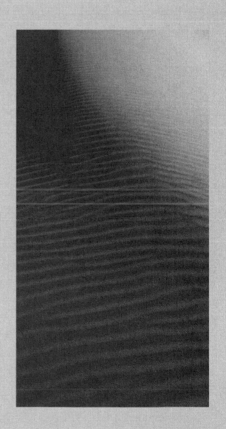

L. Frye. (Spring 2001), CAOHC *UPDATE*, P. 3.

Hard to Test Workers

By Linda Frye, COHN-S/CM MPH RN
Representative of the American Association of
Occupational Health Nurses

OHC Corner

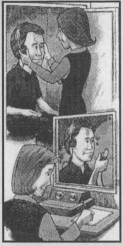

Illustration provided courtesy of E•A•R Hearing Protection Products

As an OHC I have been challenged by some workers during the audiometric procedure. I am sure many of you have your own stories to share as well. Employees who already suffer from hearing loss such as those with tinnitus or a sensorineural hearing loss such as presbycusis frequently arrive for testing with a heightened level of anxiety. Individuals who have difficulty hearing are often times self-conscious or embarrassed and they may "act out" in order to conceal the truth. Let's take a few minutes to consider the hard to test worker's perspective and alternatives that might help us as OHC's accomplish our objectives.

Hard-to-test workers have often had a negative experience during testing. This might be due to being in the booth for extended periods of time, or frustration because they have difficulty distinguishing the audiometric tones from the sounds they hear in their head. If such an employee presents with an "attitude" and is greeted by an OHC with an "attitude" because of the employee's reputation for being difficult to test, you can imagine the outcome is not going to be the desired one.

Over the years I, and other OHCs I know, have developed a few tricks for getting the best results during audiometric testing, even under difficult circumstances. These tips are not based on research and may not be appropriate in every situation, but I hope you will find them helpful. If you have others that you want to share please contact me through the CAOHC office and we will pass them on to you in future UPDATE newsletters.

Testing Tips For the Hard-To-Test Employee:

1. When a worker becomes difficult to deal with, try to pause before responding and look at things from their perspective. Perhaps they have had a bad day at work or they are concerned about the job while they are away for the testing.

2. Remember that not everyone will test well with a microprocessor. I suggest that you test an occasional employee using the manual mode to maintain your skills. If you have an agitated worker who does not test well in the microprocessor mode and you as the OHC are not comfortable and efficient in switching to the manual mode, the testing process will not go smoothly. It is essential for all OHCs to remain very familiar with the manual testing procedure. Unfortunately, some employers believe that when they purchase a microprocessor that they don't need a trained OHC such as those who attend a CAOHC approved course and become CAOHC certified.

3. If an employee has a chronic problem such as tinnitus and needs to be tested manually, mark their audiogram "test manually" to avoid wasted time and frustration next time they come in for testing.

4. If a listener has tinnitus, it's often helpful to use a "pulsed" tone rather than a continuous tone for testing (listeners often report that there is less tendency for the pulsed tone to "blend in" with the tinnitus).

5. When you have a known difficult employee to test and you have more than one OHC in your department, match the employee with the OHC who has the best rapport right from the start.

6. Keep in mind that management has the ultimate responsibility for the hearing conservation program. Should you encounter a worker who is disrespectful or non-compliant in spite of your best efforts to accommodate them, stop the testing process and call the appropriate management contact for further assistance.

7. Avoid leaving a worker in the testing booth for extended periods of time during the manual testing procedure. After a reasonable time period (e.g. 10 minutes) allow the worker to come out of the booth to rest, have a drink of water, etc. before proceeding. For those of us who have been tested ourselves, you know that after awhile you begin to hear your own heart beat and are afraid you will miss a tone if you swallow, etc.

8. Those who wear hearing aids must remove them before testing. For those of us dependent on reading glasses, it can be frustrating to be told to read without them. Now imagine being told to hear without your hearing device. Be sure to explain what, why, and when to win support for the testing procedure. Point out beforehand that the test will not be valid with the hearing aid in place because of possible acoustic feedback for example; remind them that the purpose of the test is to find out about their hearing, not their hearing aid. Then, share the results in a positive way with the worker after they have put the hearing device back on.

9. If the only reason for your interaction is to "get the test done" you may be missing the big picture. Inspiring workers to be proactive managers of their own health and well being will have far reaching benefits.

I remember a saying that goes something like, "Isn't it great to love what you're doing and doing what you love." Sometimes it takes a difficult worker to remind us what and why we are doing what we do. Being an OHC is a privilege I value and I hope you feel the same way, too.

Do you have experience with hard-to-test workers? Send your advice to CAOHC, and we'll share it with other OHCs.

Appendix K
NHCA Professional Guide for Audiometric Baseline Revision

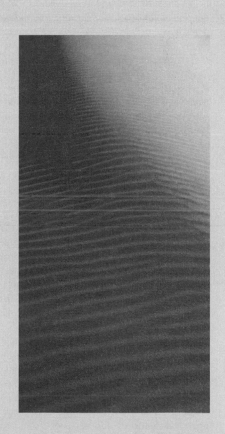

National Hearing Conservation. *Spectrum*.
(January 2001). *Vol. 1*, Suppl. 2, Pp. 1–2.

Spectrum

A PUBLICATION OF THE NATIONAL HEARING CONSERVATION ASSOCIATION

January 2001   *Volume 1, Supplement 2*

NHCA Professional Guide for Audiometric Baseline Revision

Editor's note: Although OSHA specifies that hearing conservation program baseline audiograms can be revised to reflect changes in hearing sensitivity, the details are left up to the professional. What may seem a relatively straightforward proposition has been fraught with confusion and divergent opinions since the promulgation of the hearing conservation amendment in 1981/83. A new professional guide from the National Hearing Conservation Association (NHCA) now provides a uniform and well-thought-out approach. CAOHC urges you to share that guide, reprinted below, with the professional supervisor of your audiometric testing program to help bring uniformity to this practice. Please note that the professional supervisor, and not the occupational hearing conservationist, must implement these baseline revision guidelines.

What Is Baseline Revision?

In a hearing conservation program (HCP), each employee's baseline audiogram gives the reference hearing thresholds for that individual. The results of later monitoring audiograms are compared to the baseline to detect significant changes in hearing thresholds. When significant shifts for the worse are identified, follow-up actions are taken to improve employee protection from noise.

As specified in the Hearing Conservation Amendment (CFR 1910.95) promulgated by the Occupational Safety and Health Administration (OSHA), the baseline may be revised by the reviewing audiologist or physician either for significant improvement in measured thresholds or for persistent standard threshold shift (STS).

Because the baseline audiogram is so important for detecting hearing change and reacting to prevent additional change, NHCA assigned a special committee to develop guidelines for revising audiometric baselines. The 16-member committee conducted research and evaluated various strategies over

several years. The guidelines given here, which were approved by the board of NHCA in March 1996, represent the consensus of the committee. Following these guidelines will provide consistency across professional reviewers and audiometric testing service providers, thereby increasing the degree of protection for noise-exposed workers.

Note: although the guidelines require persistence of hearing changes before the baseline is revised, protective follow-up actions for the employee are needed as soon as significant changes for the worse are first shown.

Definitions

OSHA STS: OSHA defines a standard threshold shift (STS) as a change for the worse in either ear of 10 dB or more in the average of thresholds at 2, 3, and 4 kHz, relative to the baseline.

Significant Improvement: OSHA does not specify a definition of significant improvement. However, an example in Appendix F of the Hearing Conservation Amendment illustrates revision of the baseline after an improvement of 5 dB in the average of hearing thresholds at 2, 3, and 4 kHz.

Baseline Audiogram: Initially the baseline is the latest valid audiogram obtained before entry into the HCP. If no appropriate pre-entry audiogram exists, baseline is the first valid audiogram obtained within six months of entry into the HCP (12 months for mobile testing). OSHA requires 14 hours of quiet prior to the original baseline.

Monitoring Audiograms: Subsequent to the baseline audiogram, new audiograms are obtained at least annually. To increase the preventive function of audiometry, many professionals suggest performing annual audiograms during the workshift in order to detect any noise-related temporary threshold shifts which may occur.

Age Corrections: OSHA permits optional application of age correction values (from

Appendix F) to annual audiograms when comparing them to baseline for detection of STS, in order to account for median values of age change. Note: many professionals feel that if intervention for threshold shifts is delayed until after age-corrected STS has occurred, then significant hearing changes will not receive needed follow-up attention.

How to Use NHCA's Guidelines

Professional Review

These guidelines are meant to be employed only by a professional reviewer (audiologist or physician). Although the guidelines can be programmed by computer to identify records for potential revision, the final decision for revision rests with a human being. Because the goal of the guidelines is to foster consistency among professional reviewers, human override of the guidelines must be justified by specific concrete reasons.

Separate Consideration of Each Ear

Each monitoring audiogram is compared to the baseline to detect improvement or OSHA STS (or other significant shifts). The two ears are examined separately and independently. If one ear meets the criteria for revision of baseline, then the baseline is revised for that ear only. Therefore, if the two ears show different hearing trends, the baseline for the left ear may be from one test date, while the baseline for the right ear may be from a different test date.

Use of Age Corrections

Age corrections do not apply in considering revisions for improvement. The audiologist or physician may choose whether to apply OSHA-allowed age corrections in evaluating baseline revision for persistent OSHA STS. Rule 2 operates in the same way whether optional age corrections are used or not.

Application Exceptions

These guidelines for baseline revision do not apply to the calculation of the 25-dB average shifts which in many states are recordable on the OSHA log for occupational illness and injury. The original baseline is the appropriate reference for that purpose. Neither do the guidelines apply to identification of other (non-STS) significant threshold shifts for the worse, which may be communicatively or medically important.

The Guidelines

Rule 1: Revision for Improvement

If the average of thresholds for 2, 3 and 4 kHz for either ear shows an improvement of 5 dB or more from the baseline value, and the improvement is present on one test and persistent on the next test, then the record should be identified for review by the audiologist or physician for potential revision of the baseline. The baseline for that ear should be revised to the improved test which shows the lower (more sensitive) value for the average of thresholds at 2, 3, and 4 kHz, unless the audiologist or physician determines and documents specific reasons for not revising. If the values of the three-frequency average are identical for the two tests, then the earlier test becomes the revised baseline.

Rule 2: Revision for Persistent OSHA Standard Threshold Shift

If the average of thresholds for 2, 3 and 4 kHz for either ear shows a worsening of 10 dB or more from the baseline value (OSHA STS), and the STS persists on the next annual test (or the next test given at least six months later), then the record should be identified for review by the audiologist or physician for potential revision of the baseline for persistent worsening. Unless the audiologist or physician determines and documents specific reasons for not revising, the baseline for that ear should be revised to the STS test which shows the lower (more sensitive) value for the average of thresholds at 2, 3, and 4 kHz. If both STS tests show the same numerical value for the average of 2, 3, and 4 kHz, then the audiologist or physician should revise the baseline to the earlier of the two tests, unless the later test shows better (more sensitive) thresholds for other test frequencies.

Following an STS, a retest within 30 days of the annual test may be substituted for the annual test if the retest shows better (more sensitive) results for the average threshold at 2, 3, and 4 kHz. If the retest is used in place of the annual test, then the annual test is retained in the record, but it is marked in such a way that it is no longer considered in baseline revision evaluations.

If a retest within 30 days of an annual test confirms an OSHA STS shown on the annual test, the baseline will not be revised at that point because the required six-month interval between tests showing STS persistence has not been met. The purpose of the six-month requirement is to prevent baseline revision when STS is the result of temporary medical conditions affecting hearing. Although a special retest after six months could be given if desired to assess whether the STS is persistent, in most cases the next annual audiogram would be used to evaluate persistence of the STS.

Example Description

The example below illustrates how the baseline revision guidelines apply to one audiometric record. The abbreviations used are: B for baseline, RB for revised baseline, STS for OSHA STS, and IMPR for improvement. Revisions are shown both without use of age corrections, as well as with use of OSHA age corrections (with the choice being up to the professional in charge of revision). In the left ear, baseline is revised in 1988 for persistent improvement, to the test of 11/12/87. Subsequently the left ear shows persistent STS, with revision after the 1993 retest to the test of 5/21/92 (without using age corrections). With age corrections, the left ear shows persistent STS in 1995, with baseline revised to the test of 6/25/94. In the right ear baseline revision for persistent STS without age corrections occurs in 1994 to the test of 5/28/93. With age corrections, the right baseline is revised in 1996 to the test of 06/01/95.

Note that the table shows values rounded to one-tenth of a decibel, resulting in some apparent errors of one-tenth in the columns showing change from baseline. For example, one comparison in the table indicates that $19.7 - 8.3 = 11.3$ because the underlying values are really $19.67 - 8.33 = 11.34$.

Also recall that age corrections are not applied to baseline tests, but only to annual tests. Therefore, in the sections showing calculations with age corrections, the "corrected change" column shows change from the STS average without age corrections for the currently applicable baseline compared to the STS average with age corrections on the current annual test.

Reprinted with permission of the National Hearing Conservation Association. (NHCA, 2000).

Male Employee "L.M." born 10/05/63 See far right column for test date.

Test	Left Ear Thresholds (dB) by frequency (kHz)							No Age Correction				With Age Correction (does not apply to improvement)			
Age Type	.5	1	2	3	4	6	8	STS avg.	Change	Reviewer decision	Baseline status	Corr. avg.	Corrected change	Reviewer decision	Baseline status
22 initial	10	5	5	10	25	40	15	13.3			B				B
23 annual	5	5	5	5	25	45	20	11.7	-1.7						
24 annual	0	-5	0	0	25	35	10	8.3	-5.0 impr		RB				RB
25 annual	0	-5	0	0	25	40	20	8.3	-5.0 impr	revise ↗					
26 annual	0	-5	-5	0	20	40	20	5.0	-3.3						
27 annual	0	0	0	5	25	30	10	10.0	1.7			9.0	0.7		
28 annual	5	5	5	5	35	40	15	15.0	6.7			13.7	5.3		
29 annual	5	0	5	10	40	40	15	18.3	10.0 STS		RB	17.0	8.7		
30 annual	5	0	5	10	45	45	20	20.0	11.7 STS			18.3	10.0 STS		
30 retest	10	0	5	10	40	40	15	18.3	10.0 STS	revise ↗		16.7	8.3		
31 annual	5	0	5	15	50	50	30	23.3	5.0			21.3	13.0 STS		
31 retest	5	5	5	10	50	50	35	21.7	3.3			19.7	11.3 STS		RB
32 annual	5	0	5	15	55	55	40	25.0	6.7			22.3	14.0 STS		
32 retest	5	0	5	15	50	55	35	23.3	5.0			20.7	12.3 STS	revise ↗	
33 annual	5	5	5	20	55	55	35	26.7	8.3			26.0	4.3		

Right Ear Thresholds (dB) by frequency (kHz)								No Age Correction				With Age Correction (does not apply to improvement)				Date of Test
.5	1	2	3	4	6	8		STS avg.	Change	Reviewer decision	Baseline status	Corr. avg.	Corrected change	Reviewer decision	Baseline status	
15	10	5	5	20	40	15		10.0			B				B	08/03/85
10	5	0	5	25	35	10		10.0	0							11/04/86
0	-5	0	5	25	40	20		10.0	0							11/12/87
0	0	0	0	30	35	15		10.0	0							10/15/88
0	-5	0	5	35	40	10		13.3	3.3			12.0	2.0			12/12/89
5	0	0	0	40	40	15		13.3	3.3			11.7	1.7			11/23/90
0	0	0	5	40	40	15		15.0	5.0			13.0	3.0			04/14/91
5	0	0	5	45	50	20		16.7	6.7			14.7	4.7			05/21/92
10	5	0	10	55	45	20		23.3	13.3 STS			21.0	11.0 STS			05/22/93
5	0	0	10	50	45	15		20.0	10.0 STS		RB	17.7	7.7			05/28/93
10	5	0	10	50	55	20		20.0	10.0 STS			17.3	7.3			06/10/94
5	5	0	10	50	55	20		20.0	10.0 STS	revise ↗		17.3	7.3			06/25/94
5	5	5	15	60	60	25		26.7	6.7			23.3	13.3 STS			05/07/95
5	0	5	15	55	65	30		25.0	5.0			21.7	11.7 STS		RB	06/01/95
10	0	5	10	60	60	25		25.0	5.0			21.7	11.7 STS	revise ↗		05/02/96

Appendix L
Tips for Fitting Hearing Protectors

E.H. Berger. (1988). *E·A·RLog #19*,
"Tips for Fitting Hearing Protectors,"
Aearo Co., Indianapolis, IN.

E·A·R·LOG 19

Nineteenth in a comprehensive series of technical monographs covering topics related to hearing and hearing protection.

Tips for Fitting Hearing Protectors

BY ELLIOTT H. BERGER,
Senior Scientist, Auditory Research

This EARLog[1] is intended to assist in improving the hearing protector fitting and dispensing skills of hearing conservationists. A number of straightforward fitting techniques that can be implemented without the need for specialized measurement equipment are discussed and an overview of certain factors that should be considered when issuing hearing protection devices (HPDs) is provided.

Preliminary Considerations
When any type of hearing protector is initially dispensed, the process is best accomplished one-on-one or in small groups with a student/instructor ratio of no more than about 5/1. This is important since the compatibility and fit of protectors must be individually checked on each employee. Also to be considered is that the smaller the group, the less likely it is that the trainee(s) will become self-conscious during the fitting process. Plan on allowing about 10 min. for each employee.

HPD training in larger groups is also useful when it occurs in addition to, but not in place of, individual or small-group work. Working with larger classes is a suitable way to provide a review and reminder during the annual educational sessions that are a required part of every hearing conservation program. An excellent discussion of the fitting process may be found in reference [2].

Prior to issuing HPDs the fitter should visually examine the pinna, earcanal, and circumaural regions to identify conditions which might interfere with or be aggravated by the use of the protector in question (see EARLog 17[1]). In the case of employees who are being refitted and/or retrained in the use of devices they are currently wearing, the condition of the HPDs must be checked as well.[3,4] All resilient parts such as earplug flanges and earmuff cushions must be intact and flexible so that a good acoustical seal can be obtained,

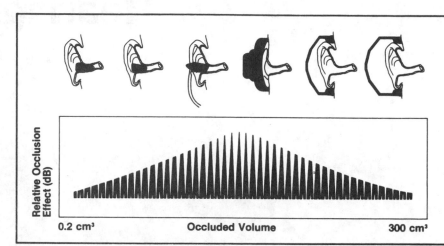

Figure 1. The **occlusion effect** and its relationship to the fit and type of hearing protector. The effect is minimized with deeply inserted plugs (left side of graph), increases in magnitude as the plugs are withdrawn, peaks when the canal is capped by a semi-aural device or the pinna is covered by a supra-aural device such as an audiometer earphone (center two drawings), diminishes as the ear is surrounded by an earmuff, and continues to reduce in magnitude as the volume of the earmuff increases (right side of graph).

(Figure axes: Relative Occlusion Effect (dB); Occluded Volume from 0.2 cm³ to 300 cm³)

and the bands on earmuffs and semi-aural devices must provide sufficient force for proper fit.

Initially, hearing protectors are typically dispensed in quiet environments away from the noisy workplace. This is primarily a matter of convenience and logistics which obviously makes it easier for the fitter to communicate with the person being fitted. The disadvantage of this approach is that in low (unobjectionable) noise levels the wearer cannot appreciate the beneficial aspects of the noise reduction provided by the HPDs. It is like trying to evaluate sunglasses by wearing them at night or in a dimly lit store.

When noise is used during the fitting process the wearer can listen to it to adjust the HPDs for the lowest perceived noise level. Recordings of broadband noise or representative industrial sounds can be presented using a portable cassette player. If a noise source is unavailable, the fitter should follow up with employees within a few days while they are in their work environment to recheck the fit and suitability of the devices that were dispensed.

The Occlusion Effect
Occluding and sealing the ear with an earmuff or earplug increases the efficiency with which bone-conducted sound is transmitted at the frequencies below 2 kHz. Called the occlusion effect,[3] this causes wearers of HPDs to experience a change in their perceived voice quality and other body-generated sounds/vibrations (breathing, chewing, walking, etc.). Of all the fitting tips that have been devised, listening for the occlusion effect is the most widely applicable, being suitable for use with nearly all types of hearing protectors.

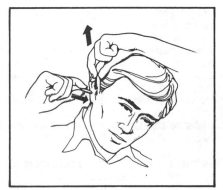

Figure 2. Pulling the pinna outward and upward while inserting an earplug.

To experience the occlusion effect, plug your ears with your fingers as you read this sentence aloud and note the change in the sound of your voice - its added fullness or resonant bassiness. Other adjectives that have been used to describe the changes in voice quality are deeper, hollow, and muffled. The effect is greatest when the earcanal is covered at its entrance. It diminishes as earplugs are inserted more deeply or with the use of earmuffs with large volume earcups (see Figure 1).

The occlusion effect can be used as a fit test for either plugs or muffs by asking the wearer to count loudly from 1 to 5 while listening for the change in voice quality which indicates an acoustical seal and the presence of the effect. With earplugs, an alternative approach is to count aloud with only one ear correctly fitted. The voice should be more strongly heard or felt in the occluded ear.[5] If this does not occur, the plug should be reseated or resized. When the second ear has been fitted correctly, the effect should be the same in both ears, causing the voice to be heard as though it were emanating from the center of the head.

Some listeners are unable to hear differences in the occlusion effect between their two ears, but most can hear a change in the overall sound of their voice when both ears are sealed. An alternative means of generating a "test signal," and one which some find

easier to detect, is to hum. It is a good way to create sounds of varying pitch and constant level that can be used when listening for the occlusion effect while adjusting the HPD.

A caveat with respect to the occlusion effect is that although it is a fine way to test the fit of HPDs, its presence is often cited as an objectionable characteristic of wearing hearing protection. As is shown in Figure 1, semi-aural HPDs will create the most noticeable occlusion effect. The amplification can be minimized by wearing earplugs that are inserted more deeply or earmuffs with larger volume earcups.

Earplug Fitting Tips

When initially dispensing earplugs the fitter should insert at least one plug into the employee's ear so that s/he can experience the feel of a properly seated device. This is especially important because of the reluctance most novice users have of placing anything deeply into their earcanals. With one earplug properly inserted, the person then has an example to try to match. Ask the wearer to insert the other plug until both of their ears feel the same and sound equally occluded. Once the two plugs have been properly inserted ask the person to remove them both and then insert them one more time for review and additional practice.

For all types of earplugs, with the possible exception of custom earmolds, insertion is easier and more effective if the outer ear (pinna) is pulled outward and upward as illustrated in Figure 2. Plugs should be inserted into the right ear using the right hand and into the left ear with the left hand. The pinna is pulled with the opposite hand by reaching behind or over the head. This allows the hand inserting the plug to have the best line of approach for proper fitting.

The fitter should determine the best direction in which to pull the pinna to access and enlarge the canal as much as possible. Merely pressing the pinna back along the side of the skull is usually not effective. Demonstrate the correct technique by guiding the user's hand to help pull his or her pinna in the proper manner. All wearers should

initially use the pinna-pull technique as they learn how to best fit their earplugs, although with time and experience some may find it no longer necessary.

Employees may also require assistance in finding the best direction in which to "aim" the plugs into their canals. Although this will usually be forward and slightly upward, it can vary substantially for different individuals, in some instances even being directed towards the back of the skull.

Once fitted, the noise reduction of earplugs can be tested subjectively by pressing firmly cupped hands over the ears while listening to a steady noise. With properly fitted plugs the noise levels should seem nearly the same whether or not the ears are covered.

When dispensing earplugs, fitters will soon learn that people are very conscious of the cleanliness of their ear canals. If cerumen (earwax) adheres to or coats trial earplugs, wearers may be embarrassed. Assure them that earplugs penetrate more deeply into their earcanals than they can or should normally reach when cleaning their ears. Furthermore, a certain amount of cerumen is necessary to provide a protective barrier for the ear (EARLog 17), and it can in fact furnish lubrication to ease and improve the fitting of earplugs.

Foam Earplugs: Foam earplugs are prepared for insertion by rolling them into a very thin crease-free cylinder. The cylinder should be as small in diameter as possible, that is, as tightly compressed as can be achieved. Crease-free rolling is accomplished by squeezing lightly as one begins rolling, and then applying progressively greater pressure as the plug becomes more tightly compressed. Be sure to roll the plug into a cylinder rather than other shapes such as a cone or a ball.

After insertion, it may be necessary to hold foam earplugs in place with a fingertip for a few moments until they begin to expand and block the noise. This is not intended to keep them from backing out of the earcanal, since properly inserted foam earplugs do not in fact exhibit such a tendency, but rather is to assure that the plugs do not move and dislodge prior to reexpanding enough to hold in place.

Unlike other types of earplugs, foam earplugs should not be readjusted while in the ear. If the initial fit is unacceptable, they should be removed, re-rolled, and reinserted. Furthermore, a large occlusion effect does not usually signify a best fit for foam earplugs since the effect is maximized when they barely enter or cap the canal, rather than when they are well inserted (see Figure 1). In fact the deeper the insertion (which for foam earplugs is usually associated with improved comfort), the better will be the fit and the attenuation, and the less noticeable and annoying will be the occlusion effect.

The simplest, but least accurate method to assess the fit of a foam earplug, is to visually (for the fitter) or with the fingertips (for the wearer), check the position of the end of the plug relative to the tragus and concha (see Figure 3). If the outer end of the plug is flush with or slightly inside the tragus, this generally indicates that at least half of the plug is in the canal and the fit is proper. If most of the plug projects beyond the tragus and into the concha, the insertion is probably too shallow. Since tragus-to-earcanal dimensions vary significantly, this check is not a foolproof indicator.

Another test that either the wearer or the fitter can perform is to remove an earplug after it has expanded in the ear for about a minute. If it was well fitted, it should appear free of creases and wrinkles, and the still partially-compressed portion of the plug will indicate that at least one-half of its length had extended beyond the entrance of the earcanal and formed a seal within the canal itself.

A comprehensive guide to all aspects of foam earplug utilization, as well as a Roll Model training aid, are available from Aearo Company.[6]

Premolded Earplugs: When initially inserting premolded earplugs the fitter should be able to easily detect gross errors in sizing. Ear gauges are available from some manufacturers of premolded earplugs to aid in this process. Plugs that are much too small will tend to slide into the canal without any resistance, their depth of insertion being limited only by the fitter's finger and not the plug itself. Overly large plugs either will not enter the canal at all or will not penetrate far enough to allow contact of their largest (outermost) flanges with the concha (see Figure 3). With certain premolded multiple-flanged earplugs, however, it is unnecessary for the outermost flange(s) to seal the ear to obtain a proper insertion and fit for those with small to extra-small earcanals.

A plug that is well seated and appears to make contact with the interior wall of the canal without appreciably stretching the tissues is a good size to begin wearing.[7] When a canal falls between two sizes the larger size plug is not necessarily the best one to choose. Even though it may provide more attenuation, if the plug is not worn or not used correctly due to discomfort, the resultant effective protection may be less than would have been achieved had the smaller more comfortable size been selected.

Experience suggests that in about 2 to 10% of the population different sizes of premolded earplugs will be required for the left and right ears. As a general rule, the more sizes in which a particular plug is manufactured, the greater will be the likelihood of this occurring.

A properly inserted premolded earplug will generally create a plugged or blocked-up feeling due to the requisite airtight seal. When a seal is present, resistance should be felt if an attempt is made to withdraw the plug from the canal, much like pulling a rubber stopper from a glass bottle. The seal can be further tested by gently pumping the plug in and out of the earcanal. When a proper acoustic/pneumatic seal is present, the pumping motion will cause pressure changes in the ear which the wearer should be able to detect.

Because of the pneumatic seal created by properly inserted premolded earplugs, suction is created if they are rapidly removed. This can be uncomfortable, painful, and/or potentially harmful to the ear. Teach wearers to remove plugs slowly, or even to use a slight twisting or rocking motion to gradually break the seals as the plugs are withdrawn.

Custom Molded Earplugs: One of the most important steps in making a custom earmold impression is the use of a cotton or foam block or eardam inside the canal. Use of eardams prevents the impression material from being forced too deeply into the canal where it could contact the eardrum or be difficult to remove.

Of equal and perhaps greater importance, an eardam helps to ensure that a better fitting impression is obtained. If the dam is absent, the impression material is permitted to flow along the canal without ever properly filling it. However, when the dam is present the flow of the impression material is blocked, which forces it radially outwards to better fill the canal, thereby providing a tighter fit and a more effective seal.

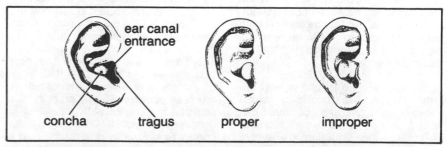

Figure 3. Key features of the external ear (pinna and ear canal) along with demonstration of a proper and improper fit of a foam earplug.

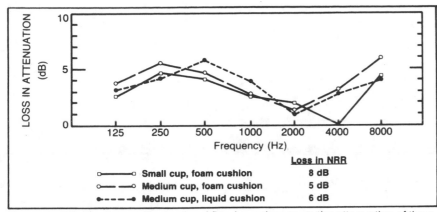

Figure 4. Effects of correctly sized and fitted eyeglasses on the attenuation of three different earmuffs.[8] 10-subject data re ANSI S3.19-1974.

Earmuff Fitting Tips

Contrary to popular belief, earmuffs are not one-size-fits-all devices. The headband may not extend or collapse enough to fit all head sizes, and cup openings may not properly accommodate the largest ears. The contours in the circumaural areas of the wearer's head may be so irregular that the cushions cannot properly seal against them. Like an earplug, an earmuff must be individually dispensed and checked for fit to acquaint wearers with its features and make sure it is compatible with their anatomy.

Place the muff on the wearer's head and be sure the cups fully enclose, and are centered about the pinnae, without resting on them. Adjust the headband so that it sits comfortably on the head and the cushions feel to the wearer as though they exert evenly distributed pressure around the ears. Instruct users about the importance of achieving the best possible seal between the earmuff cushions and the side of the head. Caps and other head-worn gear must not interfere with this seal, and excess hair should be pulled back and out from beneath the cushions.

Eyeglass temples should fit close to the side of the head and be as thin as practical in order to reduce their effect on the ability of cushions to seal around the ear. The loss in attenuation that temples create, with cushions in good condition, is normally 3 to 7 dB. The effect varies widely among earmuffs and also depends upon the fit and style

of the eyeglasses. Representative data are plotted in Figure 4.

Wearing eyeglasses in combination with earmuffs may be uncomfortable for some wearers since earmuff cushions press the eyeglass temples against the skull. The pressure can be relieved by fitting foam pads over the temple pieces, but the increase in comfort may be at the expense of attenuation as has been demonstrated for one commercially available pad product.[8] Also, pads do nothing to reduce acoustic leaks caused by overlength temples which break the cushion-to-skull seal behind the ear. However, temple pads should still be considered for use, since the improved comfort they can provide may be crucial in motivating certain employees to wear their HPDs.

Earmuff protection can be roughly checked by asking wearers to listen with earmuffs on while in the noisy environment in which they work. They should be able to detect a considerable difference in the overall apparent noise level if they lift both earmuff cups, or between their two ears if they lift only one cup. If not, the earmuffs were either grossly misfitted, are in very poor condition, or the noise in which the persons work is predominated by the lower frequency sounds for which earmuffs generally give less protection. Most listeners will not be able to detect small to modest degrees of misfit with this test since earmuffs will usually provide enough noise reduction, even when moderately misfitted, to be clearly dis-

tinguishable from the no-attenuation (i.e. the lifted-cup) condition.

Final Comments

Years of hearing conservation experience have shown that hearing protectors are often misused, and that in general their real-world performance falls far short of the protection that properly-worn and maintained HPDs can provide. To improve the situation employers must develop effective group *and individual* training sessions in which employees are provided clear and accurate guidance in the fitting and use of their HPDs. The tips described herein will be useful in that regard; training and motivational concepts have been elaborated elsewhere.[1,3,5,7,9]

Remember, it takes time to get used to hearing protectors, both how they feel and how they sound. A break-in period is advisable for new wearers, especially in the case of earplugs. It may take a week or two for some persons to fully adapt to the feeling of wearing hearing protectors and to begin to recognize and appreciate the auditory as well as the non-auditory benefits that their use provides.

Fitting hearing protectors is largely a common-sense affair. With time, commitment, and the experience gained from careful observation, nearly all ears can be successfully fitted and real-world problems overcome.

References

1. Berger, E.H. The EARLogs, complete series available upon request from Aearo Company.
2. Royster, L. H. and Royster, J. D. (1985). "Hearing Protection Devices," in *Hearing Conservation in Industry*, edited by A. S. Feldman and C. T. Grimes, Williams and Wilkins, Baltimore, MD, 103-150.
3. Berger, E. H. (1986). "Hearing Protection Devices," in *Noise and Hearing Conservation Manual, 4th edition*, edited by E. H. Berger, W. D. Ward, J. C. Morrill, and L. H. Royster, Am. Ind. Hyg. Assoc., Akron, OH, 319-381.
4. Gasaway, D. C. (1984). " 'Sabotage' Can Wreck Hearing Conservation Programs," *Natl. Saf. News* 129(5), 56-63.
5. Ohlin, D. (1975). "Personal Hearing Protective Devices Fitting, Care, and Use," U.S. Army Environmental Hygiene Agency, Report No. AD-A021 408, Aberdeen Proving Ground, MD.
6. Manual (33002) and Roll Model training aid, are available from Aearo Company at the address shown below.
7. Guild, E. (1966). "Personal Protection," in *Industrial Noise Manual, Second Edition*, Am. Ind. Hyg. Assoc., Akron, OH, 84-109.
8. Berger, E. H. (1986). Unpublished research notes on measurements taken at E•A•RCAL℠ Laboratory.
9. Royster, L. H. and Royster, J. D. (1986). "Education and Motivation," in *Noise and Hearing Conservation Manual, 4th edition*, edited by E. H. Berger, W. D. Ward, J. C. Morrill, and L. H. Royster, Am. Ind. Hyg. Assoc., Akron, OH, 383-416.

Aearo Company
5457 West 79th Street, Indianapolis, IN 46268
(317) 692-6616 FAX (317) 692-6675
www.e-a-r.com

Appendix M
Engineering Noise Control

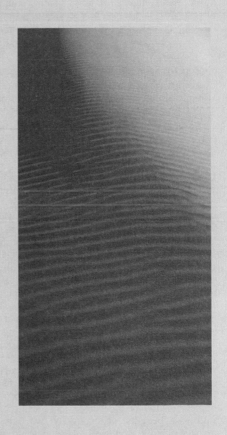

Beth Cooper. (Winter 2000/2001). "Considering an Engineered Noise Control Solution." CAOHC *UPDATE*, P. 1.
(Spring 2001). "Selecting an Engineered Noise Control Approach: Controlling Noise at the Source, Path or Receiver." CAOHC *UPDATE*, P. 4.
(Fall 2001). "Developing and Implementing an Engineered Noise Control Solution." CAOHC *UPDATE*, P. 5

Considering an Engineered Noise Control Solution

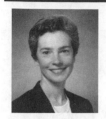

By Beth A. Cooper,
PE INCE. Bd. Cert.
Representative of the Institute of Noise Control Engineering

(Part 1 in a series on engineering approaches to reducing noise exposure.)

As an OHC, your days may be filled with audiometric testing and employee training. You may also find it within your job description to solve problems associated with high noise levels in your workplace. Perhaps you are fortunate enough to work as part of a hearing conservation team that includes a noise control engineer who is able to recommend, develop and implement engineered controls that reduce employee noise exposure. But what if YOU are the hearing conservation program? Even if you have other professional resources at your disposal, you may be responsible for managing those resources and making overall program decisions. In any case, an understanding of fundamental noise control concepts and techniques will be helpful as you approach the following tasks:

· identify specific problems that would be realistic candidates for successful engineered noise control solutions;
· anticipate, understand and be able to evaluate the range of possible solution approaches recommended by a noise control professional;
· advocate for the funds necessary to implement the recommended changes;
· properly make use of and maintain the engineered noise controls; and
· avoid worsening the problem, either before or after the controls are implemented, by making changes to the process, equipment or work area that increase the noise level and/or employee noise exposure.

Since noise control engineering *should* be a part of any effective corporate hearing conservation program, a basic familiarity with noise control concepts and techniques will be helpful to all OHCs who work in a corporate or plant setting. This article, which is the first in a series on engineering approaches to reducing occupational noise exposure, will discuss the benefits of engineered noise controls and present a process that OHCs may follow to assess any noise exposure problem prior to involving a noise control engineer. The remainder of the series will cover concepts that are the critical to the solution of every noise control problem: the three general approaches to engineered noise controls and the basic properties of acoustical materials. Specific examples of each type of approach will be discussed, including "do-it-yourself" noise control solutions that every OHC can easily implement to fix some very common noise exposure problems.

Within the context of the hearing conservation program, engineered noise controls should have a stature equal to that of audiometric testing, employee training and the wearing of personal protective equipment. Although engineered noise controls are often perceived as being a peripheral element of the hearing conservation program, in fact, well-designed engineered controls offer benefits beyond what can be achieved with even the most comprehensive and well-managed implementation of non-engineered approaches. The aggressive implementation of engineered noise control solutions can offer the following benefits, depending on whether the particular solution reduces only the employee's noise exposure or the actual sound level in the work area as well:

· reduced cost and administrative burden of the hearing conservation program;
· hearing loss prevention as well as regulatory compliance;
· reduced reliance on employee participation in other program elements (e.g., audiometric testing and use of personal hearing protection) as an essential factor in hearing loss prevention (or regulatory compliance);

· improved productivity, speech communication, concentration and safety; and
· removal of noise-related operational restrictions that limit the hours of operation and/or the total duration of operation, including those imposed for reasons other than hearing conservation (e.g., community noise issues).

When evaluating noise exposure problems as potential candidates for an engineered noise control solution, the above factors can serve as a checklist to help the OHC determine, for each problem, whether an engineered solution will be more cost effective than other alternatives. In particular, determining which of the above factors are relevant (and which are the most important) issues in each situation is an important first step in assessing and selecting the most effective noise control approach for that particular situation.

For instance, some approaches will reduce employee noise exposure but may not necessarily reduce the amount of noise that is generated by the equipment or process. Such an approach may be quite effective in one situation while not adequate in other cases. That assessment should take into account considerations such as:

· the number of employees who work in the (noisy) area;
· the specific tasks, locations, and movement within the work area that is required in order to perform the job;
· the amount of time in the noisy area that is associated with the above activity;
· whether employees are expected to communicate with each other or on radios or telephones while working in the noisy environment;
· the nature and frequency of other auditory signals that employees must be able to hear clearly (e.g., paging, alarms, etc.);
· existence and location of any nearby quiet spaces where employees may rest, perform other tasks and communicate with each other or use the telephone;
· the size and physical characteristics of the (noisy) building or room where the work activity takes place;
· whether the noise is adequately contained in the work area or also poses a hazard (or an annoyance) for passersby, adjacent work areas or the community;
· the nature of the equipment or process that is generating the noise; and
· the characteristics of the noise itself (e.g., sound level, time characteristics, frequency spectra).

The last item on the list is clearly the responsibility of the noise control engineer, who will undoubtedly acquire detailed noise measurements at the outset of the project. The recommendations he or she makes will depend as much on the information the OHC provides about the first nine items as on the characteristics of the noise. The OHC will be best prepared to discuss the range of solution options and the relative benefits of each option after spending some time researching and documenting all of the items on the above list.

An essential part of the OHC's preparation for initiating a noise control project is a productive liaison with the exposed employees and their management. The process of developing an engineered noise control solution is really a collaborative activity that relies heavily on the support and contribution of the employees who will be expected to work with or near the particular noise control equipment after it is installed. The installed controls will be most effective, and the process by which those effective controls are developed will be most valuable, if the input of the exposed employees is sought and given a high priority early on, *before* a solution approach is selected. Ideally, the exposed employees and their management should be brought into the planning activity prior to involving a noise control engineer. It is important that the noise-generating equipment and the work process are well understood, along with any other factors that may constrain the selection, design or implementation of the noise control solution. If the expectations and limitations of the engineered controls are agreed to beforehand, it is more likely that the controls will be functional, compatible with the operation and accepted by the employees who must accommodate and maintain those controls.

Selecting an Engineered Noise Control Approach: Controlling Noise at the Source, Path or Receiver

By Beth A. Cooper, PE INCE. Bd. Cert.
Representative of the Institute of Noise Control Engineering
(Part 2 in a series on engineering approaches to reducing noise exposure.)

Ideally, the selection of an engineered solution to a noise exposure problem is the product of a collaborative planning process that involves, at a minimum, the OHC, the exposed employees and their management, and a noise control engineer. The OHC plays a very important role in this process by bringing the members of the team together to develop a solution to the problem in a participative but very organized and systematic manner. Although the development of the technical specifics of the solution is clearly the responsibility of the noise control engineer, the *selection* of the *approach* should be based on a variety of factors that are best identified and documented by the OHC during field visits and employee interviews prior to bringing the noise control engineer into the discussions. The first installment in this series, "Considering an engineered noise control solution," (Winter 2000/2001 issue of *UPDATE*) presented two checklists that OHCs may use to identify and clarify the objectives as well as the relevant parameters and physical restrictions that will govern the operation of the installed solution. Only when that information is well documented and agreed to by the members of the in-house team, will the involvement of an outside noise control engineer be both helpful and cost effective.

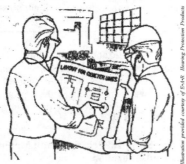

Illustration provided courtesy of E•A•R Hearing Protection Products

Although not nearly as important as an understanding of the noise exposure problem itself, a familiarity with the basic approaches to engineered noise control will help the OHC and the other decision-making members of the team better understand the noise control engineer's recommendations. In turn, the OHC will be in a stronger position to advocate for funds to implement the recommended solution and to ensure that any equipment installed as part of the solution will be used and maintained by the exposed employees in a manner that preserves its intended (noise control) function. This article will discuss the basic approaches to engineered noise control and some of the factors that influence their selection and implementation.

Since noise exposure is a function of both the noise level *and* the duration of time over which employees are exposed, exposure may be controlled by reducing either, or both, of these elements. Reducing the duration of exposure is the basis of what is referred to as "administrative controls," which typically does not involve any engineered reduction in the noise level (although certain engineered solutions actually do accomplish their goals by reducing the duration of exposure). Since we are concerned here with *engineered* approaches to reducing noise exposure, let's concentrate on how we might control noise exposure by reducing the *level* of the noise to which employees are exposed. There are three general approaches, two of which are discussed below, along with examples of typical applications. The third approach will be the focus of the next installment in this series.

Source noise control. Noise control at the source is accomplished by changing the noise-generating equipment or process, which results in a reduction in the amount of noise that is produced by that particular source. Accordingly, the noise level associated with the treated source(s) is lowered in the entire surrounding area, and the noise exposure of all persons who happen to be in the area is reduced. If there are multiple noise sources that contribute substantially to employee noise exposure, each of these sources must be treated in order to realize a measurable reduction in the sound level in the work area. Examples of source noise control include, but are not limited to, the examples presented above.

- Changing or eliminating the basic mechanism of sound generation in a way that accomplishes the same task with less noise output. This is often the most ambitious type of noise control project and one that requires specialized expertise beyond a general understanding of noise control engineering. The potential benefits make it an option worth considering, however.

- Replacing noisy equipment by intentionally purchasing or designing newer, quieter equipment. Needless to say, implementation of a corporate "Buy Quiet" policy can prevent today's purchases from becoming tomorrow's noise control projects.

- Retrofitting the noise-generating machinery with parts that are expected to lower the noise emission, such as a different motor or fan.

- Performing maintenance and repairs to reduce noise generated by problems like worn parts (e.g., bearings), unbalanced rotating machinery and equipment that is being operated at an off-design condition. A good noise control engineer will be able to diagnose this type of problem by identifying characteristic symptoms in the noise signature of a particular piece of equipment.

Ideally, noise is best controlled at the source, since reducing the generation of noise usually has more widespread benefit than approaches that treat only specific locations in the work area or specific receivers (employees). But, source noise control solutions are typically expensive and may require modifications to the source that are not technically feasible. Additionally, in areas where there are multiple sources contributing to the noise level, treating all of the sources (which is required to achieve an appreciable reduction in noise level) is often simply impractical.

Path noise control. This approach to reducing noise exposure acts along the path between the source and the intended receiver (the exposed employees) without interfering with the source itself. By inserting a noise control device in the path, the transmission of sound to the receiver is prevented or greatly reduced. This approach does not change the amount of noise that is produced, but it reduces the sound level due to the source(s) located upstream of the device and, thus, the exposure of employees who happen to be in the area *downstream of the noise control device*. Some examples of path noise control follow.

- Installing a noise control "device" such as a silencer (muffler) in the flow stream of gas or fluid flow systems to reduce the noise produced by venting, exhaust flow or turbomachinery located upstream of the silencer.

- Enclosing a noisy machine with a complete or partial enclosure to prevent or reduce the transmission of sound to the surrounding area. One example that might not come to mind immediately is acoustical pipe lagging, which prevents noise in the piping from radiating through the pipe wall to the surrounding environment.

- Repairing existing equipment enclosures and replacing missing parts. Noise "leaks" into or out of a structure that encloses either the source (or the receiver, for that matter) may be reduced by identifying and repairing gaps and openings in the enclosure. Often, these leaks can be easily identified and repaired without any specific knowledge of noise control engineering. Some guidance for "do it yourself" noise control will be the subject of a future installment in this series.

- Adding absorption to the surrounding space to reduce the buildup of reverberant sound in the work area. Although this will not reduce the noise level near the source (nor the noise exposure of employees in the vicinity of the source, such as at the "operator" position of a piece of machinery), it *will* prevent noise generated in one area of the plant from reverberating throughout the space and *causing* a problem in areas remote from the original noise source.

Receiver noise control. Control of noise at the receiver prevents or reduces the *reception* of noise by enclosing the affected employee(s) in a sound-attenuating structure. Receiver noise control treatments do not reduce the amount of noise produced by high-noise equipment, nor do they lower the sound level in any part of the work area (other than inside the sound-attenuating structure). This particular type of engineered solution works by reducing the *duration* of the affected employees' exposure to the noise produced by high-noise equipment in the work area. Protecting the receiver is typically the least elegant approach to retrofit engineered noise controls and one that may impose cumbersome operational restrictions. Receiver noise control has its place, however, and is often the easiest, most affordable and most accessible option, particularly in environments where multiple pieces of high-noise equipment contribute to the overall sound level. Here, source or path noise control approaches are likely to be unreasonably expensive, whereas enclosing noise-exposed employees in a sound-attenuating structure (when they are not specifically required to be working in the equipment area) effectively reduces the employees' exposure to *all* noise sources. Below are a few examples of this kind of approach.

- Constructing a "quiet" room (e.g., office, breakroom, control room, lunchroom) within the high-noise work area, where employees may spend time between operations, maintenance or monitoring tasks that require them to work on and around the high-noise equipment. Often, sound-attenuating structures are custom-designed by a noise control engineer and are constructed in the field from standard materials, much like any other building. There

are also high-quality prefabricated units that may be purchased directly from a reputable vendor; these should be selected to provide the required amount of noise reduction. Although it sounds deceptively simple, the design of noise-attenuating structures is a fairly technical matter that requires the involvement of a noise control professional to ensure the acoustical integrity of the structure. A future installment in this series will explore the characteristics of properly designed noise-attenuating structures, both traditional and prefabricated.

- Smaller versions of the above "quiet" rooms, communication booths are prefabricated sound-attenuating structures placed strategically around high-noise work areas in locations where there are no other quiet spaces. These booths are sized to accommodate one or two employees, who may safely remove personal hearing protectors and communicate with each other or, via telephone or radio, with remote dispatch or control stations.

- Wearing personal hearing protectors, including communication headsets, is a form of receiver noise control that is mentioned here for completeness.

The effectiveness of a receiver noise control approach depends on the willingness of the receiver to intentionally take advantage of the availability of the controls at every opportunity. An appreciation of the advantages and disadvantages of the three approaches will provide the OHC with a basis for evaluating the tradeoffs between the goals of the project and the potential effectiveness of each approach being considered. The next installment in this series will illustrate some examples of simple noise control techniques that may be easily implemented by the OHC to solve minor noise problems *without* the need for formal engineering. To assist the OHC with the solution of more complicated projects, the last installment of the series will describe resources and suggested procedures for obtaining and benefiting from professional noise control engineering support.

Developing and Implementing an Engineered Noise Control Solution

By Beth A. Cooper, PE INCE. Bd. Cert.
Representative of the Institute of Noise Control Engineering

(Part 3 in a series on engineering approaches to reducing noise exposure.)

The implementation of engineered noise control solutions is a responsibility that is shared by the entire hearing conservation team. The OHC is often the focal point of this effort, bringing the other members of the team together with the affected employees and their management to work with a noise control professional who will develop the detailed technical solution.

In the first article in this series, "Considering an Engineered Noise Control Solution," (Winter 2000/2001 issue of UPDATE), we discussed the role of the OHC in the identification and solution of noise exposure problems. Several checklists were provided to guide the OHC through the process of assessing noise exposure problems prior to involving a noise control professional. The second article, "Selecting an Engineered Noise Control Approach: Controlling Noise at the Source, Path or Receiver," (Spring 2001 issue of UPDATE) described the three basic approaches to controlling noise exposure and provided some typical examples.

This third and final installment will acquaint you with two basic noise control principles: *transmission loss* and *sound absorption*. Some suggestions for do-it-yourself solutions will be discussed, and, finally, resources will be provided to help you identify and engage a noise control professional for projects that require specialized skills.

Noise Control Principles and Materials: Transmission Loss and sound absorption

There are two basic principles that may be employed, either separately or together, to effect reduction in noise exposure: *transmission loss* and *sound absorption*. A general understanding of these principles, the differences between them, and the applicability of each to specific classes of problems is helpful in developing solutions to noise exposure problems and in understanding the recommendations of a noise control professional. It will also assist the OHC in facilitating discussions among employees, management, and the hearing conservation team as possible solutions are proposed. Misunderstandings regarding the concepts of transmission loss and sound absorption are undoubtedly the cause of many failed or less-than-successful engineered noise control attempts.

The most fundamental principle related to noise control materials is that of *transmission loss*, which may be thought of as "stopping" an unwanted sound from traveling between one space and another. Hazardous noise that exists in a plant area is "stopped" or prevented from entering a plant office or break room by the transmission loss properties of the room's structure. Likewise, noise generated by a machine housed in a sound-attenuating enclosure is "stopped" from entering the adjacent area by the transmission loss properties of the enclosure. As you might expect intuitively, transmission loss is typically provided by massive and continuous materials that completely enclose either the noise source or the receiver, depending on whether the objective of the solution (as discussed in the first article in this series) is to contain the noise inside a machine housing or to protect employees inside a quiet room. In general, as the frequency of the unwanted sound decreases, it takes more mass to "stop" the transmission of noise. Lead, loaded vinyl, concrete block, and drywall are examples of materials used for their transmission loss properties. Materials are rated for their performance using a metric called Sound Transmission Class or STC, expressed in units of decibels. An STC curve is a graph of transmission loss as a function of frequency, where each curve is named for its value at 500 Hz.

Sound absorption is the principle that complements transmission loss in most noise control constructions. Although sound that is contained within an enclosure is "stopped" from entering an adjacent space by the enclosure walls, if the inside surfaces of the enclosure are reflective, sound will reverberate inside the enclosure. This increases the sound level inside the enclosure such that its transmission loss properties may no longer be sufficient. For this reason, the interior surfaces of machinery enclosures are usually lined with absorptive material. These materials absorb incident sound and prevent it from reflecting back into the space but do not stop the absorbed sound from passing through into the adjacent space. Fiberglass, acoustical foam and standard architectural treatments like draperies and fabric office partitions are examples of absorptive materials. In the case of a "quiet" room or office where the unwanted sound is located in the adjacent space (outside the "quiet" room), absorptive material on the inside surfaces of the room is helpful, as in general building construction, for achieving a comfortable working environment with favorable conditions for speech communication. Materials that provide acoustical absorption are rated using an absorption coefficient, which may be interpreted as the percentage of incident energy that is absorbed by the material. Absorption coefficients are listed as dimensionless values of the parameter alpha (α) between 0 and 1 (sometimes slightly higher than 1 due to an artifact of the testing procedure).

Most noise control constructions will employ a combination of transmission loss and absorptive materials. Often, specialized materials or devices are also part of machine or personnel enclosures. For instance, pre-fabricated (acoustically-rated) wall and ceiling panels, doors, windows, ventilation or exhaust silencers and acoustically treated (wrapped) ventilation/exhaust ductwork are typical features of both employee and machine enclosures. Although an enclosure that is constructed for noise control purposes may not look much different than a typical office or room, the design and construction is quite specialized. It is important that construction personnel pay very close attention to the integrity of the structure during the construction process so that there are no weak spots, cracks or gaps that allow sound to inadvertently be transmitted between the enclosure and the adjacent space(s). Penetrations for electrical, ventilation and plumbing access should be minimized and properly sealed, and the structure should be vibration-isolated from the adjacent space to prevent noise from being transmitted through the floor or other structural members.

"Do-it-Yourself" Noise Control for the OHC

As an OHC, you are the first line of defense in protecting the acoustical integrity of the noise control enclosures that currently exist in your work environment. For instance, as you respond to employee inquiries about noise exposure, perform noise monitoring and begin to consider and prioritize noise exposure problems, you may be able to identify some problems that may be easily solved by your own personnel using the principles discussed here. Among these opportunities are the following, which may be implemented using materials available at a local hardware store:

- Caulk or re-cement cracks, gaps and leaks in walls, ceilings and floors where noise enters or leaves the space. A good rule of thumb is to look for places where light is visible coming from the opposite side of the wall or where an airflow path is evident. These are likely paths for sound transmission as well.
- Install acoustical seals to close gaps under doors.
- Install perimeter seals around doors.
- Replace abraded door seals.
- Replace lightweight doors in an otherwise intact structure with solid-core or acoustically rated doors.

Resources for Professional Noise Control Engineering Assistance

For the large majority of noise exposure problems for which an engineered solution is desired, the services of a noise control professional are appropriate and recommended. The following organizations are resources you may want to consider when shopping for professional assistance:

Institute of Noise Control Engineering (one of CAOHC's Component Professional Organizations - individual members may become Board Certified by passing an eight-hour exam). Members who are Board Certified and those who provide consulting services are listed on the INCE website: http://ince.org.

National Council of Acoustical Consultants (a trade organization of member firms - these are advertised by their specialties and geographic locations). A directory of firms is published for the use of potential customers on the NCAC website: http://www.ncac.com.

As an OHC, you are a key member of the hearing conservation team. Although you may not *develop* engineered solutions to noise exposure problems, you will no doubt be called on at some point to identify problems, suggest possible solutions, evaluate technical recommendations and possibly even prioritize projects. Your familiarity with the benefits, procedures, approaches and materials involved in engineered noise controls will be invaluable to the members of your team, and it will certainly make the experience more enjoyable. Most importantly, it will help ensure a properly designed solution that is well thought out and therefore effective, practical, maintainable and cost-effective for the employees whose noise exposure it is intended to reduce.

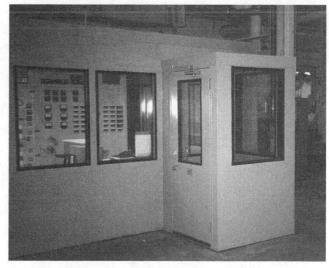

Example of a specially designed, well-sealed acoustical enclosure.

Appendix N
American National Standard Methods for Manual Pure-Tone Threshold Audiometry

ANSI S3.21-1978
(ASA 19-1978)

Reaffirmed by
ANSI in 1997

AMERICAN NATIONAL STANDARD
Methods for Manual Pure-Tone
Threshold Audiometry

Standards Secretariat
Accoustical Society of America
35 Pinelawn Road, Suite 114E
Melville, New York 11747-3177

Published by the American Institute of Physics for the Acoustical Society of America

AMERICAN NATIONAL STANDARDS ON ACOUSTICS

The Acoustical Society of America is the Secretariat for American National Standards Committees S1 on Physical Acoustics, S2 on Mechanical Shock and Vibration, and S3 on Bioacoustics. Standards developed by these committees, which have wide representation from the technical community (manufacturers, consumers, and general-interest representatives alike) are published by the Acoustical Society of America as American National Standards after approval by its standards committee.

These standards are developed as a public service to provide standards useful to the public, industry, and consumers, and to Federal, State, and local governments.

This standard was approved by the American National Standards Institute as ANSI S3.21-1978 on 7 June 1978.

An American National Standard implies a consensus of those substantially concerned with its scope and provisions. An American National Standard is intended as a guide to aid the manufacturer, the consumer, and the general public. The existence of an American National Standard does not in any respect preclude anyone, whether he has approved the standard or not, from manufacturing, marketing, purchasing, or using products, processes, or procedures not conforming to the standard. American National Standards are subject to periodic review and users are cautioned to obtain the latest editions.

Caution Notice: An American National Standard may be revised or withdrawn at any time. The procedures of the American National Standards Institute require that action be taken to reaffirm, revise, or withdraw this standard no later than five years from the date of publication.

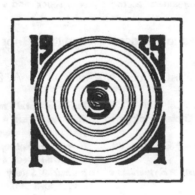

FOREWORD

[This Foreword is not a part of American National Standard Methods for Manual Pure-Tone Threshold Audiometry, S3.21-1978.]

This Standard has been developed under the jurisdiction of American National Standards Committee S3 using the American National Standards Institute (ANSI) Standards Committee Procedure. The Acoustical Society of America holds the Secretariat for Committee S3. This standard has been approved for publication by ANSI and by the Acoustical Society of America Committee on Standards (ASACOS).

This American National Standard presents procedures for accomplishing manual hearing-threshold measurement with pure tones that are applicable in a wide variety of settings. No standard has previously existed. This standard is meant to provide a procedure of pure-tone audiometry that will serve the needs of persons conducting threshold measurements in industry, schools, medical settings, and other areas who wish to work from a baseline model in the conduct of their tests. Although the standard has been written to aid in the accomplishment of a measurement, it is appropriate to point out that it differs from other measurement techniques in that it deals with human behavior. Rigid adherence to the procedure in every circumstance will not necessarily produce effective results. Certain individuals such as infants, children with severe physical and mental retardation, highly uncooperative persons, those with central nervous system disorders, many elderly persons, and numerous other members of society who fall into special groups will not be good subjects for the standard procedure and will necessitate a variety of modifications. In any instance where response behavior is apt to veer from the usual, the procedure should be modified; however, the modification shall be readily identified and specified by the user. Another kind of modification is exemplified as follows: The user of the standard who functions in a work setting which requires monitoring audiometry or diagnostic audiometry will use instrumentation which pertains to that particular setting and the frequencies at which threshold is measured will be dictated by that situation. The choice of frequencies will depend on the purpose for which the procedure is being used.

American National Standards Committee S3, under whose jurisdiction this standard was developed, has the following scope:

> Standards, specifications, methods of measurement and test, and terminology in the fields of psychological and physiological acoustics, including aspects of general acoustics, noise, shock, and vibration which pertain to biological safety, tolerance, and comfort.

At the time this standard was submitted to Standards Committee S3 for approval, the membership was as follows:

W. Melnick, *Chairman*   W.A. Yost, *Vice-Chairman*   A. Brenig, *Secretary*

Acoustical Society of America ● W. Melnick, W.A. Yost

American Academy of Ophthalmology and Otolaryngology ● R.F. Naunton, L.A. Michael *(Alt)*

Air Conditioning and Refrigeration Institute ● A.C. Potter, R.J. Evans *(Alt)*

American Conference of Governmental Industrial Hygienists ● D. C. Gasaway

Association of Home Appliance Manufacturers ● (representation vacant)

American Industrial Hygiene Association ● P.L. Michael, T.B. Bonney *(Alt)*

American Insurance Association ● M.W. Blachman

American Iron and Steel Institute ● E.H. Toothman, J.B. Masaitis *(Alt)*

American Mutual Insurance ● A.L. Cudworth

American Otological Society, Inc. ● J. Tonndorf

American Petroleum Institute ● W.R. Thornton, W. Ward *(Alt)*

American Society of Heating, Refrigerating, and Air Conditioning Engineers ● P.K. Baade, N.A. LaCourte *(Alt)*

American Society for Testing and Materials ● R.M. Guernsey, R. Huntley *(Alt)*, J.A. Thomas *(Alt)*

American Society of Mechanical Engineers ● D.K. Van Zile, S.I. Roth *(Alt)*

American Speech and Hearing Association ● L.E. Feth

Audio Engineering Society ● R. Campbell, M.R. Chial *(Alt)*

Canadian Standards Association (liaison) ● T.D. Northwood, B. Brownlee *(Alt)*

Electric Light and Power Group ● C.E. Hickman, J.P. Markey *(Alt)*

Electronic Industries Association ● F.X. Worden, W.W. Lang *(Alt)*

Environmental Protection Agency (liaison) ● R. Marrazzo

Food and Drug Administration (liaison) ● M. Gluck

Hearing Aid Industry Conference, Inc. ● W.G. Ely

Home Ventilating Institute ● J.W. Harper, W.H. Bumpus *(Alt)*

Industrial Medical Association ● J. Sataloff, H.N. Schulz *(Alt)*

Industrial Safety Equipment Association, Inc. ● F. Lotito, R. Campbell *(Alt)*, F.E. Wilcher *(Alt)*

Institute of Electrical and Electronics Engineers ● H. Silbiger, J.D. Griffiths *(Alt)*, W.D. O'Brien, Jr. *(Alt)*

Motor Vehicle Manufacturers Association ● P.E. Toth, A.M. Kooiman *(Alt)*

National Bureau of Standards ● E.L.R. Corliss, F.R. Breckenridge *(Alt)*

National Electrical Manufacturers Association ● R.J. Wells, J.B. Moreland *(Alt)*

National Hearing Aid Society ● W.F.S. Hopmeier, C.A. Murdock *(Alt)*

Society of Automotive Engineers, Inc. ● R.N. Janeway, R.K. Hillquist, W.J. Toth *(Alt)*

Telephone Group ● L.A. Strommen, L.A. Berry *(Alt)*

Ultrasonics Industry Association ● E.J. Murray

U.S. Army Medical Corps ● Major R.K. Sedge

U.S. Army Human Engineering Laboratory ● G.R. Price, D.C. Hodge *(Alt)*

U.S. Army Electronics Command ● H.S. Bennett

U.S. Department of the Air Force ● H.E. von Gierke, C. Nixon *(Alt)*

U.S. Department of Housing and Urban Development ● G.E. Winzer, R.H. Broun *(Alt)*

211

CONTENTS

American National Standard
Methods for Manual Pure-Tone Threshold
Audiometry

1. SCOPE

1.1 Purpose of standard

Pure-tone threshold audiometry is the procedure used in the assessment of an individual's threshold of hearing for pure tones. Pure-tone threshold audiometry includes manual air-conduction measurements at octave intervals from 250 through 8000 Hz and at intermediate frequencies as needed. When abrupt differences of 20 dB or more occur between adjacent octave frequencies, additional frequencies may be included at the discretion of the tester. Bone-conduction measurements may be carried out if indicated by the test requirements at octave intervals from 250 through 4000 Hz. Also, when required, masking is to be used. The purpose of this standard is to present procedures for conducting manual pure-tone threshold audiometry whose uses will minimize intertest differences based on test method.

1.2 Limit of standard

This standard is limited to a description of the measurement method of manual pure-tone threshold audiometry. Hearing screening techniques are outside its purview.

1.3 Modifications of standard procedures

The procedures described in this standard are usable in a wide variety of circumstances. However, certain individuals, such as young children, mentally retarded persons, uncooperative persons, or neurologically handicapped persons may require modifications of the procedures. If so, the modifications shall be noted in the reporting of results.

1.4 Source

The procedures detailed in this standard are adapted from those described in the Draft Guidelines for Manual Pure-Tone Audiometry (Wilson *et al.* 1974) and the Guidelines for a Training Program for Audiometric Technicians (NASNRC, 1973).

2. DEFINITIONS

NOTE: Standard definitions have been used where they exist (ANSI Standard S3.20-1973).

2.1 Air conduction

Air conduction is the process by which sound is conducted to the internal ear through the air in the external acoustic meatus (ear canal) as part of the pathway.

2.2 Bone conduction

Bone conduction is the process by which sound is conducted to the internal ear through the cranial bones.

2.3 Threshold of hearing

The threshold of hearing for a specified signal is the minimum effective sound pressure level of the signal that is capable of evoking an auditory sensation in a specified fraction of the trials. The characteristics of the signal, the manner in which it is presented to the subject, and the point at which the sound pressure level is measured must be specified.

NOTE 1: Unless otherwise indicated, the ambient noise reaching the ears is assumed to be negligible.

NOTE 2: The threshold of audibility is usually given as a sound pressure level in decibels, relative to $20~\mu\text{N/m}^2$.

NOTE 3: Instead of the method of constant stimuli, which is implied by the phrase "a specified fraction of the trials," another psychophysical method (which should be specified) may be employed.

2.4 Reference equivalent threshold sound pressure level

The reference equivalent threshold sound pressure level is the modal value, at a specified frequency, of the equivalent threshold sound pressure levels of an adequately large number of ears of otologically normal subjects within the age limits of 18–30 years inclusive.

NOTE 1: The equivalent threshold sound pressure level for monotic earphone listening is the sound pressure level set up by the specified earphone at a specified frequency in a specified artificial ear or coupler when the earphone is actuated by a voltage that would correspond to the threshold of audibility, if the earphone were applied to the ear concerned.

NOTE 2: The values for air conduction of reference equivalent threshold sound pressure levels are specified in ANSI Standard S3.6-1969.

NOTE 3: The values for bone conduction of reference equivalent threshold vibration levels are specified in ANSI Standard S3.13-1972.

2.5 Otologically normal subject

An otologically normal subject is a person in a normal state of health who is free from all signs or symptoms of ear disease and from occlusive wax in the ear canals and has no history of undue exposure to noise.

2.6 Hearing level for pure tones

Hearing level (HL) of a given ear (for a pure tone) at a specified frequency is the equivalent threshold sound pressure level for that ear minus the reference equivalent threshold sound pressure level.

2.7 Masking

Masking is the process by which the threshold of audibility for a signal is raised by the presence of a second sound. Masking is used in manual pure-tone threshold audiometry, when necessary, to exclude the nontest ear.

214

2.8 Effective masking

Effective masking occurs when the masker is just strong enough to prevent the test subject from hearing the test stimulus when stimulus and masking signals are presented simultaneously to the same ear.

2.9 Manual pure-tone threshold audiometry

Manual pure-tone threshold audiometry is the measurement of an individual's threshold of hearing for pure tones in which the signal presentations, frequencies, and levels are controlled manually by the person administering the test.

2.10 Screening audiometry

Screening audiometry is a method of testing in which a selected hearing level is held constant while frequency is varied. Screening audiometry separates test subjects into only two groups, those who respond at or below a certain hearing level, and those who do not.

2.11 Pulsed tone

A pulsed tone is a tone which is pulsed automatically by the audiometer during stimulus presentation.

2.12 Warble tone

A warble tone results from frequency modulation, usually in a sinusoidal pattern, above and below the test-tone frequency.

2.13 Audiogram

The audiogram is the graphic representation of the results of a pure-tone threshold audiometric test.

2.14 Pure-tone audiometer

An electroacoustical generator which provides pure tones of selected frequencies and of calibrated output (ANSI Standard S3.6-1969).

3. GENERAL REQUIREMENTS

3.1 Ear canal

The ear canal opening shall be inspected for blockage by cotton or other foreign objects and to recognize soft-walled canals that may "collapse" with or without earphones.

NOTE: Collapse of canal if suspected may be obviated by placing a small rigid sound conducting nipple into the opening of the canal before the test and removing it afterwards; the maneuver should be noted on the audiogram form.

3.2 Earphone placement

(1) Earphones should be held in place by a headband.

(2) The earphone should be centered over the ear and its position should be adjusted by test subject for most comfortable listening (or loudest signal) at 250 Hz.

(3) The space under the earphone should be clear of long hair, glasses, hearing aids, and other obstacles.

3.3 Instructions

The instructions shall be phrased in language appropriate to the test subject. The subject shall be told that smoking and gum chewing interfere with the test and are not allowed.

(1) Indicate the purpose of the test—to find the faintest tone that can be heard.

(2) Indicate the need to respond whenever the tone is heard, no matter how faint it may be.

(3) Indicate the need to respond overtly as soon as the tone comes on and also to respond overtly immediately when the tone goes off.

(4) Indicate that each ear is to be tested separately.

3.4 Response task

Overt responses are required from the test subject to indicate when he hears the tone go on and off; any response task meeting this criterion is acceptable. Examples of commonly used responses are (1) raising and lowering the finger, hand, or arm, and (2) pressing and releasing an indicator-light switch.

3.5 Interpretation of response

The primary parameters used in determining threshold are presence of on and off responses, latency of responses, and number of false responses.

3.5.1 On response and off response

Each suprathreshold presentation should elicit two responses—one at the start and one at the end of the test tone.

3.5.2 Latency of response

The latency of the on response varies usually with the level of presentation. The first response to a test tone in an ascending series may be hesitant, but the response to a test tone presented 5 dB higher should be without hesitation.

3.5.3 False responses

False responses may be of two types: (1) a response when no tone is presented (false positive) or (2) failure to respond on presentation of a tone which the tester believes to be audible to the test subject (false negative). Either type complicates the measurement procedure. Reinstruction may reduce the occurrence rate of either type.

4. DETERMINATION OF THRESHOLD

4.1 Familiarization procedure

The test subject shall be familiarized with the listening task by a signal presented at 1000 Hz at estimated hearing level such as to evoke a prompt and clear response. One of the following methods should be used:

(1) Beginning with the tone continuously on but completely attenuated, gradually increase the sound pressure level of the tone until a response occurs. Switch the tone off for at least 2 s and present it again at the same level. If there is a second response proceed to threshold measurement. If there is no second response, repeat the familiarization procedure.

(2) Present the tone at a hearing level of 30 dB. If a clear response occurs, commence threshold measurement. If no response occurs, present the tone at 50 dB HL and at successive additional increments of 10 dB until a response is obtained.

Familiarization is preliminary to threshold determination.

4.2 Determination of threshold

The method described is considered the standard procedure for manual pure-tone threshold audiometry.

4.2.1 Tone duration

Threshold exploration is carried out by presenting tones of 1–2-s duration.

4.2.2 Interval between tones

The interval between successive presentations shall be varied, but shall not be shorter than the test tone.

4.2.3 Level of first presentation

The level of the first presentation of tone for threshold measurement is 10 dB below the level at which test subject responded during the familiarization procedure.

4.2.4 Levels of succeeding presentations

The level of succeeding presentation is determined by the preceding response. After each failure to respond to a signal, the level is increased in 5-dB steps until the first response occurs. After the response, the intensity is decreased 10 dB and another ascending series is begun.

4.2.5 Threshold of hearing

Threshold is defined as the lowest hearing level at which responses occur in at least one-half of a series of ascending trials, with a minimum of two responses out of three required at a single level. If variation occurs, limits must be set as noted in Appendix B.

5. STANDARD PROCEDURES FOR AIR-CONDUCTION MEASURES

5.1 Test environment

The test environment shall meet the specification detailed in ANSI Standard S3.1-1977.

5.2 Instrumentation and calibration

Air-conduction audiometry shall be accomplished with an audiometer and earphones that meet the specifications of American National Standard Specifications for Audiometers S3.6-1969.

5.3 Frequency

Threshold measurements shall be made at octave intervals from 250–8000 Hz and at intermediate frequencies as required to satisfy the purposes for which the procedure is being used.

5.4 Order

When appropriate information is available, the better ear shall be tested first. The frequency of the first test stimulus shall be 1000 Hz. Higher frequencies shall then be assessed in ascending order followed by a retest of 1000 Hz, and finally the lower test frequencies, 500 and 250 Hz, shall be tested. If the retest results of 1000 Hz differ from the first test by more than 5 dB, the lower of the two thresholds may be accepted and at least one other test frequency should be retested.

NOTE: Presentation order of frequencies does not significantly influence test results; the above order is based on an arbitrary choice which will ensure consistency of approach to each test subject and minimize the risk of omissions.

5.5 Masking in air-conduction audiometry

When the air-conduction hearing level obtained in one ear exceeds the apparent or obtained bone-conduction hearing level in the contralateral (nontest) ear by 40 dB or more, masking shall be applied to the nontest ear. The type and magnitude of the masking sound should be noted on the form on which the test results are recorded.

NOTE: A standard for procedures in masking does not exist.

5.6 Recording of results

Results shall be recorded in graphic or tabular form or both, and separate forms to represent each ear may be used.

5.6.1 Audiogram form

When the graphic form is used, the abscissa should be frequency on a logarithmic scale and the ordinate should be hearing level in decibels on a linear scale. It is recommended that 1 octave on the frequency scale be linearly equivalent to 20 dB on the hearing scale. The vertical scale is to be labeled: "Hearing Level in Decibels (dB)"; the horizontal scale is to be labeled: "Frequency in Hertz (Hz)." Conventionally, normal hearing is at the top of the graph and hearing loss is plotted downward. (See Appendix A.)

5.6.2 Audiogram symbols

When the graphic form is used, the symbols presented in Appendix A are recommended for use.

5.6.3 Other information

Other pertinent information describing the test situation should be reported on the audiogram form.

6. STANDARD PROCEDURES FOR BONE-CONDUCTION MEASURES IN DIAGNOSTIC AUDIOMETRY

6.1 Instrumentation

The testing shall be accomplished with a wide-range audiometer as defined by the American National Standard Specifications for Audiometers S3.6-1969.

6.2 Calibration

The bone-conduction vibrator is to be calibrated in the interim-threshold calibration values (Appendix A, Table IV) of the American National Standard Specifications for Artificial Head-Bone for the Calibration of Audiometer Bone Vibrators S3.13-1972 and should incorporate the appropriate calibration for either mastoid or frontal placement.

NOTE: In addition to this standard, one may use comparison values for other artificial mastoids. (Wilber, 1972; Dirks and Kamm, 1975).

6.3 Vibrator placement

Vibrator and support construction shall allow mastoid or forehead placement with appropriate calibration.

6.4 Covering of ears

The test ear should not be covered for standard bone-conduction measurements. The nontest ear should be covered with an earphone for contralateral masking.

6.5 Frequencies

Threshold should be obtained at octave intervals from 250–4000 Hz.

6.6 Order

The initial frequency tested shall be 1000 Hz which shall be followed by the higher test frequencies (2000 and 4000 Hz) in ascending order and finally, by the lower test frequencies as for air conduction.

6.7 Masking

Since the threshold values on which the calibration of bone vibrators is based were measured monaurally, i.e., with masking noise in the contralateral ear, masking should be used in the testing procedure also.

6.8 Recording of results

Results may be recorded in tabular or graphic form, and separate graphic forms may be used to represent each ear. The set of symbols illustrated in Appendix A is recommended for use with the graphic form (audiogram).

7. REVISION OF AMERICAN NATIONAL STANDARDS SPECIFICATIONS REFERRED TO IN THIS DOCUMENT

7.1 General

When the following American National Standards Specifications referred to in this document are superseded by a revision approved by the American National Standards Institute, Inc., the revision shall apply:

(1) American National Standard Specifications for Audiometers, S3.6-1969;

(2) American National Standard Specifications for Artificial Head-Bone for the Calibration of Audiometer Bone Vibrators, S3.13-1972;

(3) American National Standard Psychoacoustical Terminology, S3.20-1973; and

(4) American National Standard Criteria for Permissible Ambient Noise during Audiometric Testing, S3.1-1977.

APPENDIX A: AUDIOGRAM SYMBOLS[a]

Air-conduction symbols

The air-conduction symbols should be drawn on the audiogram so that the midpoint of the symbol centers on the intersection of the vertical ruling and horizontal axis at the appropriate hearing level.

Bone-conduction symbols

The bone-conduction symbols, with one exception, should be placed adjacent to, but not touching, the frequency coordinate ruling and centered vertically at the appropriate hearing level. The symbol for the left ear should be placed to the right of the vertical ruling and that for the right ear to the left of the vertical ruling. The symbol for unmasked forehead bone conduction should be centered on the vertical ruling at the appropriate hearing level.

Symbols representation

Unless otherwise specified, symbols are to indicate that the test signals used were pure tones. The same symbols may be used for warble tones and narrowband noise, if so noted on the audiogram.

Multiple notation

When the two ears are being represented on the same graphic form and when the left-ear unmasked air-conduction threshold is the same as the right-ear air-conduction threshold, the left air-conduction symbol should be placed inside the right air-conduction symbol. When bone-conduction thresholds (except unmasked forehead bone conduction) occur at the same hearing level as air-conduction thresholds, the bone-conduction symbols should be placed beside but not touching the air-conduction symbols. The midline bone-conduction symbol in this circumstance should be placed with the point of the carat barely entering the region of the air-conduction symbols.

When bone conduction is measured at the mastoid with unmasked and masked thresholds occurring at the same hearing level, the unmasked symbol should be placed closest to the vertical ruling. The masked symbol should surround, but not touch, the unmasked symbol.

ᵃModified from "Guidelines for Audiometric symbols" (American Speech and Hearing Association, 1974).

No response

To indicate "no response" at the maximum output

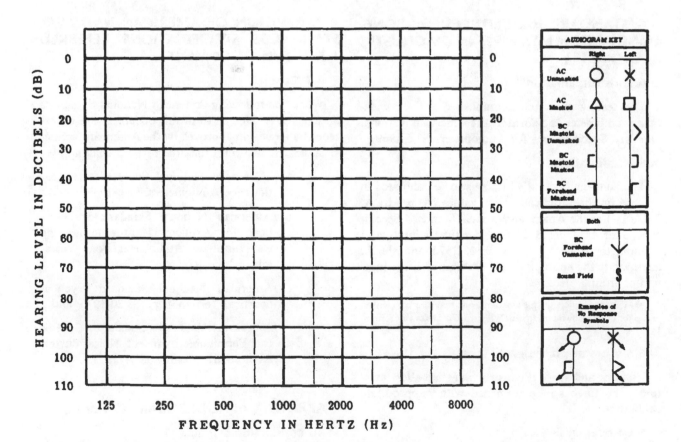

FIG. 1. Recommended form of audiogram and audiogram symbols.

of the audiometer, an arrow should be attached to the lower outside corner of the appropriate symbol and drawn downward and at about 45 degrees outward from the vertical ruling—to the right for left-ear symbols and to the left for right-ear symbols. The arrow for sound-field or unmasked forehead bone-conduction symbols should be attached at the bottom and drawn straight downward.

The "no response" symbol should be placed on the audiogram at the Hearing Level representing the maximum output limit for the particular test frequency, test modality and audiometer.

Separate forms

A separate graphic form may be used to represent each ear.

Lines connecting symbols

Lines may be used to connect symbols on an audiogram. When used, a solid line should connect the air-conduction threshold values. Bone-conduction symbols may be connected by a dashed line when an air-bone gap exists. Symbols representing "no response" for air conduction or bone conduction should not be connected to each other or to any of the response symbols.

Color coding

Color coding is not necessary to transmit information about sidedness in this symbol system. In practice, it may be desirable to avoid color coding because of the increasing use of multiple-copy audiograms and photoduplication of audiograms. However, if color is employed, red should be used for the right-ear symbols and connecting lines and blue for the left-ear symbols and connecting lines, with a third color used for the "both ears" symbols.

APPENDIX B: VARIABILITY OF THRESHOLD MEASURES

Upon retest, if a test subject shows variable threshold, a limitation should be set on the acceptable variation. If the responses do not fall within the limitations, then the test subject should be referred to an outside source since special methods and greater time may be necessary to obtain accurate results.

Several investigators have reported standard deviations for air-conducted signals of from 5 to 10 dB. If the audiometer in use has a 5-dB-step attenuator, 10 dB is considered the outside limit, attributable to causes other than hearing.

In a study of reliability of pure-tone measures Harris (1946) concluded that audiograms will be consistent to at least 5 dB. Reasonably low noise levels, cooperative test subjects, and intelligent trained operators are mandatory. The time between test and retests can affect consistency of the results. In a five-year study of persons not exposed to damaging noise, Pell (1973) found some variation related to aging, but a great deal of variation arose from test error and random fluctuations. If the variation is always in the same direction of lower or higher thresholds, then one may attribute more significance to a small shift.

Steinberg and Munson (1936) found variability related to the fit of the earphone with standard deviations of 5-7 dB. The place and the method of measurement may contribute to variability. However, under carefully controlled conditions, Myers and Harris (1949) found less than 1 dB of variability, when 1-dB steps of attenuation were used.

Bone-conduction measurements were studied for stability and found to have good inherent test-retest reliability similar to that of air conduction. For a complete and detailed discussion see Dirks (1964).

REFERENCES

American National Standards Institute (**1973**). American National Standard Psychoacoustical Terminology S3.20-1973.

American National Standards Institute (**1970**). American National Standard Specifications for Audiometers S3.6-1969.

American National Standards Institute (**1973**). American National Standard Specifications for Artificial Head-Bone for the Calibration of Audiometer Bone Vibrators S3.13-1972.

American National Standards Institute (**1977**). Criteria for Permissible Ambient Noise during Audiometric Testing S3.1-1977.

American Speech and Hearing Association (**1974**). Am. Speech Hear. Assoc., "Guidelines for Audiometric Symbols."

Dirks, D.D. (**1964**)."Factors related to bone conduction reliability," Arch. Otolaryngol. 79, 551-558.

Dirks, D.D., and Kamm, C.(**1975**)"Bone-vibrator measurements: Physical characteristics and behavioral thresholds," J. Speech Hearing Res. 18, 242–260.

Harris, J.D.(**1946**). "Free voice and pure tone audiometer for routine testing of auditory acuity," Arch. Otolaryngol. 44, 452–467.

Myers, C.K., and Harris, J.D. (**1949**). "The inherent stability of the auditory threshold," Nav. Med. Res. Lab. Rep. No. 3.

NASNRC Publ. (**1973**). "Guidelines for a Training Program for Audiometer Technicians," Rep. Working Group 66, Committee on Hearing, Bioacoustics, and Biomechanics.

Pell, S. (**1973**). "An evaluation of a hearing conservation program—a five year longitudinal study." Am. Ind. Hyg. Assoc. J. 82–91 (February).

Steinberg, J.C., and Munson, W.A. (**1936**). "Deviations in the loudness judgments of 100 people," J. Acoust. Soc. Am. 8, 71–80.

Wilber, L.A. (1972). "Comparability of Two Commercially Available Artificial Mastoids," J. Acoust. Soc. Am. 52, 1265–1266.

Wilson, W.R., Graham, J.T., Chaiklin, J.B., Sonday, F.L.,

Schoeny, Z.G., Byers, V.W., and Hopkinson, N.T. (1974). American Speech and Hearing Association," Draft Guidelines for Manual Pure-Tone Threshold Audiometry."

ACOUSTICAL SOCIETY OF AMERICA
STANDARDS SECRETARIAT

The Standards Program of the Acoustical Society of America is the responsibility of the ASA's Committee on Standards (ASACOS) and is executed by ASA's Standards Secretariat headed by its Standards Manager.

The Acoustical Society of America is the Secretariat for three standards committees of the American National Standards Institute (ANSI): S1 on Physical Acoustics, S2 on Mechanical Shock and Vibration, and S3 on Bioacoustics, and is also responsible for the international activities of ISO/TC 43 on Acoustics, for which S1 and S3 serve as the technical advisory groups. ASA also administers the international secretariat of ISO/TC 108 on Mechanical Vibration and Shock (on behalf of the American National Standards Institute) and provides the U.S. input via the technical advisory group for ISO/TC 108, which is Standards Committee S2.

Standards are produced in three broad areas: physical acoustics, mechanical shock and vibration, and bioacoustics, and are reaffirmed or revised every five years. The latest information on current ANSI standards as well as those under preparation is available from the Standards Secretariat.

This standard, ANSI S3.21-1978 (ASA Catalog No. 19-1978), is available at a single-copy price of $7.00 prepaid (a handling charge of $2.00 is required if payment does not accompany order). Make checks payable to the ASA Standards Secretariat. When ordering ANSI S3.21-1978, please also use ASA Catalog No. 19-1978 for easy reference. This standard and other standards listed in the ASA Standards Catalog may be ordered from the following address:

Back Numbers Department, Dept. STD
American Institute of Physics
335 East 45th Street
New York, New York 10017
Telephone: (212) 681-3800

If you wish to have further information on the Standards Publication Program of the Acoustical Society, address your inquiries to

Standards Secretariat
Accoustical Society of America
35 Pinelawn Road, Suite 114E
Melville, New York 11747-3177
Telephone: (631) 390-0215
Fax: (631) 390-0217
Email: asastds@aip.org

Appendix O
American National Standard Methods for Measuring the Real-Ear Attenuation of Hearing Protectors

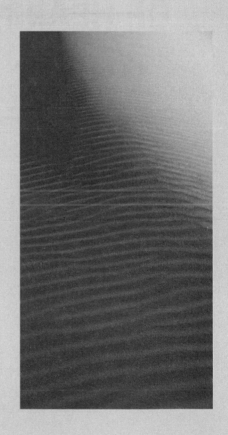

AMERICAN NATIONAL STANDARD
METHODS FOR MEASURING THE REAL-EAR ATTENUATION OF HEARING PROTECTORS

ANSI S12.6-1997

Accredited Standards Committee S12, Noise

Standards Secretariat
Accoustical Society of America
35 Pinelawn Road, Suite 114E
Melville, New York 11747-3177

The American National Standards Institute, Inc. (ANSI) is the national coordinator of voluntary standards development and the clearing house in the U.S. for information on national and international standards.

The Acoustical Society of America (ASA) is an organization of scientists and engineers formed in 1929 to increase and diffuse the knowledge of acoustics and to promote its practical applications.

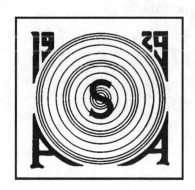

American National Standard

Methods for Measuring the
Real-Ear Attenuation of Hearing Protectors

Secretariat
Acoustical Society of America

Approved 21 February 1997
American National Standards Institute, Inc.

Abstract

This Standard specifies laboratory-based procedures for measuring, analyzing, and reporting the noise-reducing capabilities of conventional passive hearing protection devices. The procedures consist of psychophysical tests conducted on human subjects to determine the real-ear attenuation measured at hearing threshold. Two fitting procedures are provided: Method A) experimenter-supervised fit, designed to describe the capabilities of the devices under ideal conditions, and Method B) subject fit, intended to approximate the protection that can be attained by groups of informed users in workplaces with representative well-managed and well-supervised occupational hearing conservation programs. Regardless of test method, the attenuation data will be valid only to the extent that the users wear the devices in the same manner as the test subjects. This Standard does not address issues pertaining to computational schemes or rating systems for applying hearing protector attenuation values, nor does it address comfort or wearability features. Portions of this Standard correspond to International Standard ISO 4869-1:1990, Acoustics—Hearing Protectors—Part 1: Subjective Method for the Measurement of Sound Attenuation, but this document includes a subject-fit procedure which the ISO document lacks.

AMERICAN NATIONAL STANDARDS ON ACOUSTICS

The Acoustical Society of America (ASA) provides the Secretariat for Accredited Standards Committees S1 on Acoustics, S2 on Mechanical Vibration and Shock, S3 on Bioacoustics, and S12 on Noise. These committees have wide representation from the technical community (manufacturers, consumers, and general-interest representatives). The standards are published by the Acoustical Society of America through the American Institute of Physics as American National Standards after approval by their respective standards committees and the American National Standards Institute.

These standards are developed and published as a public service to provide standards useful to the public, industry, and consumers, and to Federal, State, and local governments.

Each of the Accredited Standards Committees [operating in accordance with procedures approved by American National Standards Institute (ANSI)] is responsible for developing, voting upon, and maintaining or revising its own standards. The ASA Standards Secretariat administers committee organization and activity and provides liaison between the Accredited Standards Committees and ANSI. After the standards have been produced and adopted by the Accredited Standards Committees, and approved as American National Standards by ANSI, the ASA Standards Secretariat arranges for their publication and distribution.

An American National Standard implies a consensus of those substantially concerned with its scope and provisions. Consensus is established when, in the judgment of the ANSI Board of Standards Review, substantial agreement has been reached by directly and materially affected interests. Substantial agreement means much more than a simple majority, but not necessarily unanimity. Consensus requires that all views and objections be considered and that a concerted effort be made towards their resolution.

The use of an American National Standard is completely voluntary. Their existence does not in any respect preclude anyone, whether he or she has approved the Standards or not, from manufacturing, marketing, purchasing, or using products, processes, or procedures not conforming to the standards.

NOTICE: This American National Standard may be revised or withdrawn at any time. The procedures of the American National Standards Institute require that action be taken periodically to reaffirm, revise, or withdraw this standard.

Standards Secretariat
Acoustical Society of America
120 Wall Street, 32nd Floor
New York, New York 10005-3993

Telephone: +1 212 248-0373
Telefax: +1 212 248-0146

Contents

Foreword

[This Foreword is not part of *American National Standard Methods for Measuring the Real-Ear Attenuation of Hearing Protectors*, ANSI S12.6-1997 (a revision of ANSI S12.6-1984).]

This standard is a revision of ANSI S12.6-1984 Methods of the Measurement of the Real-Ear Attenuation of Hearing Protectors. This standard does not pertain to physical attenuation measurements using acoustical test fixtures or microphones mounted in human earcanals; those procedures are covered by ANSI S12.42-1995. The principal difference between this standard and its predecessor, ANSI S12.6-1984, lies in the addition of an alternative to experimenter-supervised fit testing, namely, a subject-fit methodology which is intended to approximate the protection that can be attained by groups of informed users in workplaces with representative well-managed and well-supervised occupational hearing conservation programs. This document relates to International Standard ISO 4869-1:1990, Acoustics—Hearing Protectors—Part 1: Subjective Method for the Measurement of Sound Attenuation. However, the ANSI document differs in that it provides two alternative fitting procedures, one of which is the subject-fit method mentioned above.

This Standard was developed under the jurisdiction of Accredited Standards Committee S12, Noise, which has the following scope:

Standards, specifications, and terminology in the field of acoustical noise pertaining to methods of measurement, evaluation, and control, including biological safety, tolerance and comfort, and physical acoustics as related to environmental and occupational noise.

At the time this standard was submitted to Accredited Standards Committee S12, Noise, for final approval, the membership was as follows:

D. L. Johnson, *Chair*

P. D. Schomer, *Vice Chair*

A. Brenig, *Secretary*

Acoustical Society of America	D. L. Johnson
	W. J. Galloway (*Alt.*)
Acoustical Systems, Inc.	R. Goodwin
	R. Seitz (*Alt.*)
Air-Conditioning and Refrigeration Institute (ARI)	S. Wang
	G. Acton (*Alt.*)
Air Movement and Control Association, Inc. (AMCA)	M. Stevens
	E. W. Neitzel (*Alt.*)
Aluminum Company of America (ALCOA)	S. I. Roth
American Academy of Otolaryngology, Head and Neck Surgery, Inc.	G. Gates
	L. A. Micheal (*Alt.*)
American College of Occupational Medicine	P. J. Brownson
	J. Sataloff (*Alt.*)
American Industrial Hygiene Association	L. H. Royster
	J. F. Meagher (*Alt.*)
American Otological Society	R. F. Naunton
American Society of Heating, Refrigeration, and Air-Conditioning Engineers (ASHRAE)	J. Pei
	J. L. Heldenbrand (*Alt.*)

American Speech-Language-Hearing Association .... J. D. Royster
    M. E. Thompson (*Alt.*)

Audio Engineering Society, Inc. .... M. R. Chial
    D. Queen (*Alt.*)

Brüel and Kjaer Instruments, Inc. .... E. Schonthal
Compressed Air and Gas Institute (CAGI) .... J. H. Addington
Council for Accreditation in Occupational Hearing Conservation
    (CAOHC) .... W. Monk
    D. Driscoll (*Alt.*)

Industrial Safety Equipment Association .... J. Birkner
    W. J. Emy (*Alt.*)

Information Technology Industry Council (ITI) .... R. Lotz
    W. F. Hanrahan (*Alt.*)

Larson Davis Laboratories. .... B. Chanaud
    L. Davis (*Alt.*)

National Council of Acoustical Consultants. .... J. Erdreich
    R. L. Richards (*Alt.*)

National Electrical Manufacturers Association (NEMA) .... D. Rawlings
National Hearing Conservation Association (NHCA) .... J. Franks
    E. H. Berger (*Alt.*)

Power Tool Institute, Inc. .... R. Callahan
    D. H. Montague (*Alt.*)

U.S. Army Aeromedical Research Laboratory .... B. Mozo
    J. H. Patterson (*Alt.*)

U.S. Army Audiology and Speech Center .... R. Danielson
U.S. Army Construction Engineering Research Laboratory
    (USA-CERL) .... P. D. Schomer
    M. White (*Alt.*)

U.S. Army Human Engineering Laboratory .... G. R. Price
    J. Kalb (*Alt.*)

U.S. Department of Transportation .... A. Konheim
U.S. Navy Environmental Health Center .... J. Page
    L. Marshall (*Alt.*)

U.S. Navy National Surface Warfare Center .... D. J. Vendittis
    J. Niemiec (*Alt.*)

Individual Experts of Accredited Standards Committee S12, Noise, were:

P. K. Baade	R. Guernsey	P. D. Schomer
R. G. Bartheld	R. K. Hillquist	W. R. Thornton
R. W. Benson	D. L. Johnson	D. J. Vendittis
L. L. Beranek	W. W. Lang	H. E. von Gierke
E. H. Berger	L. F. Luttrell	L. A. Wilber
S. H. P. Bly	G. C. Maling	G. Winzer
K. M. Eldred	A. H. Marsh	G. S. K. Wong
S. Gales	J. Pope	R. W. Young
W. J. Galloway	L. H. Royster	

Working Group S12/WG11, Field Effectiveness and Physical Characteristics of Hearing Protectors, which assisted Accredited Standards Committee, S12, Noise, in the preparation of this Standard, had the following membership:

E. H. Berger, Chair

A. Behar	J. R. Franks	D. Ohlin
J. G. Casali	B. T. Mozo	J. D. Royster
C. Dixon-Ernst	C. W. Nixon	L. H. Royster

Suggestions for improvement of this Standard will be welcomed. Send suggestions for improvement to Accredited Standards Committee S12, Noise, in care of the ASA Standards Secretariat, 120 Wall Street, 32nd floor, New York, New York 10005-3993, USA. Telephone +1 212 248-0373; FAX: +1 212 248-0146.

American National Standard

Methods for Measuring the Real-Ear Attenuation of Hearing Protectors

0 Introduction

0.1 Background

Since the development of ANSI Z24.22-1957, real-ear attenuation at threshold (REAT) methods for the measurement of the noise reduction of hearing protection devices (HPDs) have been widely utilized and described in the literature. In subsequent years, many additional procedures have been devised and tested, and in some cases standardized, but the real-ear attenuation procedure has remained the most common and accepted (Berger, 1986). It is generally recognized that REAT data yield the most accurate measure of the noise reduction provided by conventional level-independent devices, for a specified test condition, i.e., *for the particular subjects who were tested for the way in which they wore the devices under test.*

A major area of contention does exist in the professional community and within the scientific literature, namely, the applicability of the laboratory-measured REAT data to real-world environments. In other words, are the data valid for application outside the laboratory? Do they provide a useful indicator of the attenuation that can be expected to be attained by groups of people wearing hearing protectors on a day-to-day basis for protection from occupational or recreational noise exposures?

Beginning in the middle 1970s and continuing up through the 1990s, studies have reported that the field-measured attenuation of HPDs was substantially less than would be predicted based upon testing conducted in conformance with the prior ANSI standards, S3.19-1974 and S12.6-1984 (Berger, Franks, and Lindgren, 1996). This divergence is especially troubling considering the importance that many hearing protector purchasers and users ascribe to published attenuation data.

Ideally, the approach to reduction of laboratory vs. real-world discrepancies would be to improve field performance to more closely match laboratory data, keeping in mind that under no circumstances can one hope to duplicate optimum laboratory data under field conditions. Regardless, most agree that industrial hearing conservation practice must be enhanced so that better real-world HPD performance can be realized (Berger, 1992). However, it is also clear that a laboratory method of measuring hearing protector attenuation that yields data which more closely correlate with existing, or even potential field performance, would be a valuable predictive tool.

The Working Group responsible for this standard embarked upon a project to develop a procedure to provide more valid estimates of field performance. In so doing various protocols were evaluated and tested via both a pilot and a full-scale interlaboratory comparison study. The results, which have been summarized and presented in three parts, provide the scientific justification for the subject-fit procedure which has been incorporated in this standard (Berger and Franks, 1996; Royster *et al.*, 1996; Franks *et al.*, 1996).

0.2 The need for a better human-factors model

Experimenter-supervised fitting of HPDs (i.e., very carefully controlled placement of the devices), which was the only option in the prior version of ANSI S12.6, is intended to describe the upper limits of hearing protector performance. This procedure can be useful for developing a better theoretical understanding of how hearing protectors block sound and interface to the head or earcanals. However, such data provide inadequate insight into the performance of HPDs when real-world human-factors considerations must be taken into account. (See Appendix A of AS 1270-1988 for additional discussion of this issue.) Since the interface between the HPD and the head or earcanal is such a critical determinant of the achieved attenuation, and because it is so strongly controlled by the subject and how the device is worn (especially for earplugs), human factors considerations must be included in the laboratory model if valid field estimates are to be obtained.

In recognition of the importance of the HPD-head/earcanal interface, standardized laboratory methods of measuring hearing protector attenuation have typically involved the use of human subjects wearing the devices under test. The value of using human subjects, as opposed to acoustical test fixtures, must not be overlooked in the development of testing procedures. Keeping the human in the equation provides the potential to develop a laboratory-based procedure that more closely models field conditions.

In spite of the importance of using of human subjects, one must also consider that an experimenter interacting with listeners may lead to variability in measured results. The experimenter can dramatically influence the data by how she/he selects, trains, supervises, motivates, and fits the subjects—in short by the experimenter's own preconceptions about how the HPD should be used and is expected to perform. The usefulness of the laboratory data in predicting field performance in a given application will be determined in large part by the degree of correspondence between the laboratory procedures for fitting HPDs and those found in the real world.

0.3 Defining validity

In order to create a procedure that generates "valid" data, the question of course has to be asked, "Valid with respect to what?" In practice, a wide range of HPD attenuation values may be observed in the work place, from essentially no attenuation at all for devices poorly fitted by untrained users who incorrectly and inconsistently wear their HPDs, to much higher levels of protection that may be obtained under ideal conditions in workplaces with the most successful hearing conservation programs. It makes no sense to excessively derate hearing protector performance to estimate worst-case attenuation values, since worst-case values are much more heavily influenced by factors other than the hearing protectors themselves. Neither is it appropriate to utilize experimenter-supervised fit values to estimate field performance, since they are in essence estimates of idealized protection obtained under laboratory conditions.

In developing a procedure to estimate field performance, the decision was made to approximate "achievable" results. Such results were defined as among the higher values of attenuation attained by groups of informed users in work places with well-managed industrial and military hearing conservation programs. It was recognized that sincerely interested and/or highly motivated individuals may obtain workplace attenuation values significantly exceeding laboratory subject-fit data, but for populations of occupational users, the subject-fit estimates will be more appropriate. The validity of the estimates was assessed and substantiated by comparing laboratory-measured values arrived at using the subject-fit protocol of this standard, to values for groups of users derived from more than 20 available real-world studies (Berger and Franks, 1996).

0.4 Why this Standard provides two options for testing

As discussed above, it is possible to demonstrate a wide range of performance with any given hearing protector, controlled in large part by the user and how she/he chooses to wear the device. It follows that, depending upon the situation one is trying to model with the laboratory test procedure, or the purpose to which one will apply the data, one or another laboratory method may be more appropriate. Thus, the choice was made in the development of this standard to maintain the experimenter-supervised fitting procedure with which much of the hearing protection community has become familiar, but also to include an alternative procedure for estimating field attenuation which has greater correspondence to most real-world situations. See annex A for additional details.

Based upon the available literature as well as the findings of the interlaboratory study which provided the foundation for this standard (Berger and Franks, 1996; Royster et al., 1996), it is anticipated that experimenter-supervised fitting will result in higher mean attenuation values and lower within-test standard deviation values than the subject-fit results. The effect will be substantially larger for earplugs than for earmuffs because of the much greater importance of fitting factors in testing insert devices. See annex B for examples of representative data.

Between-test and between-laboratory variability is anticipated to be similar for both procedures. See annex C for information on the precision of the subject-fit procedure.

The choice of the method will be determined by the application which the user intends. For guidance, see clause 1.2 Applications.

0.5 Beyond laboratory testing

The subject-fit method described in this standard was developed to approximate the real-world attenuation achieved in actual hearing conservation programs. However, for a particular workplace, the best way to estimate the attenuation actually attained by employees is to measure real-ear attenuation for a sample of workers (Berger, 1986). Ultimately, the audiometric data base for the noise-exposed employees will demonstrate whether their hearing has been protected, but this bottom-line indicator depends upon the effectiveness of the entire hearing conservation program, not hearing protector use alone (ANSI S12.13-1991).

1 Scope and applications

1.1 Scope

This standard specifies laboratory-based procedures for measuring, analyzing, and reporting the noise-reducing capabilities of hearing protection devices. The methods consist of psychophysical tests conducted on human subjects to determine real-ear attenuation at threshold.

Two methods are provided, differing in their subject selection, training, hearing protector fitting procedures, and experimenter involvement, but corresponding in all electroacoustic and psychophysical aspects. One method, designated *experimenter-supervised fit* is intended to describe the upper limits of hearing protector performance. The second method, designated *subject fit*, is conducted with persons naive with respect to the use of hearing protection. It approximates the attenuation that has been achieved by groups of users as reported in real-world occupational studies (Berger and Franks, 1996).

1.2 Applications

The selection of test method, experimenter-supervised fit or subject fit, is based upon the intended application. Experimenter-supervised fit will correspond most closely to tests using the prior version of this standard, ANSI S12.6-1984, and its predecessor, ANSI S3.19-1974. Such values are useful in the design of hearing protectors, to provide a theoretical understanding of their performance limitations, and for routine testing for quality assurance purposes.

The subject-fit procedure is intended to provide an approximation of the upper limits to the attenuation that can be expected for *groups* of occupational users. Properly trained and motivated *individuals* can potentially attain larger amounts of protection, in closer agreement with the experimenter-supervised fit data, especially for earplugs, than the subject-fit values found using this standard. However, subject-fit values provide a closer correspondence to real-world performance for groups of users than do the experimenter-supervised fit data.

Regardless of the test method which is selected, experimenter-supervised fit or subject fit, the attenuation values will be generally applicable only to the extent that:

(1) the hearing protectors are worn in practice in the same manner as did the subjects during the laboratory test;

(2) the hearing protectors are properly maintained;

(3) the anatomical characteristics of the subjects involved in the laboratory test are a reasonable match to the population of actual wearers.

The methods of this standard apply to conventional passive hearing protectors, as well as to electronic devices when the electronics are turned off. Hearing protectors can also take the form of communications headsets, helmets, pressure suits, and other systems with sound-attenuating features. Devices can be used in combination with one another, such as earplugs worn in conjunction with earmuffs or helmets.

The methods of this standard yield data which are collected at low sound pressure levels (close to the threshold of hearing) but which are also representative of the attenuation values of hearing protectors at higher levels. One exception occurs in the case of active and passive amplitude-sensitive hearing protectors for sound pressure levels above the point at which their level-dependent characteristics become effective. At those levels the methods specified in this standard are inapplicable; they will usually underestimate sound attenuation (Berger, 1986). Another exception exists with respect to predicting the noise reduction of impulsive sounds from weapons' fire and blasts, for which many questions remain with respect to the use of the results for the assessment of hazard.

The low-frequency (below 500 Hz) real-ear attenuation at threshold data resulting from this standard may be spuriously high by a few decibels, with the error increasing as frequency decreases. This results from masking of the occluded-ear thresholds caused by physiological noise during testing (Berger and Kerivan, 1983; Schroeter and Poesselt, 1986). The errors are largest for semi-insert and supra-aural hearing protectors, for small-volume earmuffs and for shallowly-inserted earplugs. The errors are smallest for large-volume earmuffs and more deeply-inserted earplugs.

This standard does not address issues pertaining to computational schemes or rating systems for applying hearing protector attenuation values, nor does it address comfort or wearability features.

2 Normative references

The following standards contain provisions which, through reference in this text, constitute provisions of this American National Standard.

ANSI S1.1-1994, American National Standard Acoustical Terminology.

ANSI S1.11-1986 (R 1993), American National Standard Specification for Octave-Band and Fractional-Octave-Band Analog and Digital Filters.

ANSI S3.1-1991, American National Standard Maximum Permissible Ambient Noise Levels for Audiometric Test Rooms.

ANSI S3.6-1996, American National Standard Specification for Audiometers.

ANSI S3.20-1995, American National Standard Bioacoustical Terminology.

ANSI S3.36-1985 (R 1990), American National Standard Specification for a Manikin for Simulated in-situ Airborne Acoustic Measurements.

NOTE – "R" stands for reaffirmed.

3 Definitions

active hearing protection device. A hearing protector which contains electronic components, including transducers, to affect the transmission of sound into the earcanal.

amplitude-sensitive hearing protection device. A hearing protector, sometimes referred to as a level-dependent hearing protector, that may be active or passive in design, which exhibits a change in insertion loss as a function of sound level.

communications headset. A device (earplug or earmuff) designed primarily for voice communication which may also provide or be used for hearing protection.

earplug. A hearing protector that is inserted into the earcanal.

earmuff. A hearing protector usually comprised of a headband and earcups with a soft cushion to seal against the head, intended to fit against the pinna (supra-aural) or the sides of the head around the pinna (circumaural). The earcups may also be held in position by attachment arms mounted on a hard hat or hard cap.

hearing protection device (HPD). A personal device, also referred to as a hearing protector, worn to reduce the harmful auditory and/or annoying subjective effects of sound.

helmet. A device, sometimes functioning as a hearing protector, that usually covers a substantial portion of the head, which may include internally mounted earcups.

occluded threshold of hearing. At a specific frequency, the minimum effective sound pressure level of the signal that is capable of evoking an auditory sensation in a specified fraction of the trials, when the hearing protector under test is worn.

open threshold of hearing. At a specific frequency, the minimum effective sound pressure level of the signal that is capable of evoking an auditory sensation in a specified fraction of the trials, when a hearing protector is not worn.

passive hearing protection device. A hearing protector which lacks electronic components, and therefore relies solely on its structural elements to block or otherwise control the transmission of sound into the earcanal.

pink noise. Noise for which the spectrum density varies as the inverse of frequency.

random incidence. Incidence of sound waves successively from all directions with equal probability.

real-ear attenuation at threshold (REAT). At a specific frequency, the mean value (in decibels) of the occluded threshold of hearing minus the open threshold of hearing on all trials under otherwise identical test conditions, either for a single listener or averaged across a group of listeners.

reference point. A fixed spatial location within the test chamber at which the midpoint of a line connecting the test subjects' earcanal openings shall be located for REAT measurements, and likewise the point to which all objective measurements of the sound field characteristics shall be referenced.

reverberation time. Of an enclosure, for a stated frequency or frequency band, the time required for the level of the time-mean-square sound pressure in the enclosure to decrease by 60 dB, after the source has stopped. Unit, second (s).

semi-insert device. An earplug-like device (also called canal cap or concha-seated hearing protector) consisting of soft pods or tips that are held in place by a lightweight band. The pods are positioned in the conchae covering the entrances to the earcanals, or fitted to varying depths within the ear-canals. Semi-inserts that cap the canal require the force of the band to retain their position and acoustic seal. Semi-inserts that enter the canal behave more like earplugs; they seal the ear to block noise with or without the application of band force.

4 Physical requirements of the test facility

4.1 Test signals

Test signals shall consist of either pink or white noise, filtered into one-third octave-bands. Center frequencies shall include at least 125, 250, 500, 1000, 2000, 4000, and 8000 Hz.

4.2 Test site

4.2.1 Diffuse sound field requirements

4.2.1.1 Uniformity. The sound pressure level measured using an omnidirectional microphone at six positions relative to the reference point, with the subject and the subject's chair absent, ± 15 cm in front-back, up-down, and left-right axes, shall remain within a range of 5 dB for each test signal. The difference between the left-right positions shall not exceed 3 dB. The orientation of the microphone shall be kept the same at each position.

4.2.1.2 Directionality. The directionality of the sound field shall be evaluated at the reference point for test bands with center frequencies greater than or equal to 500 Hz, with the subject and the subject's chair absent. The measurements shall be conducted with a directional microphone that exhibits in its free-field polar response at the one-third octave test bands, at least 10 dB front-to-side rejection for a cosine microphone, or at least 10 dB front-to-back rejection for a cardioid microphone.

The sound field shall be considered to approximate a random incidence field if, when the microphone is rotated about the center of the test space through 360 degrees in each of the three perpendicular planes of the room, the observed sound pressure level in each test band in each plane remains within the variation allowed in table 1. The sound pressure levels may also be obtained by measuring at fixed 15-degree increments as the microphone is rotated 360 degrees in each plane.

4.2.2 Reverberation time. The reverberation time at the reference point, with the subject and the subject's chair absent, shall not exceed 1.6 s for each test signal.

Table 1 – Allowable variation of sound-field sound pressure levels within each plane, for corresponding directional microphone free-field rejection.

Microphone free-field rejection, dB	Allowable variation, dB [a]
>25	6
20	5
15	4
10	3
<10	microphone not suitable

[a]For directional microphones whose free-field rejection values fall between the tabled values, the allowable variation shall be computed by linear interpolation.

NOTE – The variation in microphone response as the microphone is rotated in a random incidence field is related to the directional characteristics of the microphone and the degree of randomness of the field being measured. Thus, allowable sound field response variations are related to the free-field directional response characteristics of the microphone. The microphone characteristics may be obtained by measurement in a free field or from the microphone manufacturer.

4.2.3 Ambient noise. The ambient noise at the reference point, with the subject absent, and with all signal presentation equipment on and adjusted to a gain of 20 dB above the levels necessary to elicit the open threshold of hearing at all test frequencies, but with no test signal present, shall not exceed the octave-band levels in table 2.

If any extraneous noise becomes audible in the test room during testing, the listener shall signal the experimenter to stop the test.

Table 2 – Maximum permissible ambient noise at the reference point.

Frequency, Hz	Octave-band SPL, dB [a]
31.5	56.0
63	42.0
125	28.0
250	18.5
500	14.5
1000	14.0
2000	8.5
4000	9.0
8000	20.5

[a]Values re 20 μPa.

NOTE – Levels are taken from ANSI S3.1-1991, table II, ears not covered, 125 to 8000 Hz. Levels at 31.5 and 63 Hz are taken from Table B1 of that same standard, ears not covered, 125 to 8000 Hz.

NOTE – Any audible noise during testing may be distracting or may cause masking over a portion of the range of test signals. This will elevate the open threshold of hearing and result in erroneously small values of real-ear attenuation for the device under test. Many rooms that cannot meet the ambient noise requirements in table 2 on a continuous basis will be suitable if test periods are selected during times that do meet the requirements.

4.3 Test apparatus

The test apparatus shall include a noise generator, one-third octave-band filter set, control circuits (on-off switch and calibrated attenuators), power amplifier(s), loudspeaker(s), and a head-positioning device. Computer emulation of noise generation, filtering, and control is also acceptable.

4.3.1 Signal source. The signal source shall generate one-third octave bands of pink or white noise, spectrally shaped by filters having frequency-response characteristics meeting the requirements of ANSI S1.11-1986, Order 3, Type 1-X or 2-X. The mode of operation in changing from one band to another shall be a discrete step function; a gradual continuously adjustable mode of change is not acceptable.

4.3.2 Dynamic range. The test apparatus shall be able to generate test signal sound pressure levels at the reference point, at any test band, that vary from at least 10 dB above the subject's occluded threshold of hearing, to 10 dB below the subject's open threshold of hearing. For most hearing protectors this is equivalent to a level of 60 dB above to 10 dB below the open threshold of hearing.

NOTE – The level of 10 dB below the threshold of audibility may be calculated on the basis of electrical calibration.

4.3.3 Distortion. When the test apparatus generates 1/3 octave-band test signals at the reference point, at sound pressure levels which comply with clause 4.3.2, the sound pressure levels shall be at least 6 dB down from the maximum level in adjacent 1/3 octave bands, at least 30 dB down in 1/3 octave bands one octave or more removed from the center frequency, and at least 40 dB down in 1/3 octave bands two octaves or more removed from the center frequency. During the test, the sounds shall be reproduced without audible buzzing, crackle, or rattle.

4.3.4 Control circuits. Attenuators shall have a range of at least 90 dB for each test signal, with a step size of $\leq$ 2.5 dB.

The difference in output between any two attenuator settings, measured with a pure-tone test signal, shall not differ from the indicated difference by more than 3/10 (0.3) of the indicated increment or by 1 dB, whichever is smaller. Corrections for departure from linearity shall be applied to the data when this requirement is not met. Where possible this test shall be performed acoustically. At low sound pressure levels it is also permissible to check the linearity by electrical measurement of the signal voltage at the terminals of the loudspeaker(s).

4.3.5 Signal pulsing. Test signals shall be pulsed between two, and two-and-one-half times per second, with a 50% duty cycle, and without audible clicks, pops, or other transients. When exciting the system with pure tones at the test signal center frequencies, the on-phase (the time the signal remains within 1 dB of its maximum level) shall be greater than 150 ms, and the output during the off-phase shall reach at least 20 dB below the maximum levels, as measured electrically at the speaker terminals.

4.3.6 Fitting noise. The fitting noise shall be a broadband random noise presented at an overall A-weighted sound pressure level of approximately 65 dB (re 20 μPa) at the reference point.

4.4 Head-positioning device

Some means, such as a plumb bob to the nose or the forehead of the subject, shall be used to maintain his or her head at the reference point. A headrest or bite bar is not acceptable. This device shall not transmit to the head any vibrations that might affect the measurements, or present a reflective or absorptive surface that might alter the level of the sound at the ears of the subject.

4.5 Observation of subjects during testing

The test room shall be equipped with a viewing window or video system to allow clear observation of the subject at all times during the test.

5 Test subjects

5.1 Anatomical features

Subjects shall be selected without respect to sizes and shapes of heads, pinnae and earcanals except that those with obvious abnormalities affecting the fitting of hearing protectors, such as might arise from birth defects or prior ear surgery, shall be excluded.

5.2 Otoscopic inspection

At the time of initial audiometric testing, subjects' ears, as determined by an otoscopic inspection, shall be free from impacted cerumen and obvious signs of irritation or infection in areas of the head and ears that would be contacted by the hearing protector being tested.

5.3 Measurement of earcanal size and head dimensions

Prior to audiometric qualification and participation in attenuation testing, the dimensions of both the right and left earcanals, and the bitragion width and head height of the test subject shall be measured per the procedure of annex D. The subject shall *not* be told that her or his earcanals are being sized, nor shall she/he be advised of the results of the size determinations until such time as she/he is no longer involved in the facility's subject-fit (Method B) hearing protector attenuation studies.

A suitable explanatory phrase to tell the subjects is:

"I am going to inspect your ears and measure your head using standard evaluation devices."

NOTE – If a laboratory is certain at the time of qualification of their subjects that they will only be participants in tests of earplugs (i.e., devices without bands), then head dimensions need not be measured. Likewise, earcanals need not be measured if subjects will only be used for tests of earmuffs and helmets.

5.4 Gender balance

Unless the hearing protector under test is designed to fit only males or only females, the gender balance of the test population should be 50/50±10%.

5.5 Hearing sensitivity

5.5.1 Minimum sensitivity. Subjects shall have pure-tone air-conduction hearing threshold levels at the octave-band center frequencies from 125 Hz to 8 kHz, as measured using a standard audiometer, that are ≤ 25 dB (ANSI S3.6-1996).

5.5.2 Maximum sensitivity. No subject shall be used whose 1/3 octave-band open thresholds of hearing measured in the sound field of the test room, averaged across three determinations, are

more than 3 dB below the octave-band ambient noise levels at any test frequency from 125 Hz to 8000 Hz.

NOTE – The limitations on open threshold sensitivity relative to test-room ambient noise levels are intended to reduce the potential for the elevation of the open thresholds due to masking. If masking occurs, it would tend to decrease the mean attenuations and possibly also increase the standard deviations.

5.6 Threshold variability

Subjects shall be trained with a minimum of five open-ear sound-field audiograms (separate from those utilized for attenuation testing), administered all in one session, the last three of which shall be checked for variability. The range in the open threshold of hearing for each frequency shall not exceed 6 dB. Additional practice audiograms can be administered in the same or subsequent sessions until the subject either meets the 6-dB requirement or is rejected.

5.7 Eyeglasses and jewelry

Subjects shall not wear eyeglasses, ear jewelry, or other accessories that might affect the ability of the hearing protector to make an acoustical seal.

NOTES

1 As an example of the loss of attenuation that can be caused by eyeglasses, see annex E.

2 It is permitted to stipulate specialized tests in which subjects are required to wear eyeglasses or other head-worn personal protective equipment during attenuation tests, as long as the results are so designated.

5.8 Number of subjects

Ten subjects shall be used for each test on earmuffs or helmets. Twenty subjects shall be used for each test on earplugs or semi-insert devices.

6 Product samples

6.1 Number of samples

At a minimum, the number of product samples shall equal the number of subjects, with a unique sample or samples being assigned to each subject. For formable earplugs, such as foam or fiberglass, a new pair shall be used for each trial. For other types of earplugs the manufacturer's guidance shall be followed regarding reuse of a plug by a single subject. When sized products are tested, different sizes may be used for each ear, but once testing has begun, subjects shall continue to utilize the same size product as initially selected for all repeat fittings in a given study.

6.2 Devices with variable band force adjustments

Earmuffs and semi-insert devices which include adjustment mechanisms that allow the band force to be varied shall be initially set to the visually-determined midpoint of their adjustment range prior to being provided to each subject. During fitting, the devices may be readjusted per the provisions of clauses 8.2 or 9.2.

6.3 Special requirements for subject-fit method

Products shall include complete on-package instructions in the *exact* format (i.e., same wording, size, color, and contrast) as would be provided to a purchaser of the product. No additional instructions are permitted unless they would normally accompany the product when sold in commerce.

7 Psychophysical procedure

7.1 Informing the subject

Subjects shall be completely informed regarding the test situation and procedure, and that they can withdraw from the test at any time for any reason.

7.1.1 Additional information for participants in subject-fit tests. Subjects participating in Method B (subject-fit) measurements shall be informed as follows:

> *"Because I do not want to influence the choices you will be making in the hearing protector evaluations, I cannot tell you any of your test results as long as you are a subject in this laboratory. After you complete your work as a participant on our subject-fit test panel, I will be pleased to share with you any of your results."*

7.2 Positioning the subject

The subject shall be seated in such a way that, using the head-positioning device (see clause 4.4), his or her head will be placed and maintained at the reference point (see clause 3) for all repeated measurements.

7.3 Threshold measurement procedure

The methods to be used in measuring the open and occluded thresholds of hearing shall be identical, and shall include any recognized psychophysical method or variants thereof capable of producing the data required in clause 11.1. The method used shall be reported in sufficient detail so that it may be reproduced by any facility otherwise qualified under this standard.

7.4 Number of open and occluded threshold measurements

The attenuation for each subject at all test frequencies shall be measured on two trials during a single visit to the laboratory. Each trial shall consist of a paired open and occluded threshold, the order being counterbalanced across subjects. An example of the sequence of threshold testing is provided below. The two thresholds which comprise a given trial for each subject are the first pair of open and occluded thresholds, and the second pair of open and occluded thresholds, respectively.

Representative Testing Sequence

	One-Half of the Subjects	One-Half of the Subjects
TRIAL 1	Occluded, Open	Open, Occluded
TRIAL 2	Occluded, Open	Open, Occluded

The hearing protector shall be refitted for each trial. Although a rest period may be provided between trials, the subject shall not leave the chamber during a trial, i.e., between pairs of open and occluded thresholds.

7.5 Special requirements for automatic recording audiometer

The audiogram produced by an automatic recording audiometer shall be scored as follows:

(1) A trace at a given frequency shall be repeated if, ignoring the first reversal following a change of frequency and occasional reversals associated with trace excursions of 3 dB or less;

    (a) There are less than six reversals.

    (b) Any peak is lower than any valley.

    (c) The range of excursions (any peak to valley difference) exceeds 20 dB.

(2) Acceptable traces should be scored by ignoring the first reversal following a change of fre-

quency and then averaging together an equal number of peaks and valleys of the tracing at a given frequency. Very similar results can be obtained more simply by "visual averaging," in which a horizontal line drawn through the center of the tracing is used to estimate the average value.

(3) The average value shall be rounded to the nearest whole number in decibels.

7.6 Quiet period prior to first threshold measurement

In order to allow for accommodation to the test situation, subjects shall be seated in the test room, without talking to the experimenter and with no signals present, for a minimum of two minutes prior to the initial trial of a test session, after which time the threshold determinations may begin.

7.7 Waiting period subsequent to fitting hearing protector

When hearing protectors are tested that require time to expand or conform to fit the earcanal or circumaural regions, such as slow-recovery foam earplugs, occluded threshold measurements shall begin a minimum of two and a maximum of four minutes after the hearing protectors have been fitted, unless otherwise specified in the manufacturer's written instructions, in which case the time specified will be followed.

8 Method A: experimenter-supervised fit

NOTE – See annex F for a checklist summarizing the specific steps and the sequence of events which are required to implement this method.

8.1 Conditions for subject dismissal

There shall be *no* subject selection criteria besides those specified in clauses 5.1 to 5.6, and the requirements in the following paragraph.

Prior to commencing attenuation testing, based upon visual and tactile evaluation by the experimenter working in conjunction with the subject, a subject shall be dismissed if she/he cannot obtain a good fit with the test product. Subjects not excluded by this criterion, who satisfy the other requirements of this standard, shall not be dismissed for attaining small amounts of attenuation, nor for being unable to obtain a subjectively assessed noise-blocking seal in the presence of the fitting noise as described in clause 8.2.

8.2 Test procedure

The experimenter shall give each subject precise instructions and practice in fitting the hearing protector in accordance with instructions from the manufacturer, and the experimenter's own knowledge in fitting the same or similar devices. When the product is supplied in multiple sizes, the experimenter shall assist the subject in selecting the proper size hearing protector. Although the experimenter shall provide verbal clarification or physical assistance, or both, as part of the instruction process, and may also utilize the subject's assessment of the relative loudness of the fitting noise (clause 4.3.6), trial sound attenuation measurements shall not be part of the sizing or fitting procedures. Once the experimenter has determined that the subject can properly fit the device, the hearing protector shall be removed.

For the actual test, the subject and the experimenter shall enter the test chamber, and the subject shall don the hearing protector without the assistance of the experimenter. After the hearing protector has been positioned, the fitting noise shall be introduced and the subject shall be instructed to manipulate the hearing protector to minimize the perceived noise.

Once the subject is satisfied with the fit, the experimenter shall check each hearing protector placement using only visual cues, to assure a good fit and acoustic seal. When the experimenter deems it necessary, the subject shall be required to reinsert or readjust the protectors, or both, as many times as necessary to obtain a "best" fit prior to testing, but not after the test has begun. Once the acquisition of audiometric data has commenced, further instruction to the subject or manipulation of the hearing protector is prohibited.

9 Method B: subject fit

NOTE – See annex F for a checklist summarizing the specific steps and the sequence of events which are required to implement this method.

9.1 Conditions for subject acceptance/dismissal

There shall be *no* subject selection criteria besides those specified in clauses 5.1 to 5.6, and 9.1.1 to 9.1.3. With the exception of illness or physical inability to participate on the day of the test, no subjects shall be rejected for any reasons other than failure to meet the specified requirements.

9.1.1 Experience level of subject re hearing protector usage. Measurements shall be conducted on subjects who are naive with respect to the use of hearing protection. Subjects shall be rejected if they answer "yes" to (a), (b), or (c), or if in response to (d) they indicate use of earplugs or semi-inserts for more than 10 days, or use of earmuffs for more than 60 days, in the prior two years.

(a) Have you *ever* received one-on-one personal instruction in the fitting of hearing protectors?

(b) Within the past two years, have you attended a lecture on, or watched videotaped or computer-based instruction about how to fit hearing protectors?

(c) Within the past two years, have you participated in an experiment designed to measure hearing protector noise reduction?

(d) Within the past two years, on how many days have you worn hearing protectors because you were exposed to noise as part of your occupation, military duty, or other activity, and for how many days have you worn earplugs while sleeping or swimming?

9.1.2 Literacy. Subjects shall possess a level of literacy sufficient to be able to read and understand hearing protector instructions and any informed consent forms required for use by the test laboratory.

9.1.3 Limitations on subject retention and reuse.

Once a subject has qualified to participate in a subject-fit evaluation in a given facility, she/he may be used for a maximum of 30 separate subject-fit tests, each test consisting of two trials. Of those 30 tests, the total number permissible for earplugs and semi-inserts or both, shall not exceed 12, and there shall not be more than 6 tests on any one product.

As a condition of reuse in subject-fit experiments, subjects shall receive *no feedback whatsoever* regarding how they have done on particular attenuation tests. If subjects inquire, they shall be reread the information statement in clause 7.1. Furthermore, to guard against subjects receiving any further training or experience during their tenure as a participant in subject-fit testing, they shall be asked prior to each day's testing to reaffirm 9.1.1 (a) and (b) and to again answer (d), excluding from consideration the use of hearing protectors during participation in laboratory subject-fit tests. Criteria for rejection shall be the same as in 9.1.1.

Once a subject has been deemed unsuitable for subject-fit testing due to the requirements of this clause, she/he may still be utilized for experimenter-supervised fit tests.

9.2 Test procedure

The instructions for the subject-fit method are explicit and shall be followed in every detail. The *italicized passages* in quotations shall be read aloud, verbatim, to the subject while she/he follows the text on a printed card.

9.2.1 Prior to entering test chamber. Prior to entering the test chamber, the subject shall be handed the hearing protector in the packaging in which it is sold, along with the manufacturer's written fitting instructions that would normally accompany the device. The subject shall be instructed as follows:

> "*The purpose of this test is to estimate the noise reduction that you would be likely to attain while wearing this hearing protector in a noisy environment. Please read the instructions and fit and adjust the hearing protector to the best of your ability. I am not allowed to assist you in that process.*"

The subject shall be advised of the existence and location(s) of all available manufacturer's fitting instructions, on and/or inside the individual product packaging or master dispenser. The subject shall fit and adjust the hearing protector in both ears without any verbal or physical assistance from the experimenter. No fitting noise shall be provided.

For hearing protectors which are supplied in multiple sizes, one pair of each size shall be placed on a table in front of the subject at the time that she/he is given the manufacturer's written fitting instructions. Before the subject reads the manufacturer's instructions, the experimenter shall say,

> "*Please try these protectors on to find the size that is best for you. This may be different for each of your ears. Begin by trying a middle or regular size. Then, based on the looseness or tightness of the fit and any guidance provided in the manufacturer's instructions, proceed to larger or smaller sizes as needed.*"

The experimenter shall not provide recommendations or physical assistance, present a fitting noise, or utilize sound attenuation measurements in the size-selection process.

The total fitting process, from the time the subject begins to read the manufacturer's instructions and to fit the hearing protector, until she/he enters the chamber for testing, shall not exceed 5 min. If necessary, subjects shall be advised after 4 min have expired that they shall make their best attempt at fitting the hearing protector within the next minute.

Once the subject indicates that the fitting has been completed, or 5 min have expired, she/he shall remove the hearing protector, and enter the test chamber. The subject shall then either be seated for the 2-min quiet period (clause 7.6), or be instructed by the experimenter for the occluded test and subsequently fit the hearing protector (clause 9.2.2), and then sit quietly for 2 min. Following the quiet period, the threshold testing will begin.

9.2.1.1 Insertion-assistance devices. If any type of insertion-assistance device or seating tool (such as a cylinder to slide over the flexible stem of a multiflanged earplug, or a rigid core to slide into an openbacked earplug) is provided by the manufacturer, its use by the subject shall be treated as any other aspect of the instructions. The subject shall be handed the insertion assistance device along with the hearing protector, and shown the manufacturer's written directions. Whether or not the insertion-assistance device is used is up to the subject, not the experimenter.

9.2.1.2 Custom-molded earplugs. With these types of earplugs, which of necessity require direct physical involvement between the experimenter and the subject in order to take the impression, the manufacturer's instructions shall be followed explicitly. Ear impressions will be made by the experimenter unless the manufacturer's instructions normally accompanying the product indicate that a manufacturer's representative must be involved in the process.

Once the earmold is completed, or received back from the manufacturer ready for testing, it will be provided to the subject as would any other earplug, with only the manufacturer's written instructions, unless those instructions specify that a fitter is required to individually fit and train the subject.

> NOTE – As with all aspects of the subject-fit procedure, the experimenter is not to augment manufacturer's instructions. If the manufacturer fails to require use of an eardam, the experimenter shall not use one in taking the impressions for testing, unless this contravenes the standard practices of the test laboratory or the licensure laws of the state in which the lab resides, in which case the test will have to be declined. Even if the test is accepted by the laboratory, the manufacturer shall be informed concerning the hazards of taking impressions without eardams and offered the opportunity to modify its instructions accordingly.

9.2.1.3 Custom-fitted helmets. With these types of helmets, which of necessity require direct physical involvement between the experimenter and the subject in order to custom fit the device, the manufacturer's instructions shall be followed explicitly. Once the helmet is properly customized and adjusted, it will be provided to the subject as would any other hearing protector, with only the manufacturer's written instructions.

9.2.2 Inside the test chamber. Immediately prior to the occluded threshold, the experimenter shall instruct the subject as follows:

> *"After I leave the chamber, please put on the hearing protector in the way you have just practiced. Refer to the manufacturer's instructions as needed. Once you indicate that you have completed fitting the protector, the test will begin, and you may not touch or adjust the protector until you are asked to remove it at the end of the test. If the device falls out of your ear during the test, please signal me. Throughout the test I will be able to observe you through the window [or, using the TV camera]."*

After reading the preceding statement to the subject, the experimenter shall leave the chamber. She/he shall not be present during the final fitting process **nor shall any assistance or additional explanations be provided at that time.** The subject shall be allowed a maximum of 5 min to fit the hearing protector.

9.2.3 After testing has begun. Once the test has begun, regardless of the fit of the hearing protector, or whether or not it changes position or breaks its acoustical seal, the data shall still be accepted. However, if a hearing protector falls out of the ear during the test, the experimenter shall terminate the test, enter the room and hand the subject the instructions and the earplugs, and ask him or her to reinsert the device for a retest. If the earplug falls out a second time, testing shall again be terminated, and the subject shall be replaced.

The subject shall remain in the chamber for the complete set of two open and two occluded thresholds. The subject shall be reminded that she/he may review the written instructions prior to refitting the hearing protector for the second set of measurements, **but verbal or physical assistance from the experimenter is prohibited at that time**. If a second type of hearing protector is tested during the same visit, the subject shall exit the chamber and begin the process in the same manner as during the test of the first hearing protector.

10 Band application force

The force shall be measured on all samples of earmuff and semi-insert devices initially prior to commencing attenuation testing. This requirement does not apply to helmets. Force shall be measured two min ±5 s after the hearing protector has been positioned on the test fixture, and the values reported in newtons (N). The temperature and relative humidity at which the band force is measured shall be recorded.

> NOTE – The laboratory may devise its own band force measuring device or may purchase a suitable unit. Suitable units are available from Michael and Associates, Inc., State College, PA, or INSPEC Laboratories, Ltd., Salford, UK.

10.1 Earmuffs

The force exerted by earmuffs shall be measured on a suitable fixture with rigid flat plates against which the earmuff cushions are pressed. The earcups shall be separated a distance of 145 mm±1 mm between the earcup cushions [median head width (bitragion width)], and to a distance of 130 mm ±1 mm between the inside of the headband and an imaginary line through the pivot points of the attachments of the headband to the earcups (median head height). The headband shall remain free during the measurement. For some types of products, such as those with headbands situated behind the neck or under the chin, other head-height dimensions may be more appropriate. The actual dimensions shall be reported.

10.2 Semi-insert devices

The force exerted by semi-insert devices shall be measured on a suitable fixture having flexible pinnae, the dimensions of which are specified in annex G. The bitragus breadth shall be 145 mm ± 1 mm. The head/neck band shall remain free during the measurement. For semi-inserts with adjustable bands, the band shall be set for a head height of 130mm ± 1 mm, or its minimum setting, whichever is greater. For devices with asymmetric pods, the devices shall be properly oriented to fit the concha and earcanal entrance.

11 Processing and reporting the data

11.1 Recording the data

The data to be recorded, from which the hearing protector attenuation values will be calculated, shall consist of either relative or absolute threshold values. Two open and two occluded threshold levels shall be recorded at each test frequency for each test subject.

11.2 Computation of real-ear attenuation

The measurements shall be summarized for at least each of the seven specified one-third octave-band test signals in terms of an arithmetic mean attenuation and a standard deviation. Real-ear attenuation at threshold for each listener shall be computed at each frequency by averaging the two trials, i.e., the two open/occluded threshold differences. The mean for the panel of subjects is the average of each of the individual two-trial subject averages. The standard deviations in decibels shall be computed as:

$$\sigma = \sqrt{\frac{\sum_{i=1}^{N}(d_i)^2}{N-1}},$$

where d is the difference between the average attenuation of each individual's two trials and the panel mean attenuation, and N is the number of subjects (10 for earmuffs and 20 for semi-insert devices and earplugs).

11.3 Information to be included in test report

The test report shall include the following:

(1) Reference to this American National Standard, and the type of test procedure, experimenter-supervised or subject fit;

(2) The type of hearing protector and its brand/product name, and in the case of subject-fit tests, a copy of the exact instructions that accompanied the product and were used in the test protocol;

(3) The number of subjects and repeat measurements per subject;

(4) The number of hearing protector samples tested, and any samples that were rejected and the reasons why;

(5) A table summarizing the mean real-ear attenuation at threshold values and the associ-

ated standard deviations, as a function of the frequency of the one-third octave-band test signals, as well as the data for each replication on each individual subject;

(6) In the case of hearing protectors with head or neck bands, the mean and standard deviation of the application force for all samples tested, the position (over head, under chin, or behind head) in which the force was tested, and the temperature and relative humidity at which the tests were conducted;

(7) In the case of sized products, an indication of the sizes that were actually tested, and how many subjects tested each size;

(8) In the case of subject-fit testing of earplugs provided with insertion assistance devices, the number of subjects who utilized those devices during earplug insertion;

(9) The age and gender of the subjects, and for tests of either earplugs or semi-inserts, the distribution of right and left earcanal sizes per annex D, and for tests of semi-inserts or earmuffs the mean and standard deviation of the bitragion width and head height per Annex D;

(10) Discussion of any subjects who were dismissed per clause 8.1 of the experimenter-supervised fit method, or clauses 9.1 and 9.2.3 of the subject-fit method, including reason(s) for dismissal and their age, gender, race, and earcanal sizes.

(11) Discussion of any specialized requirements that were included in the test procedures like requiring subjects to wear personal protective equipment such as safety glasses during testing of earmuffs.

11.4 Graphical presentation of the data

When attenuation data are presented graphically, the frequency scale along the abscissa shall use equal intervals for each octave band, and the ordinate shall be linear in decibels. Attenuation shall be plotted so that it increases towards the bottom of the graph. A decade in frequency shall equal from 25 to 50 dB on the ordinate, which is equivalent to ratios of from 7.5 to 15 dB/octave.

Annex A
(informative)
Features of the subject-fit protocol including rationale for use
of naive hearing protection test subjects

[This annex is not part of American National Standard Methods for Measuring the Real-Ear Attenuation of Hearing Protectors, ANSI S12.6-1997, but is included for information purposes only.]

The subject-fit protocol of this standard consists of providing hearing protection devices (HPDs) and their accompanying manufacturers' fitting instructions to test subjects, who are then directed to fit devices to the best of their ability in a way in which they would be likely to wear them in a noisy environment. Experimenter involvement is kept to an absolute minimum.

The subject-fit method was developed in order to best estimate achievable field attenuation values for groups of users. The test subjects are persons well trained in audiometric test taking, but naive with respect to use of hearing protection. The subject-fit method, which is described in detail in clause 9, is summarized in this annex, along with the rationale for the limitations it places on subject experience

with respect to use of hearing protection.

During the development of the subject-fit method the Working Group examined a multitude of procedures for conducting laboratory-based REAT measurements. Two of the primary concerns of the Working Group were to:

(1) produce a method that would yield valid estimates of field performance attained by groups of informed users,

(2) reduce as much as possible all sources of inter-laboratory variability.

Examination of existing real-world data led to a review of the importance of the experience level of subjects with respect to use of hearing protectors. Because a subject-fit procedure was selected in which the experimenter's input was limited, much depended upon the subjects' skill in reading and interpreting instructions, which in turn would be substantially affected by their prior experience with

HPDs and any previous training they may have received. The literature strongly suggested that under such conditions it was important to select subjects with as little prior practice and training in HPD usage as possible. Otherwise their performance on the current tests would likely be strongly influenced by their preconceptions and acquired level of skill (Berger, 1992).

With respect to item (2), the choice was unequivocal. Discussions among the working group members made it clear that no single definition of subject experience was consistent across laboratories. Some laboratories would select a new panel of listeners for each test, whereas others retained what they termed an "experienced" panel of test subjects. Even within the category of experienced listeners there was a wide range of background and practice. One well-known facility in the U.S. almost exclusively utilizes audiology graduate students, whereas another uses clerical staff and blue-collar workers, many of whom have residence times on the test panel exceeding five years.

To assure consistent experience levels across subject panels, which the Working Group deemed a critical variable for subject-fit type testing, the only common denominator that was feasible to define was that of a naive user of hearing protectors. This is not to be confused with lack of experience in audiometric testing. In fact, subjects with previous experience in *audiometric* test taking are welcome. The requirements for audiometric variability for the subject-fit method are no different than for the experimenter-supervised fit method, and the required ability to consistently track audiometric thresholds (range across 3 successive open thresholds of hearing ≤ 6 dB) is the same for both procedures and for the related international standard (ISO 4869-1).

The initial naiveté of subjects is defined in the standard in clause 9.1.1. Once a subject is accepted, the Working Group decided that in order to reduce the need for continuous acquisition of new listeners, subjects could be retained for tests on more than one product, as long as consistent rules were applied across all laboratories. The requirements for retention differ depending upon the type of device under test, for example, an earmuff or an earplug (see clause 9.1.3). The justification for these decisions was based upon empirical test results (Berger and Franks, 1996; Royster *et al.*, 1996).

Although the employment of naive hearing protection users for the subject-fit procedure, and the maintenance of records of their participation in tests conducted by a particular facility, may be a minor hardship for some laboratories, the benefits were deemed to far outweigh the disadvantages. With a goal of maximum validity of test results it was unacceptable to sacrifice the quality of the data by allowing the participation by subjects with varying levels of experience in the use of HPDs. For those facilities unable to comply with such requirements, an alternative is to conduct only the experimenter-supervised fit type of tests for which the subject's level of experience in HPD utilization is a less critical issue, and is not specified in the standard.

Additional key features of the subject-fit method are summarized in the remainder of this Annex.

Subject-selection criteria. With the small number of subjects that can typically be tested in any one REAT evaluation, it is not feasible to require any specific distributions based upon subject age, size, anatomical features, or race. However, a gender balance of 50/50 $\pm$ 10% is required unless the hearing protector under test is designed to fit only one gender. Additionally, subjects are required to meet hearing sensitivity and threshold variability specifications, to be free from obvious aural abnormalities, and to be literate. No other selection or rejection criterion is specified or allowed.

Explicit instructions. One of the most likely sources of interlaboratory variability is the experimenters themselves—how their experience and judgement influence the guidance they give to, and the control they exert over, the test subjects. To limit this effect, explicit instructions for working with, training, and fitting the subjects are written into the protocol, including a number of statements that experimenters are required to read, verbatim, to the subjects.

Test of the HPD-plus-its-instructions. Since the goal in modeling real-world performance is to estimate what can be achieved in practice, assessment of the HPD is accomplished in such a way as to include a test of the instructions, i.e., that which is being tested is the product the customer purchases. The product consists of the HPD *and* the instructions which accompany it. Therefore, the protocol limits instructions to only those items explicitly provided to the end user, i.e., that which would be provided to the customer upon purchase of the device being tested.

These requirements mean that if the instructions available to the consumer are small, hard-to-read letters molded into the bottom of a plastic earplug carrying case, then that is all that will be introduced into the test scenario. As a further example, if the instructions fail to indicate that the pinna should be pulled during insertion of earplugs, or neglect to mention the exact positioning or rotation of the earplug within the earcanal, the experimenter is restricted from clarifying the instructions even though his or her own experience might dictate otherwise.

Annex B
(informative)
Differences between experimenter-supervised and subject-fit attenuation data

[This annex is not part of American National Standard Methods for Measuring the Real-Ear Attenuation of Hearing Protectors, ANSI S12.6-1997, but is included for information purposes only.]

This annex provides in figure B.1 an example of the differences which can be anticipated between experimenter-supervised fit and subject-fit attenuation testing of earplugs and earmuffs. The data are taken from one of the four laboratories that participated in the interlaboratory study which was used to evaluate the protocol upon which this standard is based. The subject-fit results are the Aearo Company's E•A•RCAL^{SM} laboratory's 24-subject data from the WG11 interlaboratory study (Royster et al., 1996). The experimenter-supervised fit data are from previous unpublished measurements con- ducted in that same facility, using a panel of ten experienced hearing protection test subjects.

Note that the differences between the two sets of test results are substantial for the earplugs, but much less so for the earmuffs. This is explained by the fact that earmuffs are much less susceptible than are earplugs to the fitting, subject selection, and other human factors aspects that differentiate the two types of test procedures. Because the experimenter-supervised fit protocol allows for the intervention of experimenter judgment and for undefined experience levels of the test subjects, the differences depicted in figure B.1 will vary between laboratories, depending upon their experimenters and subject populations.

Annex C
(informative)
Precision of subject-fit real-ear attenuation measurements

[This annex is not part of American National Standard Methods for Measuring the Real-Ear Attenuation of Hearing Protectors, ANSI S12.6-1997, but is included for information purposes only.]

There is imprecision in the measurement of sound attenuation of a hearing protector according to this or any other standard. The variability arises from many sources such as: (1) uncertainty in the threshold measurement of subjects, either occluded or unoccluded, (2) variations in fitting the hearing protectors from time to time and laboratory to laboratory, (3) differences in the anatomy of the head and ear from subject to subject, and (4) differences in the acoustic test environments and test equipment from facility to facility. Data taken from four laboratories in one case and from two in another were analyzed to examine uncertainty for the subject-fit method of this standard.

For any hearing protector for which REAT is determined using the methods in this standard, it is possible to calculate the reproducibility, defined as the value below which the absolute difference between two single test results obtained with the same method on identical hearing protectors, under differ- ent conditions (different operators, different apparatus, different laboratories and/or different time), may be expected to lie. Of most interest is the reproducibility for the worst-case frequency; the test frequency for which there is the highest within- and between-subject variability.

Reproducibility can be calculated from data pooled across laboratories for a given hearing protector on a specified number of subjects, with a selected number of repeat measurements per subject. This approach was used to generate the uncertainty data in Annex A of ISO 4869-1:1990.

Another approach is to set the level of reproducibility desired, and then calculate the necessary sample size and number of repeated measurements. That is the approach taken for this standard. There are two methods for performing such calculations, one based on inferring population characteristics from available data, the other based on using confidence intervals calculated from available data. The reproducibility for the worst-case frequency can be used to infer how many subjects and repetitions per subject are required.

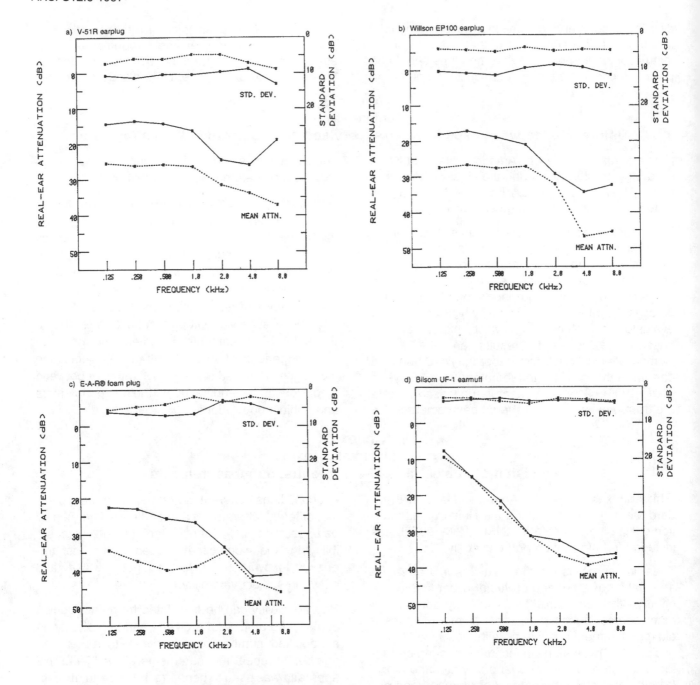

Figure B.1 – **Representative data for three types of earplugs and one earmuff, illustrating the differences to be anticipated between subject fit (————) and experimenter-supervised fit data (. . . . . . .). All test results are from one laboratory, using different listener panels for the two different fitting techniques.**

In developing the subject-fit method described in clause 9 of this standard, data collected in an inter-laboratory study (Royster *et al.*, 1996) were analyzed to determine the number of subjects and the number of repetitions per subject necessary to have reproducibility of 6 dB, i.e., a range of ±3 dB. This method, based on a hypothesis test using the F distribution, requires the desired difference, the alpha level (α), and the standard deviation, to calculate sample size. It is possible to use data collected on a few subjects to extrapolate to the larger set. When this method was applied to the inter-laboratory study with an α of 0.05, a desired reproducibility of 6 dB, and with the standard deviations from the study sample, the number of subjects for earmuff testing at the worst-case frequency (8000 Hz) was

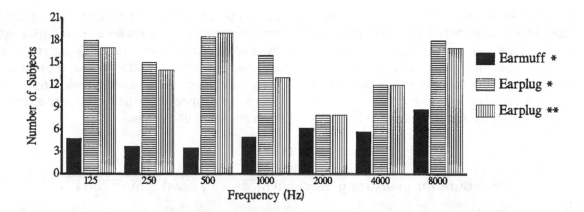

Figure C.1 – Number of required subjects with two determinations of subject-fit REAT per subject, for a reproducibility of 6 dB, for earmuffs and earplugs.
* determined using the _F_ distribution (inferential method);
** determined using a confidence interval method (confidence interval of 84%, α=0.05).

calculated to be 9, with two measurements per subject (solid bars in figure C.1). For earplug testing (worst-case frequency is 500 Hz, horizontally-hatched bars in figure C.1), the number of subjects was calculated to be 19, also with two measurements per subject.

Another way to calculate the number of subjects and number of repetitions per subject is based on a confidence interval using the _t_ distribution. A sample size is chosen such that

$$N=[S(t_{1-\alpha/2,(N-1)})/D]^2,$$

where D is the desired difference and S is an estimate of the standard deviation. In this case, _t_ is selected for the desired confidence interval, such as 84%. For the case of earplugs, the data used were taken from a follow-up to the inter-laboratory study, in which each of two laboratories tested a panel of 24 subjects three times each. The number of subjects required to achieve a reproducibility of 6 dB for earplugs was 20, with two measurements per subject (worst-case frequency is 500 Hz, vertically-hatched bars in figure C.1).

Neither approach can be applied to hearing protection devices for which the distributions of mean attenuation values are not normal. Figure C.2 shows the distributions of REATs at 125 through 8000 Hz for a foam earplug and for a single-flange pre-molded earplug. The distributions for the premolded earplug are bimodal instead of normal. Therefore, neither of the methods for calculating sample size

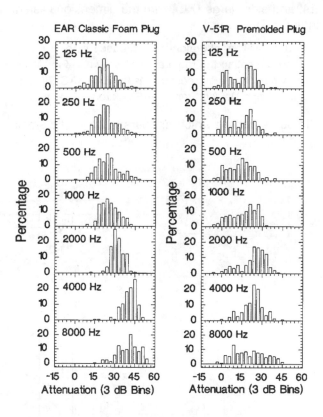

Figure C.2 – Distribution of subject-fit REATs for a foam earplug (EAR Classic—left column) and a premolded single-flange (V-51R—right column). Shown are the percentage of REATs clustered in groups of 3 dB. Data for 51 subjects were pooled from two laboratories after statistical tests show no statistical difference between the two data sets for either of the earplugs.

and number of REAT determinations per subject can be applied with any confidence, meaning that it is not possible to reliably specify the number of subjects or the number of repeat measurements per subject that will be required. Neither is it possible in this instance to calculate reproducibility.

The data analyzed for this Annex reflect best laboratory practice. It should not be assumed that such reproducibility will always be achieved. Repeatability, that is repeat measurements under the same conditions (same operator, same apparatus, and same laboratory, within a short time interval), is expected to demonstrate better values of precision than shown in this Annex.

Annex D
(normative)
Procedure for measuring earcanal sizes and head dimensions

[This annex is a mandatory part of American National Standard Methods for Measuring the Real-Ear Attenuation of Hearing Protectors, ANSI S12.6-1997.]

The device to be used for sizing earcanals is shown in figure D.1. It consists of 5 plastic spheres denoted as extra small (XS), small (S), medium (M), large (L), and extra large (XL), with the dimensions listed in figure D.1.

> NOTE – The laboratory may produce its own sizing device meeting the requirements shown in Fig. A1 or may purchase a device, such as the EARGAGE™ Earplug Sizing Device, from E-A-R/Aearo Company.

Choose a sphere which appears to be a little small for the earcanal being measured. Pull the pinna outward and upward to assist in placing the gauge in the earcanal opening until the tab of the gauge touches the floor of the concha. Release the pinna and observe if all of the earcanal opening conforms to the sphere. Then pump the gauge in the earcanal with a slight, gentle movement of about 1-2 mm. Ask the subject if she/he feels a suction or pressure. Move up in gauge size until the subject feels suction, the earcanal opening appears to conform to the sphere, *and* the gauge tab still lies on the concha floor, indicating a fully inserted sphere. The sphere accommodating these requirements represents the size of the earcanal.

If suction can only be achieved with a partial inser-

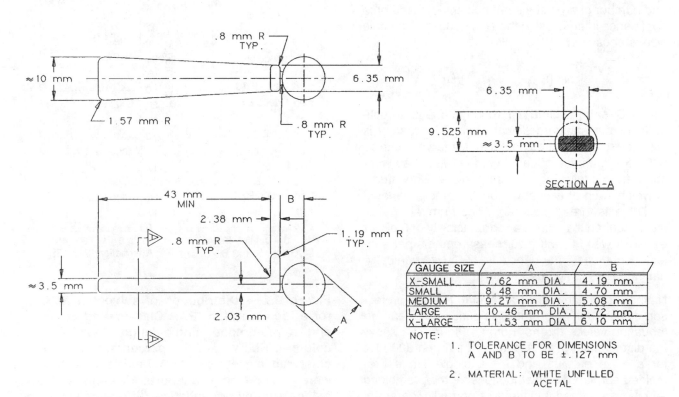

GAUGE SIZE	A	B
X-SMALL	7.62 mm DIA.	4.19 mm
SMALL	8.48 mm DIA.	4.70 mm
MEDIUM	9.27 mm DIA.	5.08 mm
LARGE	10.46 mm DIA.	5.72 mm
X-LARGE	11.53 mm DIA.	6.10 mm

NOTE:

1. TOLERANCE FOR DIMENSIONS A AND B TO BE ±.127 mm

2. MATERIAL: WHITE UNFILLED ACETAL

Figure D.1 – Dimensions of a tool to size earcanals.

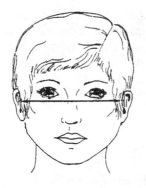

Figure D.2 Bitragion width.

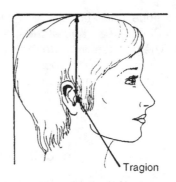

Tragion

Figure D.3 Head height.

tion, recheck the next smaller size to confirm. The assigned size will be the size that achieves a suction.

The head dimensions requiring measurement are bitragion width (commonly called head width) and

head height as illustrated in figures D.2 and D.3. The tragion (see figure D.3) is the superior point on the juncture of the tragus of the ear with the head, i.e., the notch just above the tragus. Bitragion width is normally measured with a caliper, and head height with a right angle and a straight edge.

Annex E
(informative)
Effect of eyeglasses on earmuff attenuation

[This annex is not part of American National Standard Methods for Measuring the Real-Ear Attenuation of Hearing Protectors, ANSI S12.6-1997, but is included for information purposes only.]

Any object that interferes with the circumaural seal of an earmuff against the side of the face will de-

grade its attenuation. In developing the subject-fit procedure for field-estimation purposes, three of the four facilities participating in the interlaboratory comparison experiment also tested the reference earmuff with a commonly available pair of safety glasses (Royster *et al.*, 1996). The effects on the

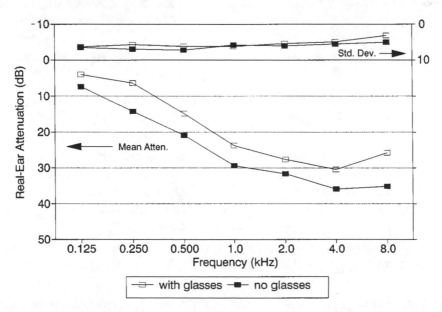

Figure E.1 – The effect of eyeglasses on the attenuation of a small-volume earmuff with foam-filled cushions, as averaged across three laboratories and 72 subjects.

mean attenuations and standard deviations, averaged across the three laboratories, are shown in figure E.1. The glasses degrade the mean attenuation approximately 5 dB across the seven test frequencies, with only a small attendant increase in variability.

For those concerned about the use of glasses with earmuffs, the data in this annex illustrate the potential magnitude of the eyeglass-effect which is both statistically and practically significant. For examples of the effects of other models of eyeglasses on a variety of earmuffs, see Nixon and Knoblach (1974).

Annex F
(informative)
Checklist for implementing Methods A and B

[This annex is not part of American National Standard Methods for Measuring the Real-Ear Attenuation of Hearing Protectors, ANSI S12.6-1997, but is included for information purposes only.]

Initial Interview and First Visit

(1) For Method B *only*, interview subject (S) prior to lab visit to verify acceptance per clauses 9.1.1. and 9.1.2.

(2) Explain study and go over informed consent (see clause 7.1).

(3) Remove jewelry and glasses if necessary.

(4) Conduct otoscopic exam (see clause 5.2).

(5) Measure earcanal sizes and head dimensions (see clause 5.3; results to be withheld from subject).

(6) Conduct screening audiogram (see clauses 5.5.1 and 5.5.2).

(7) Conduct training with minimum of 5 open-ear sound-field audiograms (see clause 5.6).

Method A: Experimenter-Supervised Fit

(1) See clauses 5.1 to 5.7 for S selection criteria and preparation. Also, S may be dismissed if a good fit cannot be obtained (see clause 8.1).

(2) **Outside chamber** (*no time limit*): help S size and fit; may give verbal and physical assistance and use fitting noise (see clause 8.2).

(3) S removes HPD and enters chamber (see clause 8.2).

(4) 2-min. quiet period, before first threshold, either before or after the HPD is fitted (see clause 7.6).

(5) **Inside chamber** (*no time limit*): Begin with open-ear test or have S fit HPD using fitting noise, but with NO ASSISTANCE from experimenter (see clause 8.2)

(6) Before actual testing, experimenter may visually check fit and require refitting for "best fit" (see clause 8.2).

(7) Measure open and occluded thresholds.

Method B: Subject Fit

(1) See clauses 5.1 to 5.7 for S selection criteria and preparation. S cannot be dismissed for any reasons pertaining to fit. Confirm S meets limitations on reuse in clause 9.1.3.

(2) **Outside chamber** (*5-min time limit*): read verbatim text to S. Hand S the HPD in original packaging to size and practice fitting with NO ASSISTANCE and no fitting noise (see clause 9.2.1).

(3) S removes HPD and enters chamber (see clause 9.2.1).

(4) 2-min. quiet period, before first threshold, either before or after the HPD is fitted (see clauses 7.6 and 9.2.1).

(5) **Inside chamber** (*5-min. time limit*): Begin with open-ear test or read verbatim text to S. Leave chamber. S fits HPD. Experimenter provides NO ASSISTANCE and no fitting noise (see clause 9.2.2).

(6) If HPD loses seal after testing begins, data are still accepted; if HPD falls out see clause 9.2.3.

(7) Measure open and occluded thresholds.

NOTE – This annex provides only an abbreviated summary of the testing requirements of this standard. The entire standard must be read and studied to properly implement the required tests.

Annex G
(normative)
Procedure for measurement of the band force of semi-inserts

[This annex is a mandatory part of American National Standard Methods for Measuring the Real-Ear Attenuation of Hearing Protectors, ANSI S12.6-1997.]

The band force for semi-inserts shall be measured with the pod separation equivalent to that observed on human heads of a median head width corresponding to that used for the earmuff measurements, namely, 145 mm. Since semi-inserts rest in the concha and not on the circumaural regions, use of flexible pinnae are required, as described in figure G.1 and table G.1, both taken from page 4 of ANSI S3.36-1985. The pinna shall have a firmness that falls between a Shore A durometer reading of 10 and 30.

> NOTE – The laboratory may produce their own pinnae meeting the requirements shown in figure G.1 and table G.1, or may purchase a device, such as the KEMAR® pinnae Models DB-065 (left ear) and DB-066 (right ear), from Knowles Electronics, Inc.

A suitable rigid plastic base in which to seat the pinna for use with typical band force measuring systems is shown in figure G.2. Note that the base includes a centrally-located recess to allow for penetration of semi-insert pods through the very shallow earcanal which is part of the flexible pinna.

Table G.1 – Pinna dimensions for force measurements of semi-insert devices, from table II of ANSI S3.36-1985.

Ear length	66 mm
Ear length above tragion	30 mm
Ear breadth	37 mm
Ear protrusion	23 mm
Ear protrusion angle	160°
Vertical tilt, front view	10°
Vertical tilt, side view	6°
Concha length	28 mm
Concha length below tragion	20 mm
Concha breadth	23 mm
Concha breadth, tragion to helix	23 mm
Concha depth	15 mm

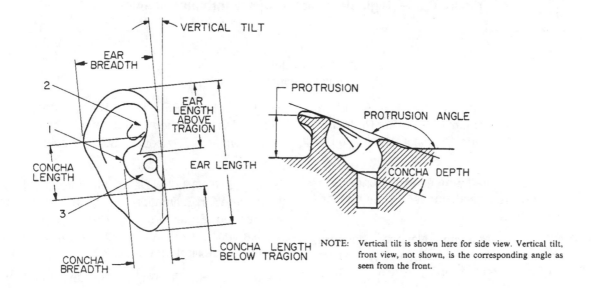

Figure G.1 – Definitions of semi-insert pinna adapter dimensions: (1) antihelix, (2) crus of helix, (3) concha.

NOTE: Vertical tilt is shown here for side view. Vertical tilt, front view, not shown, is the corresponding angle as seen from the front.

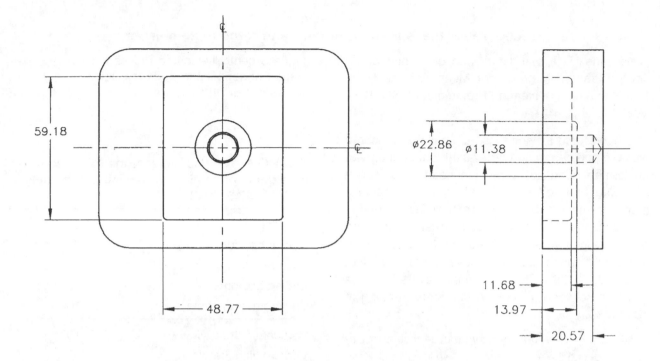

NOTES:

1. ALL DIMENSIONS IN MILLIMETERS

2. MATERIAL: POLYCARBONATE SHEET

3. BREAK ALL SHARP CORNERS AND EDGES

4. TOLERANCE TO BE ±.127 mm UNLESS OTHERWISE SPECIFIED

Figure G.2 – Rigid base plate suitable for pinna adapter.

Annex H
(informative)
Bibliography

ANSI S3.19-1974, American National Standard, Method for the Measurement of Real-Ear Protection of Hearing Protectors and Physical Attenuation of Earmuffs.

ANSI S12.13-1991, Draft American National Standard, Evaluating the Effectiveness of Hearing Conservation Programs.

ANSI Z24.22-1957, American National Standard, Method for the Measurement of the Real-Ear Attenuation of Ear Protectors at Threshold.

AS 1270-1988, Australian Standard, Acoustics—Hearing Protectors.

Berger, E. H. (1986). "Review and Tutorial - Methods of Measuring the Attenuation of Hearing Protection Devices," J. Acoust. Soc. Am. **79**(6), 1655-1687.

Berger, E. H. (1992). "Development of a Laboratory Procedure for Estimation of the Field Performance of Hearing Protectors," in *Proceedings, Hearing Conservation Conference*, Off. Eng. Serv., Univ. Kentucky, Lexington, KY, 41-45.

Berger, E. H., Franks, J. R., and Lindgren, F. (1996). "International Review of Field Studies of Hearing Protector Attenuation," in *Scientific Basis of*

Noise-Induced Hearing Loss, edited by A. Axelsson, H. Borchgrevink, R. P. Hamernik, P. Hellstrom, D. Henderson, and R. J. Salvi, Thieme Med. Publ., Inc., New York, NY, 361-377.

Berger, E. H. and Kerivan, J. E. (1983). "Influence of Physiological Noise and the Occlusion Effect on the Measurement of Real-Ear Attenuation at Threshold," J. Acoust. Soc. Am. **74**(1), 81-94.

Berger, E. H. and Franks, J. R. (1996). "The Validity of Predicting the Field Attenuation of Hearing Protectors from Laboratory Subject-Fit Data," J. Acoust. Soc. Am. **100**(4), Pt. 2, p. 2674.

Franks, J. R., Murphy, W. J., and Simon, S. D. (1996). "Repeatability and Reproducibility in Hearing Protector Testing," J. Acoust. Soc. Am. **99**(3), Pt. 2, p. 2464.

ISO 4869-1:1990, *International Organization for Standardization Acoustics - Hearing Protectors - Part 1: Subjective Method for the Measurement of Sound Attenuation.*

Nixon, C. W. and Knoblach, W. C. (1974). "Hearing Protection of Earmuffs Worn Over Eyeglasses," Aerospace Medical Research Laboratory, Rept. AMRL-TR-74-61, AD785386, available from National Technical Information Service, 5285 Port Royal Road, Springfield, VA, 22161.

Schroeter, J. and Poesselt, C. (1986). "The Use of Acoustical Test Fixtures for the Measurement of Hearing Protector Attenuation. Part II: Modeling the External Ear, Simulating Bone Conduction, and Comparing Test Fixture and Real-Ear Data," J. Acoust. Soc. Am. **80**(2), 505-527.

Royster, J. D., Berger, E. H., Merry, C. J., Nixon, C. W., Franks, J. R., Behar, A., Casali, J. G., Dixon-Ernst, C., Kieper, R. W., Mozo, B. T., Ohlin, D., and Royster, L. H. (1996). "Development of a New Standard Laboratory Protocol for Estimating the Field Effectiveness of Hearing Protection Devices, Part I: Research of Working Group 11, Accredited Standards Committee S12, Noise," J. Acoust. Soc. Am. **99**(3), 1506-1526.

STANDARDS SECRETARIAT
ACOUSTICAL SOCIETY OF AMERICA

The Standards Publication Program of the Acoustical Society of America (ASA) is the responsibility of the ASA Committee on Standards (ASACOS) and the ASA Standards Secretariat, headed by its Standards Manager.

The Acoustical Society of America provides the Secretariat for four Accredited Standards Committees of the American National Standards Institute (ANSI): S1 on Acoustics, S2 on Mechanical Vibration and Shock, S3 on Bioacoustics, and S12 on Noise.

These four Accredited Standards Committees also provide the United States input to various international committees (IEC and ISO). Standards Committees S1 Acoustics and S3 Bioacoustics provide the United States input to ISO/TC 43 Acoustics, and IEC/TC 29 Electroacoustics, as the Technical Advisory Groups. S12 on Noise serves as the U.S. Technical Advisory Group for ISO/TC 43/SC1 Noise, and for ISO/TC 94/SC12 Hearing Protection. S3 is the Technical Advisory Group for ISO/TC 108/SC4 Human Exposure to Mechanical Vibration and Shock. S2 serves as the U.S. Technical Advisory Group for ISO/TC 108/SC1, Balancing, including Balancing Machines, ISO/TC 108/SC2 Measurement and Evaluation of Mechanical Vibration and Shock as Applied to Machines, Vehicles, and Structures; ISO/TC 108/SC3 Use and Calibration of Vibration and Shock Measuring Instruments; ISO/TC 108/SC5 Condition Monitoring and Diagnostics of Machines; and ISO/TC 108/SC6 Vibration and Shock Generating Equipment.

ASACOS and the ASA Standards Secretariat provide the Secretariat for the U.S. Technical Advisory Groups listed above and administer the international Secretariat for ISO/TC 108 Mechanical Vibration and Shock, ISO/TC 108/SC1 Balancing Machines, and ISO/TC 108/SC5 Condition Monitoring and Diagnostics of Machines.

Standards are produced in four broad areas: physical acoustics, mechanical shock and vibration, bioacoustics, and noise, and are reaffirmed or revised every five years. The latest information on current ANSI standards as well as those under preparation is available from the ASA Standards Secretariat. For information, please contact:

Standards Secretariat,
Acoustical Society of America
35 Pinelawn Road, Suite 114E
Melville, New York 11747-3177
Telephone: (631) 390-0215
Fax: (631) 390-0217
Email: asastds@aip.org

MEMBERSHIP OF THE ASA COMMITTEE ON STANDARDS (ASACOS)

T. F. W. Embleton, *Chair and ASA Standards Director*

80 Sheardown Drive
Box 786, Nobleton
Ontario, Canada L0G 1N0

Tel: +1 905 859-1136
Fax: +1 905 859-1136

D. L. Johnson, *Vice Chair*

EG & G MS1
P. O. Box 9100
Albuquerque, NM 87119

Tel: +1 505 846-4252
Fax: +1 505 255-2985

A. Brenig, *Standards Manager*

Standards Secretariat
Acoustical Society of America
120 Wall Street, 32nd Floor
New York, NY 10005-3993

Tel: +1 212 248-0373
Fax: +1 212 248-0146

Representation S1, Acoustics
J. Seiler, *Chair, S1*
   ASA Representative, S1
G. S. K. Wong, *Vice Chair, S1*
   ASA Alternate Representation, S1

Representation S2, Mechanical Vibration and Shock
D. J. Evans, *Chair, S2*
   ASA Representative, S2
R. F. Taddeo, *Vice Chair, S2*
   ASA Alternate Representative, S2

Representation S3, Bioacoustics
T. Frank, *Chair, S3*
   ASA Representative, S3
R. F. Burkard, *Vice Chair, S3*
   ASA Alternate Representative, S3

Representation S12, Noise
P. D. Schomer, *Chair, S12*
   ASA Representative, S12
B. M. Brooks, *Vice Chair, S12*
W. J. Galloway, *ASA Alternate Representative, S12*

Technical Committee Representation
A. I. Tolstoy, *Acoustical Oceanography*
A. Bowles, *Animal Bioacoustics*
G. E. Winzer, *Architectural Acoustics*
S. J. Bolanowski, Jr., *Bioresponse to Vibration and to Ultrasound*
M. D. Burkhard, *Engineering Acoustics*
W. D. Ward, *Musical Acoustics*
A. S. Bommer, *Noise*
R. A. Roy, *Physical Acoustics*
R. S. Schlauch, *Psychological and Physiological Acoustics*
A. Schmidt-Nielsen, *Speech Communication*
L. A. Herstein, *Structural Acoustics and Vibration*
A. L. Van Buren, *Underwater Acoustics*

***Ex Officio* Members of ASACOS (nonvoting)**

P. Kuhl, *Chair, ASA Technical Council*
W. W. Lang, *ASA Treasurer*
A. Brenig, *ASA Representative to the Acoustical Standards Board (ASB) of the American National Standards Institute (ANSI)*
K. M. Eldred, *Past Chair ASACOS*
C. E. Schmid, *ASA Executive Director*

U. S. Technical Advisory Group (TAG) Chairs for International Technical Committees (nonvoting)
P. D. Schomer, *Chair, U. S. TAG, ISO/TC 43 and ISO TC 43/SC1*
E. H. Berger, *Chair, U.S. TAG, ISO/TC 94/SC12*
V. Nedzelnitsky, *Chair, U. S. TAG, IEC/TC 29*
D. Muster, *Chair, U. S. TAG, ISO/TC 108*

Appendix P
ANSI Technical Report
Evaluating the Effectiveness of Hearing Conservation Programs through Audiometric Data Base Analysis

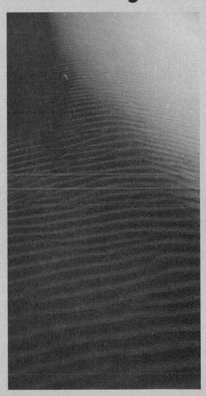

ANSI TECHNICAL REPORT

Evaluating the Effectiveness of Hearing Conservation Programs through Audiometric Data Base Analysis

ANSI S12.13 TR–2002

Accredited Standards Committee S12, Noise

Acoustical Society of America
Standards Secretariat
35 Pinelawn Road, Suite 114E
Melville, New York 11747-3177

The American National Standards Institute, Inc. (ANSI) is the national coordinator of voluntary standards development and the clearinghouse in the U.S.A. for information on national and international standards.

The Acoustical Society of America (ASA) is an organization of scientists and engineers formed in 1929 to increase and diffuse the knowledge of acoustics and to promote its practical applications.

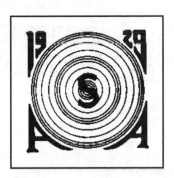

ANSI Technical Report

Evaluating the Effectiveness of Hearing Conservation Programs through Audiometric Data Base Analysis

Secretariat

Acoustical Society of America

ANSI Technical Report Registered: 26 August 2002

American National Standards Institute, Inc.

ABSTRACT

This ANSI Technical Report describes methods for evaluating the effectiveness of hearing conservation programs in preventing occupational noise-induced hearing loss by using techniques for audiometric data base analysis. The rationale is given for using the variability of threshold measurements in annual monitoring audiograms as the basis for judging effectiveness. Guidelines are discussed concerning how to select a restricted data base to which the analysis procedures will be applied. Specific procedures for data analysis are defined, and criterion ranges are given for classifying program effectiveness as acceptable, marginal, or unacceptable. Sample results for industrial audiometric data bases contributed to Working Group S12/WG12 are included as an annex for reference and illustration.

AMERICAN NATIONAL STANDARDS ON ACOUSTICS

The Acoustical Society of America (ASA) provides the Secretariat for Accredited Standards Committees S1 on Acoustics, S2 on Mechanical Vibration and Shock, S3 on Bioacoustics, and S12 on Noise. These committees have wide representation from the technical community (manufacturers, consumers, trade associations, general-interest and government representatives). The standards are published by the Acoustical Society of America through the American Institute of Physics as American National Standards after approval by their respective standards committees and the American National Standards Institute.

These standards are developed and published as a public service to provide standards useful to the public, industry, and consumers, and to federal, state and local governments.

Each of the Accredited Standards Committees [operating in accordance with procedures approved by American National Standards Institute (ANSI)] is responsible for developing, voting upon, and maintaining or revising its own standards. The ASA Standards Secretariat administers committee organization and activity, and provides liaison between the Accredited Standards Committees and ANSI. After the standards have been produced and adopted by the Accredited Standards Committees, and approved as American National Standards by ANSI, the ASA Standards Secretariat arranges for their publication and distribution.

An American National Standard implies a consensus of those substantially concerned with its scope and provisions. Consensus is established when, in the judgment of the ANSI Board of Standards Review, substantial agreement has been reached by directly and materially affected interests. Substantial agreement means much more than a simple majority, but not necessarily unanimity. Consensus requires that all views and objections be considered, and that a concerted effort be made toward their resolution.

The use of an American National Standard is completely voluntary. Their existence does not in any respect preclude anyone, whether he has approved the standards or not, from manufacturing, marketing, purchasing, or using products, processes, or procedures not conforming to the standards.

NOTICE: This Technical Report may be revised or withdrawn at any time. The procedures of the American National Standards Institute require that action be taken periodically to reaffirm, revise, or withdraw a standard.

Standards Secretariat
Acoustical Society of America
35 Pinelawn Road, Suite 114E
Melville, New York 11747-3177
Telephone   631-390-0215
FAX   631-390-0217
E-mail   asastds@aip.org

Contents

Figures

FOREWORD

[This foreword is for information only and is not an integral part of ANSI S12.13 TR - 2002 *ANSI Technical Report Evaluating the Effectiveness of Hearing Conservation Programs through Audiometric Data Base Analysis*]

This ANSI Technical Report is a revision of Draft American National Standard S12.13-1991, which was published for a period of trial use and comment regarding the validity and usefulness of the recommended procedures for evaluating the effectiveness of hearing conservation programs (HCPs) through audiometric data base analysis (ADBA), and later unsuccessfully balloted for approval as a full standard. The ADBA procedures described are those recommended by the members of S12 Working Group 12 (S12/WG12) based on the results from their original research in applying suggested procedures to actual audiometric data bases (see Annex C), as well as the additional experience and feedback obtained from S12/WG12 members and other interested users following publication of the draft standard.

In spite of the unsuccessful ballot to convert the draft standard to a full standard, S12 deemed the contents of the document of substantial value for the hearing conservation community, and hence decided to publish them for guidance as an ANSI Technical Report. The substantive negative comments during the balloting involved the following issues:

a) the possibility that gradual hearing loss in excess of that due to aging may occur in subgroups of the population evaluated in spite of acceptable ADBA criteria results on a year-to-year basis,

b) objections to the year-to-year nature of ADBA evaluations, which intentionally provide a set of indicators with values that vary annually to reflect current HCP status changes to alert personnel to incipient problems (in contrast to a single overall indicator across a long period of time),

c) concern that an inadequate selection of restricted groups for analysis by the evaluator might lead to failure to detect that different subgroups of the HCP population may show lesser degrees of protection from noise than the group selected for analysis,

d) the derivation of the numerical ranges for the criteria,

e) the fact that this results-oriented method does not address failures of omission by the HCP (such as failure to identify and include all noise-exposed individuals in the program) or failures of implementation by the HCP (such as failure to provide annual educational programs).

The Working Group chair did not elect to pursue reversal of the negative votes because the scope of changes desired by negative voters would have fundamentally altered the nature of the document. The ADBA method was developed as a tool for evaluating HCP effectiveness in terms of audiometric data variability from year to year. Other types of methods that reflect cumulative hearing loss over time are briefly described in Annexes A and B, but the intent of this document was to describe only the ADBA method.

Publication of this ANSI Technical Report has been approved by the Acoustical Society of America. This document is registered as a Technical Report in a series of publications according to the Procedures for the Registration of ANSI Technical Reports. This document is not an American National Standard and the material contained herein is not normative in nature. Comments on the content of this document should be sent to the following address:

Acoustical Society of America
Standards Secretariat
35 Pinelawn Road, Suite 114E
Melville, New York 11747-3177
Tel: 631-390-0215
Fax: 631-390-0217
E-Mail: asastds@aip.org

This ANSI Technical Report was developed under the jurisdiction of Accredited Standards Committee S12, Noise, which has the following scope:

Standards, specifications, and terminology in the field of acoustical noise pertaining to methods of measurement, evaluation, and control, including biological safety, tolerance, and comfort, and physical acoustics as related to environmental and occupational noise.

At the time this ANSI Technical Report was submitted to Accredited Standards Committee S12, Noise, for final approval, the membership was as follows:

P.D. Schomer, *Chair*
R.D. Hellweg, *Vice Chair*
S. Blaeser, *Secretary*

Abbott Labs . . . . .D. Walton, B.Muto (Alt.)
Acoustical Society of America (ASA) . . . . .B.M. Brooks, W.J. Galloway (Alt.)
Air-conditioning & Refrigeration Institute . . . . .R. Seel, M. Darbeau (Alt.)
Aluminum Company of America (ALCOA) . . . . .W.D. Gallagher
American Academy of Otolaryngology–Head & Neck Surgery, Inc. (AAO–HNS) . . .R.A. Dobie, L.A. Michael (Alt.)
American Industrial Hygiene Association (AIHA) . . . . .D. Driscoll, J. Banach (Alt.)
American Otological Society (AOS) . . . . .R.F. Naunton
American Speech-Language-Hearing Assoc. (ASHA) . . . . .G. Linn, R. Levinson (Alt.)
Audio Engineering Society, Inc. (AES) . . . . .M.R. Chial, D. Queen (Alt.)
Brüel & Kjaer Instruments, Inc. . . . . .M. Alexander, J. Chou (Alt.)
Caterpillar, Inc. . . . . .K.G. Meitl, D. Roley (Alt.)
Compressed Air and Gas Institute . . . . .J.H. Addington, D.R. Bookshar (Alt.)
Council for Accreditation in Occupational Hearing Conservation (CAOHC) . . . . .R.D. Bruce, E.H. Berger (Alt.)
E-A-R/Aearo Company . . . . .E.H. Berger
Howard Leight Industries . . . . .V. Larson, E. Woo (Alt.)
Information Technology Industry Council (ITI) . . . . .R.D. Hellweg, W.H. Johnson (Alt.)
Institute of Noise Control Engineering (INCE) . . . . .B. Tinianov, M. Lucas (Alt.)
International Safety Equipment Association (ISEA) . . . . .J. Birkner, J.C. Bradley (Alt.)
James, Anderson & Associates (JAA) . . . . .L.D. Hager, R.R. Anderson (Alt.)
Larson·Davis, Inc. . . . . .L. Davis, L. Harbaugh (Alt.)
National Council of Acoustical Consultants (NCAC) . . . . .J. Erdreich
National Hearing Conservation Association (NHCA) . . . . .K. Michael
Noise Pollution Clearinghouse . . . . .L. Blomberg
North American Insulation Manufacturers Association . . . . .R. Godfrey, R. Moulder (Alt.)
Power Tool Institute, Inc. . . . . .S. Broadbent, J. Nosko (Alt.)

U.S. Air Force . . . . .R. McKinley
U.S. Army Aeromedical Research Lab . . . . .W. Ahroon, D. Ostler (Alt.)
U.S. Army Center For Health Promotional and Preventative Medicine . . . . .G.A. Luz, W.A. Russell (Alt.)
U.S. Army Construction Engineering Lab (USCERL) . . . . L. Pater
U.S. Army Human Research & Engineering Directorate (HRED) . . . . .J. Kalb, T.R. Letowski (Alt.)
U.S. Department of Transportation . . . . .A. Konheim
U.S. Naval Surface Warfare Center (NSWC) . . . . .S.A. Fisher, J. Niemiec (Alt.)

Individual Experts of Accredited Standards Committee S12, Noise, were:

P.K. Baade	R.D. Hellwig	P.D. Schomer
R.W. Benson	R.K. Hillquist	J.P. Seiler
L. Beranek	D.L. Johnson	L.C. Sutherland
E.H. Berger	W.W. Lang	W.R. Thornton
S.H.P. Bly	G.C. Maling	H.E. von Gierke
B.M. Brooks	A.H. Marsh	L.A. Wilber
K.M. Eldred	R.J. Peppin	G.E. Winzer
L.S. Finegold	J. Pope	G.S.K. Wong
W.J. Galloway	L.H. Royster	R.W. Young

Working Group S12/WG12, Evaluation of Hearing Conservation Programs, which assisted Accredited Standards Committee S12, Noise, in the preparation of this ANSI Technical Report, had the following membership:

J.D. Royster, *Chair*

E.H. Berger, *Vice-Chair*

A. Behar	M.M. McDaniel	T.Y. Schulz
C. Dixon-Ernst	S.C. Megerson	A.P. Stewart
J.R. Franks	W. Melnick	A. Suter
J.W. Jabara	M. Roberts	E. Toothman
D.L. Johnson	L.H. Royster	

When preparation of this ANSI Technical Report was begun, Larry H. Royster was WG chair.

Suggestions for improvement will be welcomed. Send suggestions for improvement to Accredited Standards Committee S12, Noise, in care of the ASA Standards Secretariat, 35 Pinelawn Road, Suite 114E, Melville, New York 11747-3177.

Telephone: +1 631-390-0215; FAX: +1 631-390-0217.

Evaluating the Effectiveness of Hearing Conservation Programs through Audiometric Data Base Analysis

0 INTRODUCTION

0.1 Need

Hearing conservation programs (HCPs) have been implemented in occupational, military, and other settings to protect noise-exposed populations from developing occupational hearing loss, which negatively affects individuals' quality of life. For industry in the U.S.A., the Occupational Safety and Health Administration (OSHA) has promulgated regulations defining minimum standards which the employer must follow in implementing an HCP. Similar requirements also exist for the mining industry (regulated by the Mine Safety and Health Administration) and HCPs in the military. However, these regulations currently give no guidance for determining program effectiveness.

Without evaluation procedures based on objective data, it is difficult for the personnel responsible for administering the HCP to determine whether the program is actually preventing occupational noise-induced hearing loss. Several authors [5–13] have discussed the need for systematic procedures to assess whether noise-exposed populations are being adequately protected and to identify any inadequacies in the HCP. The goal of standardizing procedures for audiometric data base analysis (ADBA) is to give objective data concerning HCP effectiveness to management, to the key individual responsible for the entire HCP, and to other personnel involved in implementing the program (safety professionals, industrial hygienists, noise control engineers, audiometric technicians, fitters of hearing protectors, audiologists, medical directors, and departmental supervisors who enforce hearing protector utilization). HCP personnel need information about the program's performance to make decisions about HCP policies, to achieve and maintain adequate employee protection, to justify resource allocations, and to motivate supervisors and employees [11,12]. In addition, a method for using audiometric data to judge HCP effectiveness could be useful to regulatory compliance officers.

0.2 Rationale

Because the purpose of HCPs is to prevent occupational hearing loss, the results of monitoring audiometry for noise-exposed personnel provide the obvious test of whether the HCP has been successful. However, audiogram results cannot alert the audiologist or physician reviewer to incipient hearing loss if the threshold measurements are so variable that beginning hearing shifts cannot be identified. Likewise, unreliable data invalidate attempts to assess long-term population hearing level trends. Even if the noise-exposed population is not developing occupational hearing loss, poor quality audiometric monitoring data render the HCP ineffective because professional audiogram reviewers cannot discriminate spurious threshold shifts from real hearing changes. The employer is penalized by having to deal with follow-up actions for shift rates which are inflated by poor quality data.

This report provides procedures for evaluating HCP effectiveness based on the variability in serial monitoring audiometry for the noise-exposed population. Year-to-year audiometric variability is selected as the basis for the ADBA procedures specified in this report because it provides an immediate indication of data problems. The evaluator is alerted by the high variability to investigate whether it results from inadequate protection from occupational noise, or from poor control of audiometric testing factors. Either way, corrective actions can be taken before many individual employees develop significant threshold shifts.

0.3 Alternative Approaches

Other valid approaches using population audiometric data to judge HCP effectiveness exist, but they are not amenable to standardization because their use requires the evaluator to make case-by-case judgments rather than applying a fixed set of criterion ranges to the results. For the reader's convenience, some of these techniques are summarized in Annex A.

Annual rates of OSHA standard threshold shifts (STSs) are frequently used as a measure of HCP effectiveness, but these rates cannot be interpreted in a meaningful way without knowing relevant characteristics of both the noise-exposed population and the audiometric data. Therefore, OSHA STS rates do not provide an indicator which is amenable to standardization. Further details are provided for the reader in Annex B.

Checklist or audit approaches to evaluating HCPs are also in common use, but these approaches usually merely tally the observed completeness of a program, or its nominal regulatory compliance, without assessing the quality of the program elements that are present. Sample checklists are available which attempt to address qualitative factors [14,15]. However, the usefulness of such audits depends on the expertise of the evaluator in recognizing the difference between cursory lip service to program requirements versus meaningful implementation.

Task-based statistics regarding HCP implementation (such as the percentage of audiograms administered on time, the percentage of retests obtained promptly, the percentage of employees observed to be wearing hearing protectors, etc.) provide information that is useful to administrators, but these data do not indicate how well employees were actually protected from noise. Likewise, exposure statistics (such as the percent of the workforce in potentially hazardous noise, or reductions in daily noise exposures) are also useful, but they do not address the effectiveness of the HCP in preventing noise-induced hearing damage for those workers who are exposed.

0.4 Brief Historical Review

Summaries of research to analyze industrial hearing data have been published [5,12,13]. The first known use of audiometric data by a regulatory agency occurred in 1971, when the North Carolina OSHA program reserved the option not to issue a noise citation to a company where workers' OSHA time-weighted average noise exposures (TWAs) exceeded 90 dBA if the company had a good safety record, had implemented a complete HCP, *and* would make available the company's audiometric records for analysis [16]. Governmental evaluation of group audiometric data is currently practiced in British Columbia, Canada, where the Worker's Compensation Board of British Columbia receives audiometric results annually from each employer, processes the records, and reports to the employer various statistics concerning the data which allow different employers' HCPs to be compared [17].

0.5 Report Development Process

The S12 Working Group 12 (S12/WG12) was reorganized during the spring of 1984 with a strong emphasis on participation by representatives of industries and organizations that would be the most likely users of any recommendations made by the committee. Working group members were selected for their experience and involvement with HCPs. To create a large data base which S12/WG12 could use for its research, all working group members with access to HCP audiometric data bases were required to make them available for study purposes. It was stipulated that only the chair and the member of S12/WG12 primarily responsible for data analysis would know the sources of the data.

As a result of the requirement for data contribution by working group members and the collection of additional industrial data bases by L.H. Royster, S12/WG12 formulated the largest known industrial audiometric data base available for research purposes in the USA. All procedures suggested by members as potentially useful analysis techniques were tested by applying them to the contributed data bases. The results from these analyses performed on behalf of the working group enabled the members to compare different techniques and develop criterion ranges for selected procedures.

S12/WG12 recommendations were published as Draft ANSI S12.13-1991, which included criterion ranges for three procedures. The research undertaken by S12/WG12 in developing their draft standard is described as Annex C, which includes summary analysis results.

Further experience with the procedures, as well as comments received from other users, led S12/WG12 to eliminate one of the draft standard procedures (standard deviation of differences in hearing threshold levels) from the current report because it proved less sensitive to data quality than the two remaining procedures, which are also simpler to use.

0.6 Benefits of ADBA

0.6.1 Enhancing Prevention of Noise-Induced Hearing Loss

In occupational HCPs in the U.S.A. today, audiometry is typically conducted only for the purpose of determining if any employees have developed a standard threshold shift (STS), defined by OSHA's Hearing Conservation Amendment [18] as a change of 10 dB or more in the average of hearing levels at 2, 3, and 4 kHz in either ear from baseline values (usually with optional age corrections applied). In the U.S. military services, audiograms are reviewed to detect both OSHA STSs and another defined shift [19]. Few HCPs review audiograms to detect and follow up on other non-regulated significant hearing shifts in individuals, and very few analyze group data to evaluate program performance except by annual STS rates (see Annex A). Therefore, the potential of the audiometric data base to indicate HCP effectiveness is largely untapped.

Annual audiometry has been criticized in the literature [20–22] based on the high variability of hearing threshold measurements and the resulting difficulty in reliably detecting the small hearing shifts expected in sensitive individuals with typical daily exposures (most OSHA TWAs are less than 90 dBA). However, this criticism of audiometry is invalid if audiometric data are used to detect increased variability from temporary threshold shift in the population before the assumed related permanent hearing loss becomes detectable. In addition, if ADBA is used to identify and correct excess variability related to testing factors, then smaller shifts can be recognized. The concept of detecting high variability in the hearing threshold level measurements before permanent hearing loss develops is fundamental to ADBA.

Consider a worker who is hired and placed in the company's HCP, as shown in Figure 1. He or she may or may not be provided hearing protection devices based on the daily time-weighted average noise exposure. If the worker must develop an OSHA STS or another significant shift before we get an indication of possible HCP ineffectiveness, then it is difficult to justify the cost of audiometry which merely documents the occurrence of hearing loss. However, if ADBA procedures are used to detect and correct HCP problems early in the worker's noise exposure history, then audiometry becomes a powerful tool in preventing significant noise-induced hearing loss.

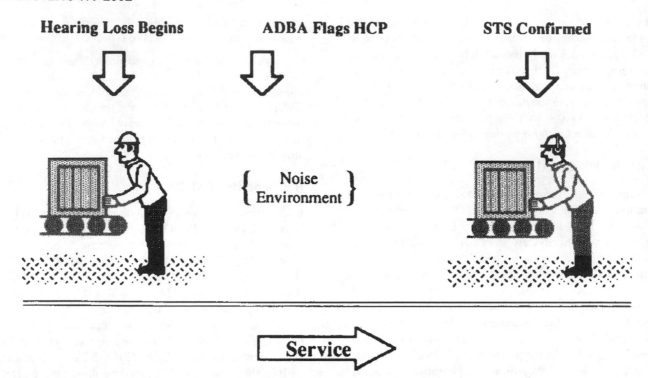

Figure 1. Sequence of events in a worker's noise exposure history showing how ADBA indicates an inadequate degree of employee protection before a confirmed OSHA STS develops.

0.6.2 Providing Cost-Effective Data for Regulatory Compliance Current federal OSHA enforcement policies may exempt an employer from implementing engineering noise controls if employees' OSHA TWA noise exposures are less than 100 dBA and an effective HCP has been established; however, there is no accepted method of making a judgment concerning program effectiveness. ADBA results could help in this decision. In the future, if OSHA implemented a method of obtaining audiometric data from employers, then compliance inspectors could use their limited time more efficiently by selectively visiting plant sites where ADBA results suggested the existence of problems in the HCP. Acceptable ADBA results for a plant could be interpreted as an overall performance indicator of an adequate program.

0.6.3 Guiding Internal Management Decisions The application of ADBA procedures provides a cost-effective method of HCP evaluation for management. If managers can determine that the HCP is ineffective, they have the opportunity to correct any problems and thereby avoid potential OSHA citations. More importantly, managers will be warned of HCP problems before many employees develop significant hearing changes which may reduce their productivity and eventually could develop into workers' compensation claims.

ADBA results not only can identify an ineffective HCP, but they also can point to the potential cause(s) of the problem. With this information, managers can make changes to prevent hearing loss. If unsatisfactory ADBA findings are similar across plant sites or departments, the existence of a shared problem or problems can be inferred. Examples include failure to enforce the use of hearing protection devices, to provide the worker with adequate instructions for fitting and wearing the hearing protection devices correctly, to allow sufficient time to obtain valid hearing threshold level measurements, or to use audiometric results to motivate employees.

In contrast, ADBA findings may show different patterns of results for population subgroups, suggesting specific problems. Examples include the relative adequacy of different hearing protection devices for the noise environment [23], differences in training for hearing protector utilization, differences in enforcement of hearing protector use, errors in audiometer calibration, or changes in audiometric methods resulting in abnormally high variability in hearing threshold level measurements.

If high variability is found to be related to testing factors rather than to noise exposure, management can take steps to improve in-house audiometry or to change mobile test service providers in order to obtain more reliable data.

In effective HCPs the total potential legal and social risk resulting from noise-induced hearing loss at the production facility would be expected to decrease over time in comparison to the risk which would have occurred for an ineffective program. The yearly ADBA results will provide objective data to show management the benefits of an effective HCP in reducing potential liability for workers' compensation by stopping the progression of occupational hearing loss.

With respect to workers' compensation claims, too often the records of companies with ineffective HCPs simply document the progression of significant hearing loss over time. If management uses ADBA procedures to guide improvement of the HCP, then records could document the overall effectiveness of the program as well as the preventive actions taken for individuals. ADBA results could provide management with information to support the quality of the company's efforts in contested compensation claims for occupational hearing loss.

0.6.4 Motivating Workers and Supervisors Some workers are more motivated by concrete data than they are by persuasive communications from management or other HCP personnel. Posting simplified summaries from yearly applications of ADBA procedures across different plant sites and/or production areas may enhance workers' interest in the HCP. If management takes the next step and uses the findings in evaluating supervisors of production areas during periodic performance appraisals, then a strong incentive is created to achieve consistent, correct use of hearing protection devices.

1 SCOPE, PURPOSE AND APPLICATIONS

1.1 Scope

This report specifies procedures for systematically assessing the effectiveness of hearing conservation programs (HCPs) in preventing noise-induced hearing loss based on the variability of regular monitoring audiometry results for noise-exposed personnel. Test-to-test variability in hearing thresholds measured in successive audiograms is used as the basis of two statistical indicators. Criterion ranges are given for the results of these indicators as applied to populations of noise-exposed personnel followed over time.

The application of the procedures specified in this report is one facet of audiometric data base analysis (ADBA), which also includes related techniques described in Annex A.

1.2 Purpose

The goal of ADBA—to evaluate the degree of protection for populations in hearing conservation programs—is complementary to the purpose of detecting hearing changes in individual noise-exposed employees. In audiogram review the records for a person are examined to detect significant cumulative hearing change from the initial or baseline audiogram and to trigger any follow-up actions needed to increase the degree of protection for that particular person. In contrast, ADBA is a separate process of evaluating group audiometric data to monitor the degree of protection provided to the noise-exposed population as a whole, or in selected subgroups such as departments or noise exposure groups. If ADBA results show undesirable trends, the follow-up action involves changes in overall HCP policies or procedures rather than changes in the treatment of individual employees [10–12].

The purpose of this report is to define objective procedures for evaluating HCP effectiveness in preventing occupational noise-induced hearing loss in a noise-exposed population through ADBA procedures which evaluate the variability of the serial audiometric data for the noise-exposed population as a whole or for selected subgroups.

The intended users of these procedures include industrial or military personnel directly responsible for HCPs, as well as related professionals providing consulting services in support of HCPs, and public health or regulatory agency personnel interested in evaluating HCP effectiveness. These personnel can use information about HCP effectiveness to reinforce good HCP implementation, or to identify deficiencies and justify program improvements, thereby increasing the degree of protection for the noise-exposed population before many individuals show significant hearing changes.

1.3 Applications

The fundamental assumptions underlying the ADBA approach to evaluating HCP effectiveness are described below. In addition, certain requirements are described that the audiometric data must meet before the approach can validly be applied.

1.3.1 Assumptions

1.3.1.1 Effective Hearing Conservation Program An effective HCP provides the noise-exposed population with adequate protection from on-the-job noise exposures so that changes in their hearing threshold levels over time are not different from those found in a properly matched control population which exhibits all of the relevant characteristics of the occupational noise-exposed population except on-the-job noise exposure. Characteristics which should be accounted for in a matched control population include age, sex, race, the incidence of ear disease, and non-occupational noise exposure.

1.3.1.2 Audiometric Variability as an Indicator The year-to-year variability in the population's hearing threshold levels as measured during approximately annual HCP audiometric evaluations is a valid indicator of the effectiveness of the HCP. For a population of noise-exposed workers who are properly protected from on-the-job noise, the year-to-year variability in their hearing threshold levels will be no larger than that for a similar population without significant occupational noise exposure. It is implied that the only way to achieve a satisfactorily low level of variability in the data base is to establish an effective HCP that prevents both temporary threshold shift and permanent occupational hearing loss [10].

The recommended ADBA procedures are based on the variability of hearing threshold level measurements between sequential pairs of audiograms, not comparison of later audiograms back to the initial test or to a revised baseline audiogram. The use of criteria involving baseline comparisons was rejected for two reasons:

1) such procedures place unmerited confidence in the validity of the baseline hearing level measurements and the comparability of baseline and later tests, and

2) after several years, comparisons to baseline hearing threshold levels require consideration of corrections for age-related hearing loss, which may be inappropriate for individuals with substantial pre-existing hearing loss on the baseline test (see ANSI S3.44-1996 [R2001]) [4], and which require selection of appropriate reference age-effects data.

1.3.1.3 Analysis of a Restricted Data Base If the ADBA results for a representative sample data base from the exposed population indicate the HCP to be effective, then it is assumed that the HCP is also effective in protecting all other workers included in the HCP but who were not included in the restricted data base (such as recently hired workers). If the workers included in the restricted data base are being properly protected from the noise, it is unlikely that on a year-to-year basis the workers not included in the analyzed data base would have received different treatment resulting in a different degree of protection. However, if there are small groups of employees with substantially higher noise exposures than the rest of the population, the evaluator may choose to analyze their data separately for a group-specific test of adequate protection from noise.

1.3.1.4 Reliance on ADBA Results ADBA techniques assess an HCP for adequacy, not for perfection. As long as the results of ADBA procedures indicate that an HCP is effective, then even if some undesirable characteristics are observed (such as inconsistent use of hearing protection devices), the overall program should still be judged as adequate in preventing noise-induced hearing loss. It is true that superior HCP implementation will be necessary to adequately protect young, previously non-noise-exposed personnel working in a high OSHA TWA, compared to those required to adequately protect older employees with pre-existing hearing loss working in a low-noise-exposure environment. In each case ADBA techniques assess the adequacy of the HCP in its own context.

1.3.1.5 Interpretation of Undesirable Results If the results from applying ADBA procedures indicate that the effectiveness of the HCP is marginal or unacceptable, the evaluator must be careful in interpreting the findings. High variability does not necessarily mean that the noise-exposed population has received inadequate protection and is developing noise-induced hearing loss. High variability may result from inadequate control of the acoustic environment for audiometry, audiometer calibration, or audiometric testing techniques. Such factors do prevent the HCP from being effective because true hearing threshold shifts for individuals cannot be detected if the audiometric data are unreliable. Therefore, it is necessary to control audiometric testing factors in order to achieve reliable data. To identify potential problems in audiometric testing the evaluator needs to examine the HCP's documentation regarding whether OSHA requirements [18] have been met, as well as to determine whether the audiometric practices have been consistent with more stringent ANSI standards (see section 2).

1.3.2 Data Requirements

Before the procedures for ADBA recommended in this report may be used to evaluate the degree of protection from noise exposure for a population, the data must meet certain requirements.

1.3.2.1 Annual Audiometry The audiograms must be administered approximately annually. If the average intervals between sequential audiograms are greater than 24 months, the criterion ranges defined in this report might not be appropriate.

1.3.2.2 Constant Restricted Population The user must restrict the population to a constant group for analysis. That is, for each year during the time period to be analyzed, the group membership must consist of the same individuals.

1.3.2.3 Minimum Number of Audiograms All members of the restricted population must have received a specified minimum number of audiograms, with this minimum number (two or more) being selected by the evaluator.

1.3.2.4 Representative Restricted Population Ideally the restricted population will include all available employees who have received the minimum number of audiograms. However, if it is necessary in a very large population to reduce the size of the group for analysis, then the selected group should be representative of the total. For example, employees from certain job categories (such as maintenance workers) should not be excluded because their compliance with requirements for utilization of hearing protection devices is more difficult to monitor.

1.3.2.5 Minimum Size of Restricted Population A minimum of 30 people per restricted group is suggested. Although ADBA procedures have been applied successfully to smaller groups, the percentage values of the statistics will be more reliable if the groups include at least 30.

1.3.2.6 Identification of Obvious Contaminants in the Data The user should examine the mean hearing threshold levels at each audiometric test frequency for the restricted group over the time period to be analyzed in order to identify any abrupt shifts which might indicate artifacts from equipment malfunction or calibration changes. Discrete calibration deviations will affect the ADBA statistics for the involved tests, but the data may still be usable if the problem is accounted for. However, if the data are completely unreliable, then they can not be used for ADBA or for hearing trend analysis.

1.3.2.7 Audiometric Testing During Workshifts Because ADBA procedures utilize the variability of annual hearing threshold level measurements as an indication of the adequacy of a population's degree of protection from noise exposure, it is essential that audiograms be obtained when there is an opportunity to observe any temporary threshold shift which might be present. Therefore, the audiometric data to which ADBA techniques are applied must be obtained at varying times during the normal course of the workshift (not prior to the beginning of the employee's workshift) except for the baseline audiogram, which should be conducted without prior noise exposure to avoid TTS. For annual audiograms, employees should wear their customary hearing protection devices in their usual manner on the day of the audiogram, not take special precautions to avoid temporary threshold shift (such as by wearing earmuffs, for example).

2 REFERENCES

At the time of approval of this ANSI Technical Report by the American National Standards Institute, the standards referenced below were valid. All standards are subject to revision, and parties to agreements based on this Technical Report are encouraged to investigate the possibility of applying the most recent editions of the standards listed below.

[1] ANSI S1.1-1994 (R1999), *American National Standard—Acoustical Terminology.*

[2] ANSI S3.20-1995 (R1999), *American National Standard—Bioacoustical Terminology.*

[3] ANSI S3.21-1978 (R1997), *American National Standard Method for Manual Pure-Tone Threshold Audiometry.*

[4] ANSI S3.44-1996 (R2001), *American National Standard—Determination of Occupational Noise Exposure and Estimation of Noise-Induced Hearing Impairment.*

[5] Melnick, W., "Evaluation of industrial hearing conservation programs: A review and analysis," *American Industrial Hygiene Association Journal,* 1984, 45: 459–467.

[6] Royster, L.H. and Royster, J.D., "Making the most out of the audiometric data base," *Sound and Vibration,* 1984, 18(5): 18–24.

[7] Royster, J.D. and Royster, L.H., "Using audiometric data base analysis," *Journal of Occupational Medicine,* 1986, 28(10): 1055–1068.

[8] Suter, A.H., "The need for and benefits of audiometric data base analysis," *Sound and Vibration,* 1989, 23(12): 14–16.

[9] Stewart, A.P., "The comprehensive hearing conservation program," in *Hearing Conservation in Industry, Schools, and the Military,* edited by D.M. Lipscomb. Boston, MA: College-Hill Publications, 1988.

[10] Royster, L.H. and Royster, J.D., "Important elements and characteristics of hearing conservation programs and determination of their effectiveness," *Environment International,* 1990, 16: 339–352.

[11] Royster, L.H. and Royster, J.D., "Getting started in audiometric data base analysis," *Seminars in Hearing,* 1988, 9: 325–338.

[12] Royster, J.D. and Royster, L.H., "Evaluating hearing conservation program effectiveness," in *The Noise Manual, 5th edition,* edited by E.H. Berger, L.H. Royster, J.D. Royster, D.P. Driscoll, and M.E. Layne. Fairfax, VA: American Industrial Hygiene Association, 2000.

[13] Dobie, R.A., "Prevention of noise-induced hearing loss," *Archives of Otolaryngology Head and Neck Surgery,* 1995, 121: 385–391.

[14] Royster, J.D. and Royster, L.H., *Hearing Conservation Programs: Practical Guidelines for Success,* Chelsea, MI: Lewis Publishers, 1990.

[15] Franks, J.R., Stephenson, M.R. and Merry, C.J., *Preventing Occupational Hearing Loss — A Practical Guide,* U.S. Department of Health and Human Services (NIOSH) Publication No. 96–110.

[16] Royster, L.H. and Creel, W.C., *A Recommended Compliance Plan for Evaluation by Industry in Developing an Effective Hearing Conservation Program,* Raleigh, NC: North Carolina Department of Labor, 1972.

[17] Roberts, M., "Hearing conservation: the British Columbia experience," *Spectrum* (the National Hearing Conservation Association Newsletter), 1989, 6(1), 10–13.

[18] Occupational Safety and Health Administration, "Occupational noise exposure; hearing conservation amendment; final rule," *Federal Register,* 1983: 48, 9738–9785.

[19] Department of Defense. DoD Instruction 6055.12 Hearing Conservation Program, dated April 22, 1996. Available at this website:
http://web7.whs.osd.mil/text/i605512p.txt

[20] Hetu, R., "Critical analysis of the effectiveness of secondary prevention of occupational hearing loss," *Journal of Occupational Medicine,* 1979, 21: 251–254.

[21] Atherley, G. and Johnston, N., "Audiometry — the ultimate test of success?," *Annals of Occupational Hygiene,* 1981, 27: 427–447.

[22] Macrae, J.H., "Improved detection of hearing threshold impairment caused by occupational noise exposure," *Australian Journal of Audiology,* 1994, 16: 25–35.

[23] Royster, L.H., Royster, J.D. and Cecich, T.F., "An evaluation of the effectiveness of three hearing protection devices at an industrial facility with a TWA of 107 dB(A)," *Journal of the Acoustical Society of America,* 1984, 76: 485–497.

NOTE — With regard to ANSI Standards, "R" stands for reaffirmed, as in [1].

3 DEFINITIONS

Throughout this ANSI Technical Report the terms and definitions given in ANSI S1.1-1994 (R2001) [1] and ANSI S3.20-1995 (R 1999) [2], as well as the definitions given below, apply.

baseline audiogram. Audiogram against which the results of later audiograms are compared during the review of the audiometric records for an individual in a hearing conservation program. This is usually the first audiogram obtained from the individual. However, a revised baseline may be established by the audiologist or physician reviewing the audiometric records if revision is needed to reflect persistent significant improvement in hearing thresholds or persistent worsening of hearing thresholds comprising an OSHA STS or other shift defined by regulatory agencies.

hearing level for pure tones. Hearing threshold of a given ear at a specified frequency and for a specified type of transducer when measured with an audiometer calibrated to reference equivalent threshold levels for air or bone conduction. Abbreviation HL.

hearing threshold. For a specified signal, the minimum sound pressure level (or vibratory force level for bone conducted stimuli) that is capable of evoking an auditory sensation in a specified fraction of trials. A pure-tone threshold measurement procedure is described in ANSI S3.21-1978 (R 1997) [3] which recommends defining threshold as the lowest signal level at which responses occur in at least 50% of a series of ascending trials.

> NOTES
>
> 1 The characteristics of the signal, the way it is presented to the subject, and the method by which the sound pressure level or force level is measured must be specified.
>
> 2 Sound pressure levels and force levels are relative to the standard reference of 20 µPa and 1 µN, respectively.

reference equivalent threshold level. At a specified frequency, for a specified type of transducer, and for a specified type of coupler or artificial ear or artificial mastoid, is the modal value, at that frequency, of the equivalent threshold levels of an adequately large number of ears of otologically normal subjects within the inclusive age limits 18 to 30 years.

temporary threshold shift. A temporary increase in the measured hearing level for an ear at a specified frequency. Temporary threshold shift is by definition reversible and does not imply destruction of inner ear hair cells but only fatigue or reversible injury. When the shift is due to noise exposure to sounds with peak sound pressure levels less than 140 dB, recovery from temporary threshold shift is usually complete within 16 hours. Temporary threshold shift may be superimposed on a permanent or persistent threshold shift. Abbreviation TTS.

4 RECOMMENDED ADBA STATISTICS

4.1 Procedures

Two indicators of variability in measured hearing levels are recommended which are based on comparisons of sequential approximately annual audiograms, such as test 1 to test 2, test 2 to test 3, test 3 to test 4, etc., excluding retest audiograms (see 5.1). The two statistics are defined as follows:

Percent Worse Sequential (%W_s): the percent of the population which shows a shift of 15 dB or more toward worse hearing at any test frequency (0.5 to 6 kHz) in either ear between two sequential audiograms.

Percent Better or Worse Sequential (%BW_s): the percent of the population which shows a shift of 15 dB or more either toward better hearing or toward worse hearing at any test frequency (0.5 to 6 kHz) in either ear between two sequential audiograms.

4.2 Criterion Ranges

The criterion ranges for the %W_s and %BW_s statistics are shown as Table 1. Criterion ranges for evaluating the results of the recommended ADBA statistics are given separately for sequential comparisons of the first four audiograms (comparisons of tests 1-2, 2-3 and 3-4) and for sequential comparisons of later audiograms (comparisons of tests 4-5, 5-6, 6-7 and higher). There are no criterion ranges shown for the %BW_s procedure over tests 1-4 because the influence of learning-effect improvement in measured hearing levels [11,12] complicates interpretation of this statistic during early tests.

Table 1. Criterion ranges (in percent) for rating HCP performance using the values of the statistics Percent Worse Sequential and Percent Better or Worse Sequential.

HCP Rating	Sequential comparisons of any of the first four tests (1-2, 2-3, or 3-4)	Sequential comparisons of any later tests (4-5, 5-6, 6-7, etc.)	
	%W_s	%W_s	BW_s
Acceptable	< 20	< 17	< 26
Marginal	20 to 30	17 to 27	26 to 40
Unacceptable	> 30	> 27	> 40

5 IMPLEMENTING THE PROCEDURES

5.1 Selecting the Restricted Data Base

Since the criterion ranges for interpreting ADBA results differ for the first three sequential comparisons versus for later audiograms, the evaluator must consider the number of available audiograms when selecting the restricted data base. In order to be able to detect potential audiometric calibration problems, the evaluator must keep audiograms from the same years together, restricting the data base to those employees whose desired audiograms (such as test 1, test 5, etc.) occurred in the same year.

The restricted data base must have constant group membership over the time period selected for analysis. That is, the same employees must be included in the restricted data base from beginning to end, with no dropouts and no new employees added.

For ADBA purposes, only one audiogram per year per employee should be included in the restricted data base. Therefore, if an employee received one or more retests in a single year, one audiogram should be selected for inclusion in the data base for ADBA. If retesting was performed due to threshold shifts consistent with temporary threshold shift on the first audiogram in that year, then the first audiogram should be included in the data base for ADBA. If retesting was performed due to non-noise-related factors, then the most valid audiogram should be included.

5.1.1 Early Tests For a HCP which has not yet accumulated many years of annual audiometric data, evaluation of the first two to four audiograms is the only choice. The data base should be restricted to the largest possible number of employees who have received the maximum number of annual audiograms all beginning in the same calendar year, and with the latest audiogram included occurring during the most recent year of testing.

For example, if an analysis is to be conducted in 1990 for a HCP which began audiometric testing in 1988, the evaluator might restrict the data base to all employees who have received three annual audiograms, with the first test in 1988 and the third test in 1990.

5.1.2 Later Tests For an HCP which has many years of audiometric data available, the evaluator can decide what type of restricted data base would yield the desired information. It might be appropriate to restrict the data to the first N tests for all employees with at least N annual tests (8 or 10, for example) and whose first test was in a selected year (such as the first year the HCP was implemented).

For an HCP with a very large number of annual audiograms, the evaluator might want to consider only the most recent few years of data for all employees with at least N tests, providing the first of the most recent few tests is test number 4 or higher. Because the criterion ranges for the results of ADBA procedures are the same for sequential comparisons of test numbers 4-5 and all later tests (see Table 1), it is acceptable to evaluate the year-to-year variability for employees with different numbers of audiograms as long as the restricted data base includes only audiograms which are test number 4 or higher. For example, the evaluator might restrict the data to all employees who received annual audiograms in 1986, 1987, 1988, and 1989 as long as the 1986 test was number 4 or higher. The advantage of this approach is that a larger number of employees can be included in the restricted data base than

if only employees who all have had exactly the same number of audiograms were selected.

5.2 Examining the Data for Contamination

Once the restricted data base has been formed, the mean (average) hearing levels at each audiometric test frequency are calculated for each year of testing included in the data base. These mean hearing levels are plotted in order to look for aberrations in the data which affect variability and which might make the data unusable for analyzing hearing trends. The most common type of data contamination is abnormal shifts in hearing levels due to inadequately controlled audiometric calibration procedures [7,11] or differences between test paradigms for different audiometers (such as self-recording versus microprocessor audiometers, or two different microprocessor audiometers).

ADBA statistics can still be applied even if this type of systematic hearing level aberration is found. The ADBA statistics will be skewed in the year of the aberration, but the impact will depend on whether the systematic change raised or lowered measured hearing levels. For example, a systematic shift toward increased hearing level values will cause increases in both $\%W_s$ and $\%BW_s$. However, a systematic shift toward decreased hearing level values will cause a decrease in $\%W_s$ and an increase in $\%BW_s$.

ADBA statistics correctly identify these aberrations as causing increased variability in hearing levels. In contrast, such systematic aberrations (especially those causing decreased hearing level measurements) may not be obvious from examination of annual STS rates, even though the aberrations do affect these rates. Long-term hearing level trend analyses are invalidated by such aberrations unless adjustments can be made (see Annex A).

5.3 Applying the ADBA Procedures

In addition to the instructions given below, an illustration for sample data is provided as Annex D to assist users in making sure they are correctly interpreting the procedures.

5.3.1 Percent Worse Sequential ($\%W_s$) For each of the desired sequential test comparisons (such as test 1 to test 2 or test 5 to test 6), count the number of individuals in the restricted data base who showed a shift of 15 dB or more toward worse hearing at any audiometric frequency from 0.5 to 6 kHz in either ear. Divide this count by the total number of individuals in the restricted data base and multiply by 100% to obtain the percentage.

5.3.2 Percent Better or Worse Sequential ($\%BW_s$) For each of the desired sequential test comparisons, count the number of individuals in the restricted data base who showed a shift of 15 dB or more either toward better hearing or toward worse hearing at any audiometric frequency from 0.5 to 6 kHz in either ear. Divide this count by the total number of individuals in the restricted data base and multiply by 100% to obtain the percentage.

6 INTERPRETING THE RESULTS

6.1 Classifying HCP Effectiveness

After the values for the two recommended ADBA statistics have been obtained for the restricted population being evaluated, the results for each sequential comparison are compared to the criterion ranges given in Table 1. For any given sequential comparison (such as test 2 to test 3), if the values obtained for both statistics fall into one range, then the effectiveness of the HCP may be classified as acceptable, marginal, or unacceptable for the year represented by that sequential comparison. However, if the results obtained for the two ADBA statistics in a given sequential test comparison do not fall within a single range, then the effectiveness of the HCP must be interpreted as spanning the criterion ranges involved (for example, marginal to unacceptable).

Over multiple years, the criterion ranges into which the ADBA statistic results fall may vary from one year to the next, reflecting changes in audiometric data variability. For example, an HCP might be rated as acceptable for several years, then marginal in the following year due to some change (such as the relaxation of HPD use requirements, or a change in audiometric testing procedures).

Identification of audiometric variability changes is an advantage of ADBA compared to historical hearing level trend analyses over many years. The ADBA statistics allow changes in data quality to be detected immediately, enabling HCP personnel to look for the causes and correct those problems identified.

6.2 Identifying Sources of High Variability

If the effectiveness of the HCP is indicated as marginal or unacceptable in any sequential test comparison, then the evaluator must determine whether the high variability for that comparison is due to:

a) poor control of the audiometric phase of the HCP (acoustic environment for testing, audiometer calibration consistency, earphone placement, testing methods, and subject instructions and motivation),

b) an inadequate degree of protection from occupational noise exposure due to deficiencies in HCP elements (employee education and motivation; hearing protection device selection, fitting, or utilization; or engineering and administrative noise control efforts), or

c) some other factor.

In interpreting ADBA results, it is highly desirable to acquire audiometric data for an internal control group of non-noise-exposed employees tested annually under the same conditions as the personnel in the HCP. Excess audiometric variability for this control group clearly implies causes unrelated to occupational noise, such as audiometric testing factors. Differences in ADBA results between the control group and noise-exposed groups implicate occupational noise as a cause.

For a detailed analysis, the evaluator may want to compare the results for separate departments or noise exposure categories, groups of employees wearing different hearing protectors, groups of employees tested by different technicians or using different audiometric equipment, or other appropriate subgroups in order to identify the reasons for the high data variability. If problems in HCP implementation are identified, the evaluator can use the ADBA results to demonstrate the need for program improvements in order to increase the degree of protection from noise exposure for the population.

ANNEX A
(Informative)

POPULATION COMPARISON ADBA TECHNIQUES

Hearing level data for noise-exposed populations may be compared to reference age-effect hearing level data either at a single point in time, or longitudinally in terms of hearing level changes. However, because noise-induced permanent threshold shift (NIPTS) develops gradually, especially at moderate noise exposures, the passage of considerable time is required before HCP success or failure can be assessed by such comparisons. In addition, the comparison may be misleading if an inappropriate reference data base is selected. For further discussion, see reference [A1] and S3.44-1996 [4].

A.1 Comparisons at One Point in Time

In this approach the median hearing levels for a noise-exposed group in the HCP are compared to the expected age-effect reference data for a population without occupational noise exposure. If the two populations are comparable in all respects except for occupational noise, then the difference in their hearing levels represents the typical amount of NIPTS present.

This approach is useful in estimating the reduction in NIPTS for employees who were hired after the initiation of an HCP, compared to employees of the same age group who worked for a given number of years prior to HCP implementation.

Examples of this type of population comparison may be found in references [A2–A7].

A.2 Comparisons of Longitudinal Hearing Level Trends

Longitudinal changes in hearing for a noise-exposed population in an effective HCP should be no greater than age-effect reference population trends. However, the rate of change in hearing is affected by the amount of pre-existing hearing loss present, as described in ANSI S3.44-1996 (R2001). Therefore, hearing change rates for HCP groups with pre-existing loss exceeding reference age-effect hearing levels cannot validly be compared to change rates for reference age-effect data bases without occupational NIPTS. Furthermore, the comparison depends upon whether an appropriate age-effect reference population has been selected to be comparable to the HCP population in all important factors other than occupational noise exposure.

For further discussion, see reference [A1].

A.3 References

[A1] Royster, J.D. and Royster, L.H., "Evaluating hearing conservation program effectiveness," in *The Noise Manual, 5th edition,* edited by E.H. Berger, L.H. Royster, J.D. Royster, D.P. Driscoll, and M.E. Layne. Fairfax, VA: American Industrial Hygiene Association, 2000.

[A2] Pelausa, E.O., Abel, S.M., Simard, J. and Dempsey, I., "Prevention of noise-induced hearing loss in the Canadian military," *Journal of Otolaryngology,* 1995, 24: 271–280.

[A3] Roberts, M., "Has the hearing conservation program worked?," in the proceedings of the 22nd annual conference of the National Hearing Conservation Association. Denver, CO: National Hearing Conservation Association, 1997.

[A4] Rosler, G., "Progression of hearing loss caused by occupational noise," *Scandinavian Audiology,* 1994, 23: 13–37.

[A5] Savell, J.F. and Toothman, E.H., "Group mean hearing threshold changes in a noise-exposed industrial population using personal hearing protectors," *American Industrial Hygiene Association Journal,* 1987, 48: 23–27.

[A6] Schulz, T.Y., "Alternative methods to evaluate hearing conservation program effectiveness," in the proceedings of the 21st annual conference of the National Hearing Conservation Association. Denver, CO: National Hearing Conservation Association, 1996.

[A7] Wolgemuth, K.S., Luttrell, W.E., Kamhi, A.G., and Wark, D.J., "The effectiveness of the Navy's hearing conservation program," *Military Medicine* 1995, 160: 219–22.

ANNEX B
(Informative)

RATES OF OSHA STS AS AN INDICATOR

B.1 Common Use of STS Rates

OSHA requires employers under its jurisdiction to perform follow-up actions to increase the degree of protection for employees whose audiometric records exhibit STS from baseline values. Therefore, the purpose of OSHA STS (to react to a defined cumulative indiv-idual hearing change) is fundamentally different from the purpose of ADBA to evaluate overall HCP effectiveness. Nevertheless, because annual rates of new OSHA STSs are available to employers and are relevant to the follow-up effort required of the employer, management often attempts to use STS rates as a measure of HCP performance.

B.2 Reasons for Excluding STS Rates from this Report

S12/WG12 rejected STS rates as a potentially standardizable indicator because such rates depend on factors including the following:

1. Whether the baseline audiogram and subsequent audiograms are obtained under comparable testing procedures (i.e., using the same test methods, types of audiometer, etc.),

2. Whether OSHA-allowed age corrections are used,

3. The amount of pre-existing hearing loss in the population at the time of the baseline audiogram,

4. The average age and years of service of the population,

5. The degree of employment turnover in the population,

6. The baseline revision practices of the audiologist or physician who reviews individual audiometric records,

7. Whether baselines have already been revised for persistent STS in a substantial percentage of employees (greatly reducing the probability of an additional STS).

In general, although high STS rates indicate problems with audiometric data and/or an ineffective HCP, low STS rates do not necessarily indicate that the HCP is effective, due to the factors listed above.

B.3 References

If the reader is interested in other research concerning STS rates, several references are provided below.

[B1] Royster, J.D. and Stewart, A.P., "What affects STS rates?," in the proceedings of the 22nd annual conference of the National Hearing Conservation Association. Denver, CO: National Hearing Conservation Association, 1997.

[B2] Simpson, T.H., McDonald, D. and Stewart, M., "Factors affecting laterality of standard threshold shift in occupational hearing conservation programs," *Ear & Hearing* 1993, 14: 322–331.

[B3] Simpson, T.H., Stewart, M. and. Kaltenbach, J.A., "Early indicators of hearing conservation program performance," *Journal of the American Academy of Audiology,* 1994, 5: 300–306.

ANNEX C
(Informative)
RESEARCH PERFORMED BY S12/WG12

This annex presents the research conducted by S12/WG12 on the HCP audiometric data bases made available to the committee for analysis.

C.1 Data Tape Availability

As a consequence of the requirement for data contribution by S12/WG12 members and the collection of additional industrial data bases by the first WG chair, S12/WG12 formulated the largest known publicly available occupational audiometric data base in the U.S.A. The two members of the working group with the primary responsibility for receiving the data and carrying out the various statistical analyses requested by S12/WG12 were able to obtain a contract from NIOSH for the purpose of checking the accuracy of the data and organizing the data on a tape to be made available to the general public. Parties interested in obtaining a copy of this data base should send their request to NTIS, Springfield, VA 22161 [(703) 487-4650] and request PB88-117916/KHX (Industrial Audiometric Data).

The NTIS audiometric data base includes data from twenty-two companies representing various types of industries from different areas of the U.S.A. and Canada. The data base contains data used by S12/WG12 from the time of its reorganization in 1984 up through 1986. The data were taken as received from the contributing sources; S12/WG12 had no way of verifying the reported data except by questionnaires to the data donors. There were 15,297 employees with at least four audiograms within the 22 data sets and 3,958 employees with at least 8 audiograms. Included on the tape are control data bases of low-noise or non-noise-exposed individuals. Note that the noise-exposure classification in the data sets applies only to the year of each audiogram; therefore, the subjects indicated as non-exposed may have had prior occupational noise exposure.

Since the summer of 1986, S12/WG12 has obtained several additional data bases and some of the earlier data bases have been updated. However, S12/WG12 has not obtained any additional funding to support updating the data base available to the general public through NTIS.

C.2 Procedures Evaluated

When S12/WG12 began considering procedures for assessment of HCP effectiveness, they evaluated not only procedures that had been previously discussed in the literature [A1-A7, C1-C8], but also newer procedures recommended by WG members. Some of the procedures studied yielded results that would not support their continued investigation or consideration.

One procedure that was dropped was the attempt to correlate the slopes of HTL trends at different test frequencies with program effectiveness. This effort may have failed due to the limited number of audiograms available (eight annual tests) for the populations studied, of which only the last four tests could provide a slope indication free of the learning-effect improvement [A1, C2, C5, C7]. Another factor which inhibited the usefulness of slope data was the existence of apparent calibration deviations in several data bases. However, a more fundamental problem with this approach is the differential susceptibility to additional NIPTS for populations with differing amounts of pre-existing hearing loss, from none to a substantial amount.

Of the various procedures investigated, the main focus of the working group's investigation was a consideration of the following procedures for comparisons of **sequential** pairs of annual audiograms:

(a) Percent Better Sequential ($\%B_s$), a 15-dB shift at any test frequency (0.5 to 6 kHz) in either ear toward better hearing [A4, A7],

(b) Percent Worse Sequential ($\%W_s$), a 15-dB shift at any test frequency (0.5 to 6 kHz) in either ear toward worse hearing [A4, A7],

(c) Percent Better or Worse Sequential ($\%BW_s$), a 15-dB shift at any test frequency (0.5 to 6 kHz) in either ear toward either better or worse hearing [C4, C7],

(d) the American Academy of Otolaryngology—Head and Neck Surgery (AAO-HNS) shift, which is a change of 10 dB or more in either ear in the average of HTLs at 0.5, 1, and 2 kHz or in the average of HTLs at 3, 4, and 6 kHz [C9],

(e) the standard deviation of differences across the population in binaurally averaged HTLs between sequential audiograms, calculated at the individual test frequencies from 0.5 to 6 kHz and for three frequency averages: 0.5, 1, 2, 3 kHz, 2, 3, 4 kHz and 3, 4, 6 kHz, and

(f) the OSHA standard threshold shift: a change of 10 dB or more in either ear in the average of HTLs at 2, 3, and 4 kHz [C10].

The use of criteria employing comparisons to the baseline or initial audiogram was rejected because such procedures place unmerited confidence in the validity of the baseline HTL measurements, and the comparability of baseline tests to later tests. They also require that the data be corrected for aging, which may be inappropriate if the individual already has substantial pre-existing hearing loss (see ANSI S3.44-1996 [R2001]) [4].

C.3 Recommended Procedures

The ADBA procedures evaluated thus far which have proved most easily applied and which yield the widest ranges of results (thereby allowing greater ability to discriminate among different HCPs) are procedures (b) and (c) as defined above.

Note that the $\%BW_s$ procedure is used only for sequential comparisons of tests higher than test number 5. During the earlier audiometric tests, improvements in measured hearing threshold levels due to the learning effect may cause the $\%BW_s$ value to be large if the population is well protected from noise exposure [C2, C7]. Therefore, this statistic can be used for ADBA purposes only after the learning effect has diminished, in sequential test comparisons 4-5 and later.

C.4 Data Base Comparisons Used to Define Criterion Ranges

S12/WG12 had available 17 data bases exhibiting a sufficient number of workers with at least eight approximately annual audiometric evaluations to be analyzed. For each data base that exhibited a sufficient number of subjects by race, the data bases were further subdivided, resulting in a total of 25 data bases. Due to the small number of females, *only male employees* were included.

Four data bases (which were divided into seven single-race study populations) were utilized as controls. Two control data bases consisted of low-noise-exposed populations with time-weighted average noise exposures (TWAs) less than 87 dBA. Two populations with higher TWAs were designated as controls because several years of personal experience with their HCPs and on-site observations indicated that the quality of HPD fitting and utilization in these programs was sufficiently strict to make them useful in control comparisons. In addition, comparison of audiometric variability for noise-exposed and non-noise-exposed subgroups within these two data bases indicated equivalent protection for the exposed HPD wearers and the non-exposed employees.

The remaining data bases available to S12/WG12 were simply designated as non-controls because less information was available about them. No assumption was made concerning the level of protection for employees in these programs.

The findings from applying the selected ADBA procedures to both the control and non-control population data bases are presented in Figures C1 through C13.

These figures show the distribution of values obtained in the control and non-control data bases, plotted as notched box and whisker plots. These plots illustrate the range of the data, the median value, and also the degree of skewness in the data. The height of the central box covers the middle 50% of the data values, between the lower and upper quartiles. The whiskers (vertical lines) generally extend out to the extremes (minimum and maximum values) of the data. When unusual values occur away from the bulk of the data (outlier points), they are plotted as separate points beyond the whiskers. The whiskers extend only to those points that are within 1.5 times the quartile range. The central horizontal line across the box is the median value. The notch indicated around the median value corresponds to the width of the confidence interval for the median. The confidence level on the notches is set to allow pairwise comparisons to be performed at the 95% confidence level by examining whether two notches overlap.

Presented in Figures C1 and C2 are the percentages of workers included in the $\%W_s$ statistic over the first three sequential test comparisons (1-2, 2-3 and 3-4) and over the last three available test comparisons (5-6, 6-7 and 7-8). The box-and-whisker plots indicate a significant difference in the median values for the control and non-control populations. However, some overlapping of the control and non-control data occurs, especially for the early tests.

The largest separation of the data between controls and non-controls occurs in Figure C3 for the $\%BW_s$ procedure over sequential comparisons of tests 5-6, 6-7, and 7-8. Almost no overlapping occurs. The findings for the $\%BW_s$ procedure over tests 1-4 are not presented since the learning effect [C2, C7] complicates interpretation of this statistic during early tests.

Presented in Figures C4 and C5 are the findings for the AAO-HNS shift procedure for sequential comparisons over the first four and last four tests.

Presented in Figures C6 through C7 are the data for the standard deviation of the differences in hearing threshold levels measured in sequential audiograms. Results for single audiometric frequencies are shown for the control data bases (Figure C6 for sequential test comparisons over tests 1-4 and Figure C7 for sequential test comparisons over tests 5-8) and for the non-control data bases (Figures C8 and C9). Similar results for frequency-averages are presented in Figures C10 and C11 (control data bases) and C12 and C13 (non-control data bases).

If the results for the standard deviations of the differences in hearing threshold levels for either the single-frequency or the frequency-average data are compared for control vs. non-control data bases, the boxes of the box-and-whisker plots are separated, while the whiskers indicate some overlap. No particular test frequencies or frequency averages appear to yield greater separation, except possibly the single frequency comparisons at 2 and 3 kHz and the average at 0.5, 1, 2 and 3 kHz over tests 5-8.

C.5 Defining the Criterion Ranges

In order to establish value ranges for acceptable, marginal and unacceptable HCP performance, the raw data utilized to generate the notched box-and-whisker plots in Figures C1 through C13 were analyzed to calculate standard deviations for the distribution of values for each ADBA statistic among *only the control data bases* available to S12/WG12. The criterion range indicating that an HCP was "Acceptable" was defined as plus or minus two standard deviations of the mean value *for these control populations*. The criterion range indicating that an HCP was "marginal" HCP was defined as more than two but no more than four standard deviations above the control populations' mean value. The criterion range for judging an HCP as unacceptable was defined as above four standard deviations from the mean value for the control data.

The criterion ranges for judging HCP effectiveness which were established using this method of defining value ranges corresponding to acceptable, marginal and unacceptable HCP performance for three ADBA procedures (%W$_s$, %BW, and the standard deviation of the differences in sequential test comparisons) were incorporated into the initial draft standard. However, trial use of the draft standard did not support continued use of the standard deviation of differences procedure, which was eliminated from the current report.

C.6 Conclusions and Recommendations

This current report recommends two ADBA procedures and associated criterion ranges for classifying HCP effectiveness as acceptable, marginal or unacceptable. The user should employ both procedures in assessing the effectiveness of a HCP.

It is important that the user of the ADBA procedures keep in mind that the failure of a HCP to meet the acceptable criterion range does not necessarily imply that on-the-job noise-induced hearing loss is occurring. Audiometric variability in excess of the guidelines could result from inconsistent audiometry procedures, inadequate calibration procedures, bad connecting cables between the audiometric test room and the audiometer, or other methodological factors. However, such a flaw in the system does render the HCP ineffective because it prevents the detection of shifts associated with inadequate use of hearing protectors, a significant change in a worker's hearing threshold levels due to noise exposure, or some other event.

The S12/WG12 members feel that the time has come to do more with the vast audiometric data base that is available than simply tallying OSHA STSs and documenting the development and progression of noise-induced hearing loss. The cost and effort involved in the audiometric phase of the HCP are not justified unless the audiogram results are used to trigger actions which prevent hearing loss. It is critical that we begin making use of the real potential of the audiometric data base—the prevention of on-the-job noise-induced hearing loss—by applying ADBA procedures and using the results to improve HCP effectiveness.

C.7 References

[C1] Lilley, D.T., "Analysis techniques for evaluating the effectiveness of industrial hearing conservation programs," Master's thesis submitted to North Carolina State University, Raleigh, North Carolina, 1980.

[C2] Royster, L.H. and Thomas, W.G., "Age effect hearing levels for a white nonindustrial noise exposed population (NINEP) and their use in evaluating industrial hearing conservation programs," *American Industrial Hygiene Association Journal,* 1979, 40: 504–511.

[C3] Royster, L.H., Driscoll, D.P., Thomas, W.G. and Royster, J.D., "Age effect hearing levels for a black nonindustrial noise exposed population (NINEP)," *American Industrial Hygiene Association Journal,* 1980, 41: 113–119.

[C4] Royster, L.H., Lilley, D.T. and Thomas, W.G., "Recommended criteria for evaluating the effectiveness of hearing conservation programs," *American Industrial Hygiene Association Journal,* 1980, 41: 40–48.

[C5] Royster, L.H. and Royster, J.D., "Methods of evaluating hearing conservation program audiometric data bases," in *Personal Hearing Protection In Industry,* edited by P.W. Alberti. New York: Raven Press, 1982, 511–539.

[C6] Royster, L.H. and Royster, J.D., "Making the most out of the audiometric data base," *Sound and Vibration,* 1984, 18(5): 18–24.

[C7] Royster, J.D. and Royster, L.H., "Using audiometric data base analysis," *Journal of Occupational Medicine,* 1986, 28(10): 1055–1068.

[C8] Royster, L.H. and Royster, J.D., "Getting started in audiometric data base analysis," *Seminars in Hearing,* 1988, 9: 325–338.

[C9] Cantrell, R.W., Catlin, F.L., Dobie, R.A., et al. *Guide for Conservation of Hearing in Noise,* Rochester, MN: American Academy of Otolaryngology, 1982.

[C10] Occupational Safety and Health Administration, "Occupational noise exposure; hearing conservation amendment; final rule." *Federal Register* 1983, 48 (March 8): 9738–9785.

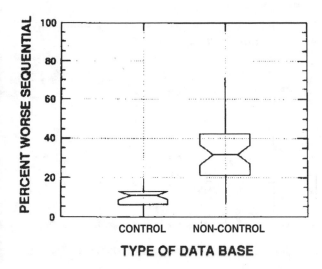

Figure C1. Distribution of %W$_s$ values in sequential comparisons of tests 1-4.

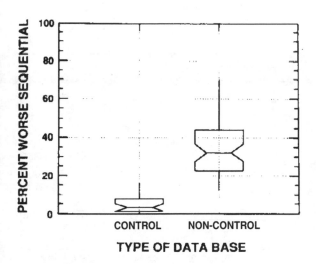

Figure C2. Distribution of %W$_s$ values in sequential comparisons of tests 5-8.

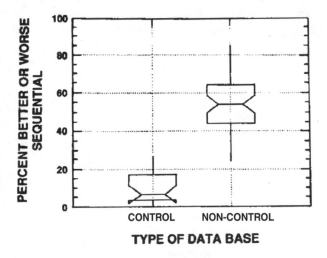

Figure C3. Distribution of %BW$_s$ values in sequential comparisons of tests 5-8.

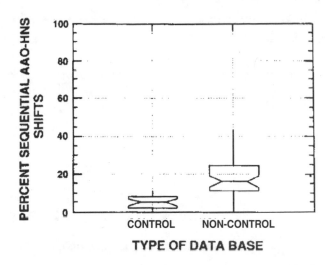

Figure C4. Distribution of percent AAO-HNS shifts in sequential comparisons of tests 1-4.

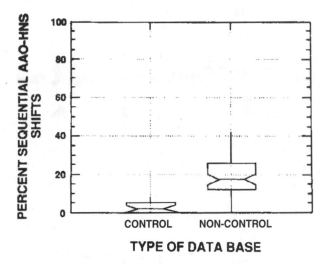

Figure C5. Distribution of percent AAO-HNS shifts in sequential comparisons of tests 5-8.

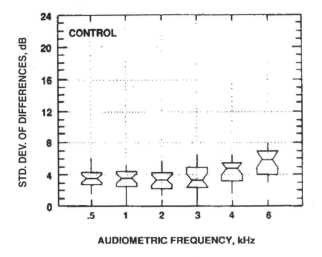

Figure C6. Distribution of standard deviations of differences in HTLs at single audiometric test frequencies in sequential comparisons of tests 1-4 for control data bases.

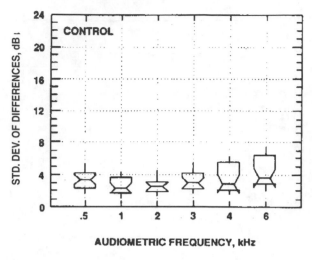

Figure C7. Distribution of standard deviations of differences in HTLs at single audiometric test frequencies in sequential comparisons of tests 5-8 for control data bases.

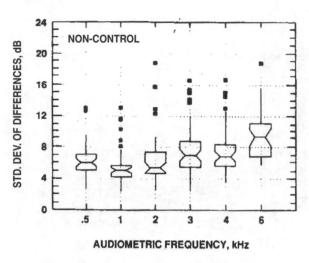

Figure C9. Distribution of standard deviations of differences in HTLs at single audiometric test frequencies in sequential comparisons of tests 5-8 for non-control data bases.

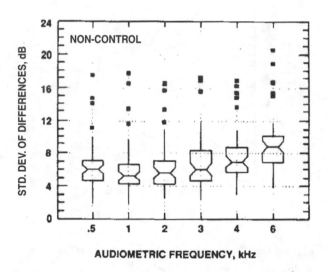

Figure C8. Distribution of standard deviations of differences in HTLs at single audiometric test frequencies in sequential comparisons of tests 1-4 for non-control data bases.

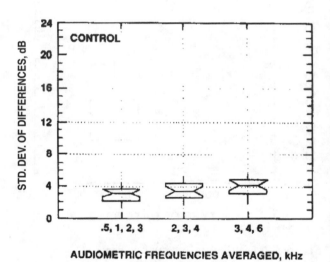

Figure C10. Distribution of standard deviations of differences in HTLs for averaged audiometric test frequencies in sequential comparisons of tests 1-4 for control data bases.

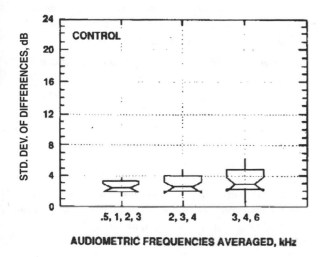

Figure C11. Distribution of standard deviations of differences in HTLs for averaged audiometric test frequencies in sequential comparisons of tests 5-8 for control data bases.

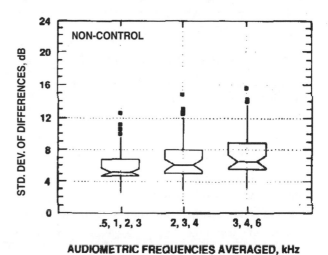

Figure C13. Distribution of standard deviations of differences in HTLs for averaged audiometric test frequencies in sequential comparisons of tests 5-8 for non-control data bases.

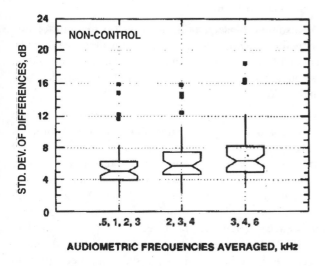

Figure C12. Distribution of standard deviations of differences in HTLs for averaged audiometric test frequencies in sequential comparisons of tests 1-4 for non-control data bases.

ANNEX D
(Informative)

ANALYSIS EXAMPLE

This annex provides a sample analysis to illustrate the process for readers. A summary of the steps to follow in performing ADBA is given as Table D1.

Table D1. Steps in Implementing ADBA

1. Compile the complete audiometric data base, including demographic information.

2. Discard all but the first valid audiogram per person per year (drop retests unless retesting was done for reasons unrelated to noise exposure).

3. Select the restricted data base of all employees with at least N tests according to the information desired, such as

   a. For recent HCP protection of senior employees, choose N=10, then look at the most recent 4 tests with the latest test being in the current calendar year.

   b. For recent HCP protection of newly hired employees, choose N=3 and look at the first 3 tests with the third test being in the current calendar year.

   c. For historical HCP performance, look at all audiograms for employees who were first tested in the year the HCP was initiated and who have been tested in every subsequent year up to the present.

   d. If possible, select an internal control group of non-noise-exposed employees for comparison to the noise-exposed restricted group.

4. Examine the mean hearing levels of the restricted group and internal control group.

5. Calculate and plot the mean hearing levels by year and by test frequency for the restricted groups over the years included in the analysis in order to determine whether any aberrations appear to be affecting measured hearing levels. As long as the data appear to be reliable, continue with the analysis.

6. Calculate the $\%W_s$ and $\%BW_s$ values for the noise-exposed group and for the internal control group, and compare the values obtained to the criterion ranges in Table 1 of this report.

7. For a given test comparison (such as 1995 to 1996), if the results for both ADBA statistics fall into the same criterion range (such as "acceptable") then that range describes the HCP's rating for that year. If the results for the two procedures span two criterion ranges, then the HCP's rating for that year is described as spanning the two ranges involved (such as "marginal to acceptable") for that year.

8. If the variability indicators indicate less than acceptable HCP effectiveness, then look for sources of high variability in hearing level measurements, including factors related to inadequate protection from noise as well as factors related to poorly controlled audiometric testing procedures.

An example of sequential audiometric records for one individual is shown as Table D2 to illustrate the identification of sequential comparisons for which the individual is counted in the percentages for variability statistics $\%W_s$ and $\%BW_s$.

The sample data base includes audiograms from 1973 to 1991 for a meat processing plant. Senior employees have accumulated many annual tests, but few current employees share the same year for test 1. In order to obtain as large a group size as possible, senior employees were included in this analysis if their 1991 audiogram was test 9 or higher (eliminating the learning-effect influence). Then the most recent five years of data (1987-1991) were evaluated. This restricted group selection yielded 63 noise-exposed employees, plus an internal control group of 29 non-noise-exposed employees who also received annual audiograms.

Table D2. Example of determining whether an individual employee will be included in the Percent Worse sequential ($\%W_s$) and Percent Better or Worse sequential ($\%BW_s$) statistics in each of three sequential test comparisons.

Test Number	Left ear HTLs (dB) by frequency (kHz)						Right ear HTLs (dB) by frequency (kHz)						Tests Compared	Employee included in...		
	.5	1	2	3	4	6	.5	1	2	3	4	6		$\%W_s$	$\%B_s$	$\%BW_s$
1	20	5	5	10	30	50	20	10	0	20	35	50				
2	0	-5	0	0	25	35	0	0	-5	-5	25	40	1-2	no	yes	yes
3	0	-5	0	0	25	50	0	0	0	0	20	45	2-3	yes	no	yes
4	0	0	0	5	25	30	5	0	0	-5	35	40	3-4	yes	yes	yes

The 1991 mean hearing levels for white and black males and females within each noise exposure group are shown as Figure D1. The mean thresholds for blacks are quite similar regardless of noise exposure, while the white exposure groups show a small mean difference of about 6 dB at 3000 and 4000 Hz. The mean audiogram for the noise-exposed whites shows high-frequency notching indicating some noise-induced damage.

The mean hearing levels by test frequency over 1987–1991 are plotted in Figures D2 and D3 for the two exposure groups, respectively. No aberrations are apparent.

The variability indicators $\%W_s$ and $\%BW_s$ tabulated separately for the non-exposed and noise-exposed groups over the most recent five tests, are plotted as Figures D4 and D5. The non-exposed group data fall well within the acceptable ranges for both indicators, while the noise-exposed group data are closer to the borderline of the marginal range (or just across the boundary) in several comparisons. These findings indicate that testing-related variability is low (since the data are good for the non-noise group). While HCP effectiveness is acceptable for the noise-exposed employees, the higher variability for exposed workers compared to the internal control group suggests that protection might still be improved.

In fact, this HCP had not required HPD utilization in a department with TWAs of 85–89 dBA. Based on these results, management decided to require HPDs in the low-noise department.

For additional examples see reference A1, which also describes a learning-based indicator which may be applied for early years of testing for restricted groups.

Figure D1. Mean hearing levels on the latest audiogram for noise exposure groups subdivided by race.

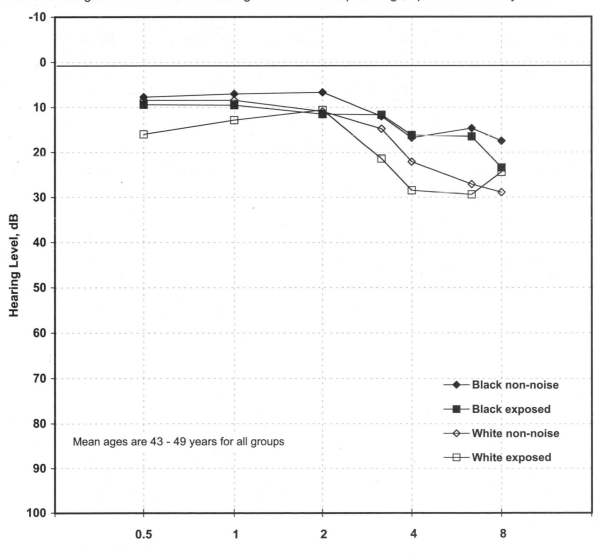

Figure D2. Mean hearing levels at 2–6 kHz on the most recent five approximately annual audiograms for noise-exposed subjects, as a function of mean age at the time of each test.

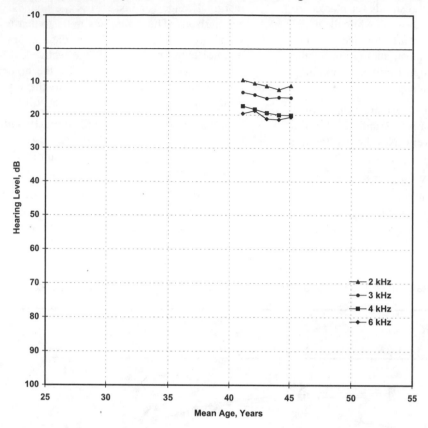

Figure D3. Mean hearing levels at 2–6 kHz on the most recent five approximately annual audiograms for non-noise-exposed subjects, as a function of mean age at the time of each test.

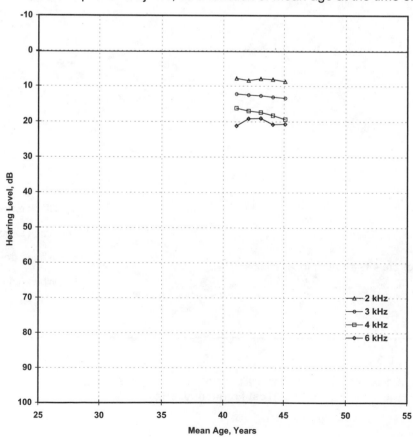

288

Figure D4. Percent Worse sequential results over the most recent four test comparisons for noise-exposed and non-noise-exposed groups.

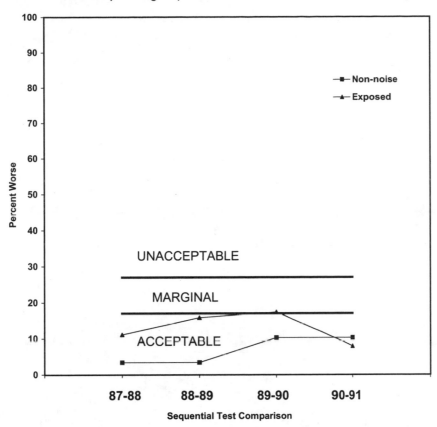

Figure D5. Percent Better or Worse sequential results over the most recent four test comparisons for noise-exposed and non-noise-exposed groups.

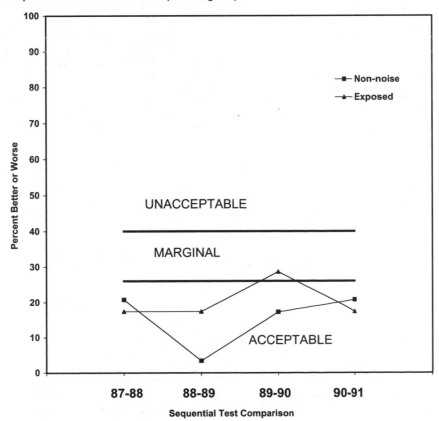

Appendix
Quiz Answers

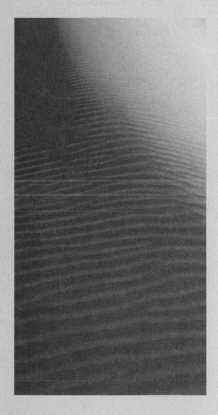

four of these:
Audiologist
Occupational health nurse
Safety specialist
Industrial hygienist
Occupational physician
Otolaryngologist
Noise control engineer

2. 5.2 million

3. Council for Accreditation in Occupational Hearing Conservation.

4. Any five of these:
American Academy of Otolaryngology—Head and Neck Surgery
American Association of Occupational Health Nurses
American College of Occupational and Environmental Medicine
American Industrial Hygiene Association
American Speech-Language-Hearing Association
Institute of Noise Control Engineering
Military Audiology Association

5. True

6. False

7. The CAOHC authorized video may be substituted for one of the three professional
disciplines required as instructors.

8. For example:
Baseline and annual audiometric testing
Visual inspection of the ear
Taking a history
Screening audiograms to select problem audiograms for review by an audiologist or
physician
Referral to appropriate sources
Recordkeeping
(For more answers see section on Role of the OHC)

9. For example:
Instruct other hearing conservationists
Interpret audiograms
Diagnose hearing disorders
Administer a hearing conservation program
(For more answers see section on Role of the Professional Supervisor)

10. The date of their certification course

11. dB

Answers to Quiz for Chapter II

1. About 1 million

2. True

3. False

4. Impulsive ("Impulse" noise would also be correct, or "impact" noise when referring to noise generated by objects striking each other)

5. Temporary threshold shift; permanent

6. Heavy metals (such as lead and trimethyl tin)
   Organic solvents (such as toluene, xylene, and carbon disulfide)
   Asphyxiants (such as carbon monoxide)
   (Naming the 3 main categories, or any three of the specific agents would be correct)

7. Wood working tools
   Chain saws
   Unmuffled motorcycles
   Loud music
   Guns

8. Tinnitus
   It often precedes the development of noise-induced hearing loss.

9. Interference with communication
   Degraded job performance
   Annoyance, fatigue
   Stress

10. Management will display leadership and support for hourly workers, showing that they feel that the hearing conservation program is important.

11. a. To determine whether they should be included in the hearing conservation program.
       To see what kind of hearing protection is needed.
       Also, to comply with regulations.
    b. Noise dosimeter or sound level meter

12. At least 14 hours away from noise exposure of any kind, and preferably pre-employment.

13. Well into the work shift

14. Better labor–management relations
    Improved employee morale
    Greater job satisfaction, productivity, safety
    Reduction in accidents, illnesses, and lost time

Answers to Quiz for Chapter III

1. Understanding speech
   Tuning in to wanted sounds
   Hearing warning signals
   Enjoying music and the sounds of nature
   Can you name others?

2. Audiogram

3. 500, 1000, 2000, 3000, 4000, and 6000
   Sometimes 8000 is included.

4. False

5. Tympanic membrane
   False

6. Cerumen
   Earplugs

7. Malleus, incus, and stapes (or hammer, anvil, and stirrup)
   Any of these answers would be correct:
       Conduct sound into the inner ear
       Transfer vibrations to the fluid of the inner ear
       Act as a mechanical transformer, increasing the sound pressure level reaching the inner ear

8. Balance

9. Cochlea

10. Hair
    Electrical

11. Eighth cranial or Auditory

12. High

Answers to Quiz for Chapter IV

1. Otolaryngologists or ENT specialists
   Otologists

2. None, unless the OHC has been trained as an otolaryngologist or audiologist

3. Prevention, assessment, diagnosis, and rehabilitation of hearing impairments

4. Examples include:
   Impacted cerumen (earwax)
   Perforated tympanic membrane (eardrum)
   Otitis media (middle-ear infection)
   Cholesteatoma
   Otosclerosis

5. External ear infections

6. Very small earcanal entrances, which tend to close with the pressure of the audiometer
   earphone

7. In the inner ear or in the nerve leading from the ear to the brain

8. Presbycusis

9. Examples include:
   Presbycusis
   Birth defects
   Rubella (German measles) in pregnant mother
   Blood incompatibility in parents
   Viral infections (usually with high fever)
   Ototoxic drugs
   Meniere's disease
   Acoustic neuromas
   Do you know any others?

10. Because a pronounced one-sided hearing loss may be an indication of a tumor on the acoustic
    nerve, which is a very serious condition.

11. False

Answers to Quiz for Chapter V

1. False, unless the OHC has been specifically trained

2. The pressure wave

3. Intensity or sound pressure level
   decibels or dB

4. Pitch

5. Because the sound pressure variations occur at only one frequency

6. It represents the weakest sound pressure level the young, normal human ear can hear in its
   most sensitive frequency range.

7. Examples:
   Home shop tools
   Power lawn mower
   Motorcycle
   Snowmobile
   Subway
   Motorboat

8. Sound level, frequency, and temporal (time) characteristics

9. Time-weighted average
   TWA

10. Exchange rate

Answers to Quiz for Chapter VI

1. NIOSH, located in the Department of Health and Human Services, conducts research, develops criteria, and performs Health Hazard Evaluations. OSHA, located in the Department of Labor, makes regulations and enforces them.

2. Regulation (Congress legislates)

3. 90 dBA
   5 dBA
   85 dBA

4. 100 dBA

5. Employers must use feasible engineering or administrative controls, and provide hearing protectors to overexposed workers. Workers must wear hearing protectors.

6. When workers are not highly mobile, there are no significant variations in the noise level, and there is no significant impulsive noise component.

7. False (audiometric tests must be *made available* to all employees exposed to TWAs of 85 dBA and above)

8. 6 months, or 1 year if company relies on mobile test services
   Before *any* exposure to potentially hazardous noise

9. Audiologist or physician

10. Average shift from baseline of 10 dB or more at 2000, 3000, and 4000 Hz.
    NIOSH: shift of 15 dB or greater from baseline in either ear at any test frequency which has been confirmed with a follow-up test (same ear and same frequency)

11. 21

12. Within 30 days of receiving evidence or confirmation of an STS:
Retrain the miner
Provide the miner with the opportunity to select a new or different hearing protector.
Review the effectiveness of any engineering and administrative controls to identify and correct deficiencies.

13. Purpose of the functional check is to make sure that the audiometer is working properly—that (a) the tone is not distorted, (b) the sound is coming out of the appropriate earphone, and (c) the sound pressure levels are accurate. This process involves more steps than the "biological check," which is basically step (c), using an electronic device or someone with known stable hearing threshold levels to check sound pressure levels.

14. An employee has not yet had a baseline audiogram and has worked in noise for more than 6 months or an employee has experienced an STS.

15. Noise Reduction Rating
NRR

16. At least once a year
Not according to OSHA, but MSHA requires a certificate of training, so one could infer that all training must be carried out at one time at least once a year

17. True

18. 105
800

19. True

20. Answers could include:
Federal Railroad Administration (in the Dept. of Transportation)
Bureau of Motor Carrier Safety (in the Dept. of Transportation)
Department of Defense (all three branches of the military)
U.S. Coast Guard
NASA
Department of Interior
Department of Energy

21. 25
92

22. False. While it is true that the employer must make a reasonable accommodation, this is only if it does not impose significant difficulty and/or expense.

23. True

1. The earphones

2. Least expensive; operator maintains control over the presentation of tones
   Most prone to human error

3. The OHC must switch to the manual override or use a manual audiometer in difficult-to-test cases or where the microprocessor is unable to test individuals whose responses are inconsistent.

4. Because there is a variety of different methods of tone presentation among these instruments that can affect the measured thresholds. Of course, calibration differences can be another source of variability.

5. To prevent masking or falsely elevating thresholds often most noticeable at 500 and 1000 Hz. Also to prevent the employee from becoming distracted while taking the audiometric test.

6. 40 dB, 21 dB

7. False

8. Pre-employment or before exposure to hazardous noise
   To prevent the baseline audiogram from being affected by TTS or permanent hearing loss

9. Well into the workshift.
   To identify TTS and take precautions before it becomes a permanent hearing loss

10. 14

11. When the OHC is unable to obtain a valid test.

12. Visually inspect the ear before inserting the otoscope. If there are signs of swelling, pain, or discharge, do not insert the otoscope. Be gentle with the employee's ear and the use of the otoscope. Possibly use a soft-flanged speculum.

13. False

14. 90

15. Better

16. American National Standard Methods for Manual Pure-Tone Threshold Audiometry, ANSI S3.21-1978 (R1997). (See Appendix N in this manual)

17. True

18. 1 to 2

19. False

20. Functional check, acoustic, and exhaustive
    Exhaustive

21. Possible correct answers:
    Make sure the signal is not leaking into the non-test earphone.
    Check the signal for the presence of distortion or hum.
    Check the cords for possible intermittencies in the signal.
    Inspect earphone cushions.

Answers to Quiz for Chapter VIII

1. False

2. In noisy backgrounds, such as when the TV is on, riding in the car, in restaurants, in reverberant rooms, in social groups, and when people speak softly or indistinctly

3. Air conduction: R = O
                                 L = X
   Bone conduction: R = <
                                 L = >

4. Unilateral
   Asymmetric

5. Conductive

6. Sloping toward the high frequencies or the "notch" configuration

7. Mixed

8. True

9. Reinstruct the subject, encouraging him or her to listen very carefully, and retest. If inconsistent responses persist, refer to an audiologist or physician.

10. A shift of 10 dB or greater

11. Current

12. When hearing threshold levels improve

13. False
    No. But there are other requirements. See both OSHA and MSHA regulations.

14. The employer *should* be responsible but the OSHA standard is unclear on this point.

15. True

1. Identify overexposed workers and quantify their exposures
   Assess the noise problem(s) for engineering or administrative controls
   Measure the background levels in audiometer rooms

2. 2

3. Logarithmically

4. Slow

5. False. Use the "peak" or "instantaneous" setting.

6. Microphone

7. To measure the sound levels of particular frequencies (or frequency bands). These measurements are used for engineering control purposes and for measuring the background noise in audiometer rooms.

8. Profile or log

9. Dosimeters

10. Before and after each period of use

11. True

12. 80; 130

13. Look in Table G-16a in Appendix A of OSHA's noise regulation or Table 62-1 in MSHA's regulation.
    87 dBA

14. Difficulty communicating at about 3 feet
    Tinnitus
    "Dullness" of hearing or TTS

15. Windscreen

16. Source, path, receiver

17. Correct answers could include:
    Reduce time and expense of other hearing conservation measures because they are no longer needed when employees' exposures are below a TWA of 85 dBA
    Prevent noise-induced hearing loss since eliminating the noise problem is the most effective solution
    Improve safety, productivity, and communication
    Eliminate any adverse effects on the neighboring community

Answers to Quiz for Chapter X

1. True

2. Low and middle

3. Short-duration, intermittent exposures where sound levels are not very high

4. About 5 dB

5. Electronic circuitry

6. Because the earphones provide little or no attenuation and the employee will be tempted to turn up the volume to override the workplace noise, adding to the possible hazard of noise-induced hearing loss.

7. False

8. Clean

9. True

10. Occlusion effect
    When plugs or semi-aurals are not deeply inserted into the earcanal and, to a lesser extent, with small-volume earmuffs

11. When the noise levels drop below about 85 dBA
    When the wearer has a hearing loss, especially in the high frequencies

12. Vertical

13. Uniform or flat

14. True

15. Loose

16. When they no longer recover to their original shape

17. 90
    85 dBA is safer, but it depends on the circumstance

18. 7
    True

19. One-third to one-half

20. 50

Answers to Quiz for Chapter XI

1. Managers and supervisors

2. 15–25 minutes

3. Seminar format

4. Hypothetical audiogram typical of a group member or a composite audiogram reflecting the average of the group's hearing threshold levels

5. While waiting for the audiometric test or during some other free time

6. Post it on the bulletin board

7. Early in the training session

8. a. Institutionalized reward and punishment programs *may* lead to:
      Destructive competition among workers
      Animosity between workers and supervisors
      Lowered worker self-esteem
      Decreased productivity
      Sabotage (i.e. modification) of hearing protectors
   b. When workers themselves design and carry out the program

Answers to Quiz for Chapter XII

1. A copy of the noise regulation, employee's baseline and most recent audiometric test results, background sound levels in audiometric test rooms, and audiometer calibration information

2. a. OSHA: Duration of the employee's employment
   b. MSHA: Audiometric test records for duration of miner's exposure plus 6 months; training certificate for length of miner's enrollment in hearing conservation program plus 6 months
   c. At least several years after separation or retirement

3. True

4. False. While it is true that OSHA requires employers to notify employees whose TWAs are above 85 dBA of the results of the monitoring, written notification is not mandatory. Some companies, however, may wish to notify workers in writing.
   Yes.

5. Good records should be accurate, thorough, well organized, and legible.

6. No
   No

7. Appendix P. The regulatory checklists are also useful—for OSHA's regulation in Appendix C and MSHA's in Appendix F

8. True

9. 30

10. (A rhetorical question) You, the OHC, of course!

exchange rate: 33, 37, 47
    EPA 3 dB: 33
    NIOSH 3 dB: 50
    OSHA 5 dB: 50
exit audiogram (see audiogram)
external auditory meatus: 19, 66
external canal: 18
external otitis: 24, 68
extra-auditory effects of noise: 11

F

feasability (see noise control)
FECA (see Federal Employee's Compensation Act)
Federal Coal Mine Safety and Health Act: 35
Federal Employee's Compensation Act (FECA): 51
Federal Railroad Administration: 50
Federal Register: 35-36, 47
Field Inspection Reference Manual (OSHA): 45
flat audiogram (see audiogram)
follow-up procedures (see audiometric testing)
Form 300 (see Occupational Safety and Health
    Administration)
frequency: 29, 32
    audiometric test frequencies: 18
functional hearing loss (see pseudohypacusis)

G

Guide to Conducting Noise Sampling (MSHA): 50
gunfire (see also impulse noise): 104-105, 111

H

hair cells: 20-21
hammer: 18-19
hearing
    characteristics: 17
    disorders: 23-26
    normal: 75
    range of human hearing: 18, 31
        as a function of frequency and SPL: 32
    sensitivity: 17-18
    threshold level: 18
hearing aid: 8, 107
hearing aids: 27
Hearing Conservation Amendment (OSHA): 2, 14, 36-45,
    142-150
    action level: 37
    comparison tables of OSHA, MSHA, and NIOSH
        hearing conservation regulations and
        recommendations: 40-42
    preamble: 36
    requirements for
        assessment of dose: 37
        audiometric testing program: 38
        audiometric tests: 43
        hearing protectors: 44
        noise exposure monitoring: 38
        recordkeeping: 45
        training program: 44
hearing conservation program: 1
    benefits of: 8, 11
    employee education and training: 13-14

establishing: 11
evaluation: 14, 129-131, 178-181, 259-290
    MSHA Program Evaluation Checklist: 131, 167-175
    OSHA Compliance Checklist: 131, 151-156
    practical survey: 131
    Program Evaluation Checklist (NIOSH): 177-181
    statistical procedures: 131
    major components of: 12-14
    motivation/rewards for wearing hearing protection:
        123-124
    MSHA Regulation Checklist: 168-175
    OSHA Noise Standard Compliance Checklist: 152-156
    recordkeeping: 14, 126-129
    worker participation: 101
hearing handicap: 8, 76
    formulas to calculate: 52
    high fence: 52
    low fence: 52
    relating the audiogram to: 76
hearing level: 30
hearing level scale (HL): 31
hearing loss
    aging process and: 18, 26
    asymmetric: 77
    conductive: 23-24
    material impairment of hearing: 7
    mixed: 26, 80
    need to prevent: 121
    noise-induced: 8
    non-occupational: 9
    non-organic: 26
    occupational: 1, 7-8
    ototoxic: 9
    permanent: 8
    sensorineural: 9, 17, 23, 25-26
    Statutes in the U.S. and Canada: 183-188
    total: 52
    unilateral: 17, 77
        audiogram: 77
    work-related: 46, 129-130
        Form 300, recording on: 46, 130
        log of: 46
        MSHA reporting requirements: 130
        OSHA reporting requirements: 129-130
hearing protection
    communication interference: 10
    dual, or double: 48, 104
    motivation/rewards for wearing hearing protection:
        123-124
    overprotection: 107
    recordkeeping: 129
    summary of: 13
hearing protectors
    (see also earplugs; earmuffs; semi-inserts)
    acceptance: 11, 101
    active noise-reduction (ANR): 105
    advantages and disadvantages of: 105-106
    amplitude-sensitive: 104-105
    attenuation: 13, 44, 92, 107
        field attenuation: 112
        List of Personal Hearing Protectors and
            Attenuation Data (NIOSH, 1975): 111
        measurement: 223-258

817 307 2768